ADVANCES IN SURGICAL PATHOLOGY
ENDOMETRIAL CANCER

ADVANCES IN SURGICAL PATHOLOGY SERIES

SERIES EDITORS: Philip T. Cagle, MD, and Timothy C. Allen, MD, JD

Advances in Surgical Pathology: Lung Cancer
Philip T. Cagle and Timothy C. Allen, *2010*

Advances in Surgical Pathology: Gastric Cancer
Dongfeng Tan and Gregory Y. Lauwers, *2010*

Advances in Surgical Pathology: Endometrial Cancer
Anna Sienko, *2012*

Advances in Surgical Pathology: Mesothelioma
Richard Attanoos, *2012*

Advances in Surgical Pathology: Prostate Cancer
Jae Y. Ro, Steven S. Shen, and Alberto G. Ayala, *2012*

Advances in Surgical Pathology: Pancreas
Vikram Deshpande and Gregory Y. Lauwers, *2013*

Advances in Surgical Pathology: Colorectal Carcinoma and Tumors of the Vermiform Appendix
Rhonda K. Yantis, *2013*

ADVANCES IN SURGICAL PATHOLOGY
ENDOMETRIAL CANCER

Anna Sienko, MD
Clinical Professor University of Calgary
Department of Pathology
Calgary Laboratory Services
Calgary, Alberta
Canada

SERIES EDITORS

Philip T. Cagle, MD
Professor of Pathology and Laboratory Medicine
Weill Medical College of Cornell University
New York, New York
Director, Pulmonary Pathology
The Methodist Hospital
Houston, Texas

Timothy Craig Allen, MD, JD
Professor and Chairman
Department of Pathology
The University of Texas Health Science
   Center at Tyler
Tyler, Texas

Wolters Kluwer | Lippincott Williams & Wilkins
Health
Philadelphia · Baltimore · New York · London
Buenos Aires · Hong Kong · Sydney · Tokyo

Senior Executive Editor: Jonathan W. Pine, Jr.
Product Manager: Marian Bellus
Vendor Manager: Alicia Jackson
Senior Manufacturing Manager: Benjamin Rivera
Senior Designer: Stephen Druding
Production Service: Absolute Service, Inc.

Copyright © 2012 Wolters Kluwer Health | Lippincott Williams & Wilkins

Two Commerce Square
2001 Market Street
Philadelphia, PA 19103

All rights reserved. This book is protected by copyright. No part of this book may be reproduced in any form or by any means, or utilized by any information storage and retrieval system without written permission from the copyright owner, except for brief quotations embodied in critical articles and reviews.

Printed in the People's Republic of China

Library of Congress Cataloging-in-Publication Data

Sienko, Anna.
  Advances in surgical pathology. Endometrial cancer / book author, Anna Sienko.
    p. ; cm. — (Advances in surgical pathology)
  Endometrial cancer
  Includes bibliographical references and index.
  ISBN 978-1-60913-178-4
  I. Title. II. Title: Endometrial cancer. III. Series: Advances in surgical pathology series.
  [DNLM: 1. Endometrial Neoplasms—pathology. 2. Endometrial Neoplasms—diagnosis. WP 458]

  616.99'466—dc23

                                                                    2011037443

Care has been taken to confirm the accuracy of the information presented and to describe generally accepted practices. However, the authors, editors, and publisher are not responsible for errors or omissions or for any consequences from application of the information in this book and make no warranty, expressed or implied, with respect to the currency, completeness, or accuracy of the contents of the publication. Application of this information in a particular situation remains the professional responsibility of the practitioner; the clinical treatments described and recommended may not be considered absolute and universal recommendations.

The authors, editors, and publisher have exerted every effort to ensure that drug selection and dosage set forth in this text are in accordance with the current recommendations and practice at the time of publication. However, in view of ongoing research, changes in government regulations, and the constant flow of information relating to drug therapy and drug reactions, the reader is urged to check the package insert for each drug for any change in indications and dosage and for added warnings and precautions. This is particularly important when the recommended agent is a new or infrequently employed drug.

Some drugs and medical devices presented in this publication have Food and Drug Administration (FDA) clearance for limited use in restricted research settings. It is the responsibility of the health care provider to ascertain the FDA status of each drug or device planned for use in his or her clinical practice.

Visit Lippincott Williams & Wilkins on the Internet at LWW.com. Lippincott Williams & Wilkins customer service representatives are available from 8:30 am to 6 pm, EST.

9 8 7 6 5 4 3 2 1

Series Overview

Expectations for the pathologist practicing today exceed those for pathologists in practice only a few years ago. In addition to the rapid growth of knowledge and new technologies in the field of pathology, recent years have seen the emergence of many trends that significantly impact the traditional practice of pathology including the subspecialized multidisciplinary approach to patient care; personalized therapeutics including targeted molecular therapies; and imaging techniques such as endoscopic microscopy, molecular radiology, and imaging multimodality theranostics that compete with conventional light microscopy. In order to remain a viable member of the patient care team, the pathologist must keep up with growing knowledge in traditional subjects as well as in new areas of expertise such as molecular testing. Additionally, the pathologist is subject to an increasing number of credentialing requirements and, for those now completing training, self-assessment modules for maintenance of certification, which require the pathologist to be examined on the recent advances in pathology in order to sustain their qualifications to practice.

Each volume in the new series *Advances in Surgical Pathology* focuses on a specific subject in pathology that has undergone recent advancement in terms of knowledge, technical procedures, application, and/or integration as part of current trends in pathology and medicine. Each book includes an accompanying Solution site with a fully searchable online version of the text and image bank. This series of books not only updates the pathologist on recently acquired knowledge but also emphasizes the new uses of that knowledge within the context of the changing landscape of pathology practice in the 21st century. Rather than information in a vacuum, the pathologist is educated on how to apply the new knowledge as part of a subspecialized multidisciplinary team and for purposes of personalized patient therapy.

Each volume in the series will be divided into the following sections: (1) Overview—updates the pathologist on the general topic, including epidemiology, bringing the pathologist generally up-to-date on a topic as a basis for the more specialized sections that follow. (2) Histopathology—reviews histopathology and specific recent changes that warrant more description and more illustration, for example, recently described entities and recent revisions in classifications. This will also emphasize histopathology figures to illustrate recently described entities and to demonstrate the basis for classification changes so that the pathologist is able to understand and recognize these changes. (3) Imaging—reviews the impact of imaging techniques on histopathologic diagnosis and on the practice of pathology. An example of the former is the use of increasingly sensitive high-resolution CT scan in the diagnosis of interstitial lung diseases. An example of the latter is the use of multimodality theranostics rather than traditional histopathology for the diagnosis and treatment of lung cancer. Figures linking the radiologic images to the histopathology will be emphasized. (4) Molecular Pathology—a review and update on specific molecular pathology as it applies to specific diseases for the practicing pathologist regarding molecular diagnostics and molecular therapeutics. An example of the former is the identification of a specific fusion gene to diagnose synovial sarcoma. An example of the latter is the identification of specific EGFR mutations in pulmonary adenocarcinoma and its relationship to treatment with EGFR antagonists. (5) For those volumes dealing with cancers (*Lung Cancer, Breast Cancer, Prostate Cancer,*

Colon Cancer, etc.), additional sections will include Preneoplastic and Preinvasive Lesions, which will emphasize histopathologic figures and staging, particularly emphasizing the new staging systems and to illustrate specific problems in staging.

These books will assist the pathologist in daily practice in the modern setting and provide a basis for interacting with other physicians in patient care. They will also provide the timely updates in knowledge that are necessary for daily practice, for current credentialing, and for maintenance of certification. As such, this series is invaluable to pathologists in practice at all levels of experience who need to keep up with advances for their daily performance and their periodic credentialing and to pathologists-in-training who will apply this knowledge to their boards and their future practice. In the latter case, this series will serve as a useful library for pathology training programs.

This book is dedicated to Dr. Fred Silva and Dr. Philip Cagle, my colleagues and friends. I thank them for their mentorship, support, encouragement, and for all the opportunities they gave me. I also want to thank and acknowledge all the contributors for their hard work and commitment.

ACKNOWLEDGMENTS

I want to extend a big thank you to all of the contributors for their time and effort in compiling this book and a very big thank you to everyone at LWW, especially Jonathan W. Pine, Jr., senior executive editor and Marian Bellus, project manager for their guidance and patience.

Preface

The aim and intent of this book was to "fill a gap" and bridge the need for a focused joint approach to endometrial carcinoma from both the pathology and clinical perspectives.

The goal for the content of this book from all of the contributors was to provide concise, useful, practical, and as current as possible information on endometrial carcinoma to practicing pathologists and gynecologic oncologists; gynecology, oncology, and pathology residents and fellows; and all clinicians in their daily practice.

Anna Sienko, MD

Contributors

Tri A. Dinh, MD
Department of Obstetrics & Gynecology/
 Gynecological Oncology
The Methodist Hospital
Houston, Texas

Martin Kobel, MD
Department of Pathology
Calgary Laboratory Services
Foothills Medical Centre
Calgary, Alberta, Canada

Ognjen Kosarac, MD
Department of Pathology
The Methodist Hospital
Houston, Texas

Cheng-Han Lee, MD
Anatomical Pathology
Vancouver General Hospital
Vancouver, BC, Canada

Anais Malpica, MD
Department of Pathology
MD Anderson Cancer Center
Houston, Texas

Dina Mody, MD
Department of Pathology
The Methodist Hospital
Houston, Texas

Anna Sienko, MD
Department of Pathology
Calgary Laboratory Services
Peter Lougheed Centre
Calgary, Alberta, Canada

Reagan Street, MD
Fellow
Department of Gynecological Oncology
The Methodist Hospital
Houston, Texas

Contents

SECTION I: Overview

1 Introduction — 3

2 Overview of Endometrial Carcinoma — 5
Anna Sienko, MD

SECTION II: Histopathology

3 Preneoplastic Conditions of the Endometrium: Endometrial Hyperplasia, the Emergent Concept of Endometrial Intraepithelial Neoplasia, and Others — 17
Anais Malpica, MD

4 Endometrial Carcinoma — 41
Anais Malpica, MD

SECTION III: Imaging

5 Diagnostic Modalities for Endometrial Carcinoma — 105
Reagan Street, MD, and Tri A. Dinh, MD

6 Current Management and Issues in Treatment of Endometrial Carcinoma — 129
Tri A. Dinh, MD, and Reagan Street, MD

SECTION IV: Molecular Pathology

7 Molecular Pathogenesis of Endometrial Carcinoma — 145
Martin Kobel, MD

8 High-Risk Endometrial Carcinoma — 163
Martin Kobel, MD

9 Endometrial Sarcomas — 181
Cheng-Han Lee, MD

SECTION V: Staging

10 Staging and Issues Related to Staging of Endometrial Carcinoma — 193
Anna Sienko, MD

SECTION VI: Role of Cytology

11 Glandular Cell Abnormalities in Pap Tests — 201
Ognjen Kosarac, MD, and Dina Mody, MD

12 Peritoneal Washings — 211
Ognjen Kosarac, MD, and Dina Mody, MD

13 Endometrial Biopsy versus Curettings versus Cytology — 217
Anna Sienko, MD

Index 227

ADVANCES IN
SURGICAL PATHOLOGY
ENDOMETRIAL CANCER

SECTION I

Overview

- **CHAPTER 1:** Introduction
- **CHAPTER 2:** Overview of Endometrial Carcinoma

Introduction

Endometrial carcinoma is the fourth most common female malignancy and accounts for 6% of all gynecologic cancers. Endometrial carcinoma is the most common cancer in women in developed and industrialized countries, with most cases occurring in postmenopausal women at an average age of 61 years. However, the incidence of endometrial carcinoma is increasing in premenopausal women and women less than 40 years of age. Most standard gynecologic pathology textbooks have sections or chapters that include a discussion of the epidemiology and risk factors of endometrial carcinoma, as does this book. However, standard gynecologic pathology books do not usually include an overview of patient treatment and management and the related issues involved, as found in this book (Chapter 2). The approach to histologic diagnosis and classification of endometrial hyperplasia and carcinoma are also discussed in most standard gynecologic textbooks and are discussed in this book in Section 2 (Chapters 3 and 4). However, to my knowledge, no book is currently available specifically dedicated to endometrial carcinoma that encompasses not only the histology, but also the broader view of clinical ramifications based on pathology. This book has unique sections that are not found in other standard gynecologic pathology textbooks such as the section entitled "The Pathologist's Responsibility" in Chapter 2. Section 3 (Chapters 5 and 6) was written by practicing gynecologic oncologists involved in the daily care of patients with gynecologic malignancies. This book also includes the most current aspects of molecular pathology of endometrial carcinoma (Section 4, Chapters 7 to 9) and is the first book to include the limitations and pitfalls of cytology of endometrial carcinoma (Section 6). Issues and current challenges, including shortcomings and pitfalls in the diagnosis of endometrial carcinoma and classification of histologic cell type based on different sampling techniques, are discussed (Chapter 13). Staging directly impacts on patient treatment and prognosis. The new revised staging for endometrial carcinoma is reviewed in the context of the most pertinent issues and difficulties encountered by the pathologist in assessment of the pathologic staging of the surgical specimens.

This book hopes to convey that communication is crucial between pathologists and gynecologic oncologists and all clinicians involved in patient care. The pathologist plays an integral part in patient management because the pathology diagnosis rendered has major clinical impact—guiding the surgeon and determining the extent of surgical resection, impacting the choice of patient management and whether or not to include adjuvant treatment, and predicting the risk of recurrence and overall patient prognosis.

Overview of Endometrial Carcinoma

▶ Anna Sienko, MD

EPIDEMIOLOGY

Endometrial carcinoma ranks as the fourth most common malignancy in women, accounting for 6% of female cancers. Endometrial carcinoma is the most common malignancy in women in developed and industrialized countries, with 75% of cases occurring in postmenopausal women at an average age of 61 years[1] (Table 2-1). The remaining 25% of cases occur in premenopausal women, with 5% of cases reported in women under age 40 years.[2] Premenopausal women who develop endometrial carcinoma usually have certain increased risk factors such as obesity, nulliparity, hypertension, anovulatory cycles, and diabetes.[3] An estimated 40,100 cases of endometrial adenocarcinoma will be diagnosed annually in the United States, with 7,470 annual reported deaths.[1] One in 20 cases of female cancers reported in Europe are endometrial carcinomas.[4] It is estimated that 4,500 new cases of uterine cancer will be diagnosed in Canada in 2010, with 790 deaths.[5] Worldwide, endometrial adenocarcinoma has been increasing over the last 20 years, and cervical carcinoma has been decreasing.[6] More than 90% of endometrial carcinoma cases are sporadic, with approximately 10% of cases associated with hereditary syndromes such as Lynch II syndrome, also known as hereditary nonpolyposis colorectal cancer. This syndrome is an autosomal dominant germ line defect in DNA mismatch repair genes and accounts for 9% of endometrial carcinomas in patients under 50 years of age (see Chapters 7 and 8). Incidence of endometrial carcinoma is higher among White women compared with Asian or Black women. However, the mortality is much higher among Black women, which is thought to be due to presentation at higher stage of disease and less adequate access to health care.[1,7]

ETIOLOGY AND RISK FACTORS

Endometrial adenocarcinoma represents a biologically and histologically diverse group of carcinomas that have traditionally been divided into two groups based on age of presentation, histologic features, and prognosis (Table 2-2). Type I endometrial carcinomas, which account for 80% to 90% of endometrial carcinomas, are seen in perimenopausal women; are estrogen-dependent, well-differentiated tumors (more often endometrioid histology type); and have a favorable prognosis. Type II endometrial carcinomas account for the remaining 10% to 20% of endometrial carcinomas; these carcinomas occur in older postmenopausal women, are estrogen-independent, histologically higher grade tumors (mostly serous

Table 2-1	Epidemiology of Endometrial Carcinoma
Incidence	6% of all invasive cancers in women 4th leading cause of cancer in women 40,100 new cases/year in United States 150,000 new cases/year worldwide 7,470 deaths/year in United States
Age range/median age	Postmenopausal/55–65 years
Geographic distribution	Worldwide but higher in industrialized countries

carcinoma, clear cell carcinoma, and other nonendometrioid histologic types), and present at a higher stage of disease with a higher incidence of metastasis at time of diagnosis.[8] Type I endometrial carcinomas are usually preceded by endometrial hyperplasia, whereas type II endometrial carcinomas are not associated with hyperplasia. The molecular pathways have also been documented to be different; type I endometrial carcinomas demonstrate mutations in the *KRAS* proto-oncogene and *PTEN* tumor suppressor gene and microsatellite instability, whereas type II endometrial carcinomas have been shown to have *p53* mutations with rarely documented microsatellite instability or *KRAS* or *PTEN* mutations (see Chapters 7 and 8 and Table 7-1).[8,9]

Mass screening for endometrial carcinoma has not been advocated or found to be cost effective.[10,11] Most patients present with postmenopausal bleeding and seek medical evaluation, with 10% of patients diagnosed with malignancy upon further investigation. As a result of early investigation and detection, 70% to 75% of patients have surgical stage I disease.[12,13]

Excess or unopposed estrogen, either from exogenous (e.g., hormone replacement therapy [HRT], tamoxifen, oral contraceptives) or endogenous sources (e.g., obesity, polycystic ovary syndrome, tumors secreting estrogen such as ovarian granulosa cell tumors), increases the

Table 2-2	Comparison between Types I and II Endometrial Carcinoma	
Type I	**Type II**	
Younger age	Older age	
Perimenopausal	Postmenopausal	
Associated with estrogen	Not associated with estrogen	
Frequently associated with endometrial hyperplasia	Not associated with endometrial hyperplasia	
Low histologic tumor grade	High histologic tumor grade	
Usually endometrioid type	Not endometrioid type	
	Usually serous carcinoma or clear cell carcinoma	
Lower stage, good prognosis	Higher stage, worse prognosis	
KRAS, PTEN mutations	*p53* mutation	

risk of developing endometrial adenocarcinoma.[14] Unopposed exogenous hormones were demonstrated to have variable risk depending on age of the patient, perimenopausal or postmenopausal status, and whether the serum levels measured represented high estrone and albumin-bound estradiol, which have been associated with increased risk. However, high levels of serum total, free, and albumin-bound estradiol were unrelated to increased risk.[14] An elevated level of androstenedione was also cited as a risk factor in both perimenopausal and postmenopausal women; however, the risk factor associated with obesity was not affected by adjustment for hormones.[15,16] Risk associated with unopposed estrogen was decreased by addition of progestin to HRT, use of oral contraceptives, and smoking.[15–20] It was found that women who took combined oral contraceptives ("the pill") for at least 1 year had a 40% to 50% reduced risk of endometrial carcinoma and were "protected" for up to 15 years after discontinuing the pill.[16,21] Postmenopausal women who were prescribed a combined estrogen–progesterone HRT regimen also had a decreased risk of endometrial carcinoma.[21]

Tamoxifen is a selective nonsteroidal receptor modulator that blocks estrogen receptors by competing for the same site as estrogen. However, tamoxifen shows "mixed" function in that in reproductive, perimenopausal women, it demonstrates an estrogenic effect, whereas in postmenopausal women, it demonstrates an antiestrogenic effect. As a result of the "dual personality" of tamoxifen, controversy exists as to its usage, with some studies showing greatly increased risk for endometrial carcinoma and high-grade endometrial carcinomas, whereas other studies have found no significant increased risk.[22–24]

Additional well-defined risk factors for developing endometrial carcinoma are obesity, nulliparity, fat-rich diet adding to weight gain, diabetes, hypertension, and early menarche/late menopause. Obesity has been shown to increase the relative risk for endometrial adenocarcinoma 3-fold in women who are 20 to 50 lb overweight and more than 10-fold in women who are ≥50 lb overweight. Increased relative risk was due to increased conversion of androstenedione to estrogen and increased unopposed estrogen in fatty tissue due to increased aromatization of androgens to estradiol.[18,25] Nulliparity, like polycystic ovary syndrome, is thought to increase unopposed estrogen as a result of anovulatory cycles and chronic anovulation. Early menarche and late menopause are considered risk factors because patients are exposed to estrogen for a longer period than women with late menarche and early menopause.

Patients with both type 1 and type 2 diabetes are at a twofold increased risk for developing endometrial adenocarcinoma compared with women without diabetes. This increased risk was independent of other risk factors such as obesity.[18,25–28]

TREATMENT

This section provides an overview of the current treatment of endometrial adenocarcinoma, as well as current issues and controversies. The approach to treatment of endometrial adenocarcinoma is based on initial assessment of the patient by endometrial sampling, with the histologic grade and tumor cell type guiding the surgeon as to extent of the resection. Additional factors taken into account are the age of the patient, overall patient health, and comorbidities. Definitive tumor histology, tumor cell type, and the stage of the tumor are confirmed by the pathologist examining the surgical resection. The pathologic postoperative findings and cytology of pelvic washings have been incorporated into three groups for risk of recurrence. Patients with low risk of recurrence are defined as having histologic grade 1 or 2 endometrioid-type adenocarcinomas with less than 50% of myometrial invasion, no endocervical involvement, no lymphovascular invasion, and negative pelvic washings on cytology or grade 3 adenocarcinomas with no myometrial invasion. Management of these patients includes surgical resection with no adjuvant therapy (radiation or chemotherapy); however, many gynecologic oncologists provide adjuvant therapy to patients with grade 3 tumors. Patients with intermediate risk of recurrence are defined as having histologic grade 1 or 2 endometrial carcinoma, with more than 50% myometrial invasion and/or endocervical involvement. Adjuvant radiotherapy to the pelvis or vagina or both has been recommended in these patients, with studies showing a decrease in local recurrence but no significant change in overall survival.[29,30] Patients with high risk of recurrence are defined as having endometrioid-type adenocarcinoma with grade 3 tumor histology, any depth of myometrial invasion (< or ≥50%), lymphovascular invasion, endocervical involvement, or nonendometrioid tumor type (serous or clear cell tumor type). In these patients, in addition to the "standard" treatment of total abdominal hysterectomy and bilateral salpingo-oophorectomy (TAH-BSO), lymph node resection is performed, and adjuvant therapy is administered, either radiotherapy or chemotherapy or both.

Usually, the accepted standard of care is surgical resection with TAH-BSO for all stages of endometrial carcinoma. Many advocated surgical resection only for stage I low-grade endometrial carcinomas and in rare cases of stage I endometrial carcinoma in young women who have not completed childbearing; medical management is advocated only after evaluation has been performed to rule out a higher grade of disease.[30-33] Series reports cited initial response rates of 50% to 75% and a pregnancy rate of 25% with conservative treatment.[31-33] After childbearing or with persistent or recurrent disease, definitive TAH-BSO is recommended.

Patients who have significant comorbidities and stage IA disease have been treated with radiation therapy alone to avoid the risks of surgery, but this strategy results in a 20% decreased survival rate compared with surgical resection.[34] Radiation therapy is added based on a given patient's assessment of increased risk factors for recurrence and metastatic potential and is recommended by many in the management of postoperative patients over age 70 and patients with high endometrial tumor grade, serous or clear cell tumor type, or deep endometrial invasion (stage IB); additional radiotherapy to the vaginal area is recommended in cases of endocervical involvement (stage II).[35-37]

Patients with recurrent or metastatic disease have a poor prognosis, with a median survival time of 12 months despite treatment with combined modalities such as addition of chemotherapy to radiotherapy.[37]

ISSUES IN MANAGEMENT AND TREATMENT

Lymph Node Resection

Surgical resection is the standard of care and management in endometrial carcinoma for all stages of tumor, with lymph node resection of pelvic and para-aortic lymph nodes performed in patients with higher stage tumors (stage III). However, there is no consensus concerning whether to perform pelvic and para-aortic lymph node resection in lower stage tumors.[38] The decision to perform lymph node resection is usually based on several factors, including tumor grade and depth of myometrial invasion because these two factors directly impact on the risk of regional lymph node metastasis. Although there are many articles published on this particular issue regarding patient management, there is no consensus approach between institutions in a given city or country or worldwide for primary surgical lymph node resection.[39] The pelvic lymph nodes are most often involved and are the most common regional node location for metastatic disease in patients in whom the tumor appears confined to the uterus. Several studies of women undergoing pelvic lymph node resection reported occult metastasis after histologic evaluation in up to 28% of patients.[40]

Preoperative assessment by magnetic resonance imaging (MRI) has been advocated by many for assessment of depth of myometrial invasion; however, there is variability in accuracy of interpretation and reporting, which has been shown to be institution dependent.[41,42] The result is inconsistency as to lymph node resection based on MRI. Overall, use of MRI has not been found to be cost effective or justified in "routine" preoperative patient assessment for endometrial carcinoma. Frozen section at the time of surgical resection is used in many institutions for assessment of the resected uterus for myometrial depth of invasion to aid in decision making for lymph node resection. Frozen section was shown to be more accurate in assessing depth of invasion; however, marked variability in reported accuracy was found among institutions that used this method.[43]

Lymph node metastatic disease directly impacts patient prognosis and staging, which directly impacts decisions regarding adding adjuvant treatment such as radiotherapy and chemotherapy to patient management. One study showed that 13% of patients who were clinically assessed as stage I, who underwent lymph node resection, had metastatic disease resulting in a higher stage (stage III), compared with 3% of patients who did not undergo lymph node resection.[44] Additional controversy exists whether lymph node resection should include the para-aortic lymph nodes as well as the pelvic lymph nodes. One study compared patient outcome with resection of pelvic lymph nodes only to outcome with pelvic and para-aortic lymph node resection and showed there is benefit in also removing the para-aortic lymph nodes in patients assessed as having intermediate and high risk of recurrence of tumor. No benefit was seen with para-aortic lymph node resection in patients with low risk of recurrence.[45,46] However, some gynecologic oncologists performed lymph node resection on all patients undergoing surgical resection for endometrial carcinoma.[39]

Adjuvant Chemotherapy Therapy and Hormonal Therapy

Adjuvant radiotherapy has been shown to increase the survival rate by 10% and decrease local recurrence in high-risk patients but not in low- or intermediate-risk patients.[47] Addition of adjuvant radiotherapy is now part of the treatment offered to patients, with patient selection based on tumor grade, tumor type, and depth of invasion.

Adjuvant hormonal therapy is only recommended to be offered for stage III endometrial carcinoma if the patient cannot undergo surgery or radiation therapy. Types of hormonal treatment include megestrol (Megace, Apo-megestrol, Nu-megestrol, Linmegestrol) and medroxyprogesterone (Provera).

Adjuvant chemotherapy in low-risk, less advanced disease remains controversial and is most often offered to high-risk patients over 70 years of age, with a reported overall increased survival rate of 89% and increased progression-free survival rate of 84% in one study.[48] High risk of local recurrence has been show to occur with single-modality adjuvant chemotherapy; thus usually, a combination of anthracyclines (doxorubicin) and platinum-based agents (carboplatin) is used.[49] Addition of the taxane paclitaxel to doxorubicin and cisplatin was found to greatly improve progression-free and overall survival in high-risk patients.[50] However, the problem with studies and trials adding adjuvant chemotherapy for patient treatment is that all "high-grade" endometrial carcinomas have been lumped together into one "high-risk" group.

Molecular studies currently have demonstrated that not only do high-grade carcinomas, such as serous carcinoma and clear cell carcinoma, have distinct features, but also endometrial carcinomas of a similar histologic type demonstrate different clinical behavior and can show different molecular profiles. It is hoped that research in the molecular pathways of endometrial carcinoma will soon lead to a better understanding of the biology of the tumors and to the development of more effective therapies and more specific "individual" targeted therapies (see Chapters 7 and 8).

Follow-Up and Prognosis

Although the management of endometrial carcinoma involves a "standard" approach to initial evaluation with surgical resection (TAH-BSO), significant variability in treatment exists by geographic location (from country to country but also regionally within a country), between institutions, and between gynecologic oncologists.[39,51,52] Recommended follow-up with routine surveillance is usually every 4 months for the first 2 years because most recurrences occur within this period, and then every 6 months for the next 3 years and annually thereafter. Each follow-up visit usually includes a physical/pelvic examination, Pap test, and lymph node survey. Chest x-ray, CT scan, or other diagnostic imaging is performed if symptoms persist or if suspicious findings are noted on the physical/pelvic examination or Pap test result.

Endometrioid adenocarcinoma is usually diagnosed in the early stage of the disease due to symptomatic presentation, with abnormal uterine bleeding and postmenopausal bleeding leading to investigation and early diagnosis with good survival rates. However, high-grade types of endometrioid carcinoma and nonendometrioid carcinoma types (serous, clear cell) have poor survival rates in stage-for-stage comparison (Table 2-3).

Table 2-3 Tumor Stage Distribution and 5-Year Relative Survival by Stage at Diagnosis, 2001–2007, All Races

Stage	Stage Distribution (%)	5-Year Relative Survival (%)
Localized (confined to primary site)	68	95.8
Regional (spread to regional lymph nodes)	19	67.1
Distant (tumor metastasis)	8	16.2
Unknown (not staged)	4	50.1

Definitions: *Relative survival* indicates net survival, which is calculated by comparing the observed (overall) survival of cancer patients with expected survival from a comparable set of people who do not have cancer to measure the mortality that is associated with a cancer diagnosis. The overall 5-year relative survival for 2001–2007 from 17 Surveillance, Epidemiology, and End Results (SEER) geographic areas was 81.8%. Five-year relative survival by race was 83.7% for White women and 60.2% for Black women.
Stage distribution: Stage is a measure of disease progression that details the extent to which cancer is presents at time of diagnosis or the extent the cancer has advanced.
Modified from Howlader N, Noone AM, Krapcho M, et al., eds. SEER cancer statistics review, 1975–2008. Bethesda, MD: National Cancer Institute; 2010. http://seer.cancer.gov/csr/1975_2008/.

THE PATHOLOGIST'S RESPONSIBILITY

This section will attempt to address the responsibility of the pathologist and the interaction with the clinician, which could include the general practitioner, obstetrician/gynecologist, and/or gynecologic oncologist. The first and most important piece of information that should be communicated to the pathologist is an accurate clinical history. The clinical history should be provided on all specimens received in the department of pathology for histologic or cytologic evaluation. The type of specimens received will vary on a case-to-case basis and from a given patient and may include endometrial tissue submitted as biopsy, curetting, or surgical resections. The cytology could consist of pelvic washings, uterine cavity aspirations, or part of a cervical examination, such as a Pap test.

The pathologist's role is not only to communicate the histopathologic findings but also to be an active participant in patient care because clinical decisions are made for patient treatment based on the diagnosis rendered by the pathologist. The pathologist's responsibility to the patient is to make the most accurate interpretation of the specimen using the histologic features present, determining whether the features are benign, preneoplastic (hyperplasia), or neoplastic (carcinoma). The lack of a clinical history with a submitted specimen or lack of an accurate clinical history can negatively impact interpretation and can lead to either undertreatment or overtreatment with adverse patient outcome. Inaccurate or incomplete clinical history can lead to misinterpretation of tissue findings, especially in patients who have had a previous history of malignancy with prior chemotherapy and/or radiation therapy or who are on exogenous hormones or hormone replacement therapy or medications that have an effect on the endometrium, such as tamoxifen (see Chapter 3).[53,54]

A biopsy or curetting specimen sample can also be limited, especially if the amount of tissue is scanty or not representative (e.g., lower uterine segment tissue or endocervical/cervical tissue in specimen submitted as endometrial biopsy), resulting in diagnostic disagreement with under- or overinterpretation. Criteria for an adequate endometrial sample have not been established, with much of the current trend for endometrial sampling performed by Pipelle technique (biopsy) and as an office or outpatient procedure rather than by curetting.[55,56] In many instances, a definite diagnosis cannot be made based on a biopsy or curetting, and a more descriptive type of interpretation or diagnosis is given (see Chapter 13).

Based on curetting, biopsy, or surgical resection, the pathologist's responsibility includes the evaluation of the tumor and identification of the most accurate histologic cell type and nuclear grade in surgical resection specimens for endometrial carcinoma.[56,57] The pathologist's responsibility will also include oversight of the surgical resection specimen examination, usually total hysterectomies, to ensure that appropriate tissue sections were submitted from the neoplasm to document size, depth of invasion into underlying myometrium, and extent of involvement of endocervical canal. Resections may include ovaries, fallopian tubes, pelvic nodes, omentum, and other tissue as part of a staging procedure (see Chapter 10).

References

1. Howlader N, Noone AM, Krapcho M, et al., eds. *SEER cancer statistics review, 1975–2008.* Bethesda, MD: National Cancer Institute; 2010. http://seer.cancer.gov/csr/1975_2008/.
2. Holland C. Unresolved issues in management of endometrial cancer. *Exp Rev Anticancer Ther.* 2011;11:57–69.

3. Soliman PT, Oh JC, Schmeler KM, et al. Risk factors for young premenopausal women with endometrial cancer. *Obstet Gynecol.* 2005;105:575–580.
4. Bray E, Dos Santos Silva J, Moller H, et al. Endometrial cancer incidence trends in Europe: underlying determinants and prospects for prevention. *Cancer Epidemiol Biomarkers Prev.* 2005;14:1132–1142.
5. Canadian Cancer Society. Statistics Canada. Public Health Agency of Canada. http://www.cancer.ca.
6. Jobo T. Cytological findings of early stage of endometrial adenocarcinoma. Prevention and early diagnosis. XV International Congress of Cytology; 2004; Santiago de Chile, Chile.
7. Allard JE, Maxwell GI. Race disparities between black and white women in the incidence, treatment and prognosis of endometrial carcinoma. *Cancer Control.* 2009;16:53–56.
8. Bokham JV. Two pathogenetic types of endometrial carcinoma. *Gynecol Oncol.* 1983;15:10–17.
9. Koul A, Willen R, Bendahl PO, et al. Distinct sets of gene alterations in endometrial carcinoma implicate alternate modes of tumorigenesis. *Cancer.* 2002;94:2369–2379.
10. Mathers ME, Johnson SJ, Wadehra V. How predictive is a cervical smear suggesting glandular neoplasia? *Cytopathology.* 2002;13:83–91.
11. Kapali M, Agaram NP, Dabbs D, et al. Routine endometrial sampling of asymptomatic premenopausal women shedding endometrial cells in Papanicolaou tests is not cost effective. *Cancer Cytopathol.* 2007;111:26–33.
12. Brand A. Diagnosis of endometrial cancer in women with abnormal vaginal bleeding. *SOGC Clin Pract Guidelines.* 2000;86:1–3.
13. Seamark CJ. Endometrial sampling in general practice. *Br J Gen Pract.* 1998;48:1597–1598.
14. Beckner ME, Mori T, Siverberg SG. Endometrial carcinoma: nontumor factors in prognosis. *Int J Gynecol Pathol.* 1985;4:131–145.
15. Potischman N, Hoover RN, Brinton LA, et al. Case-control study of endogenous steroid hormones and endometrial cancer. *J Natl Cancer Inst.* 1996;88:1127–1135.
16. The Cancer and Steroid Hormone Study of the Centers for Disease Control and the National Institute of Child Health and Human Development. Combination oral contraceptive use and the risk of endometrial cancer. *JAMA.* 1987;257:796–800.
17. Ulrich LS. Endometrial cancer, types, prognosis, female hormones and antihormones. *Climacteric.* 2011;14:418–425.
18. Heller DS, Mosquera C, Goldsmith LT, et al. Body mass index of patients with endometrial hyperplasia: comparison to patients with proliferative endometrium and abnormal bleeding. *J Reprod Med.* 2011;56:110–112.
19. Austin H, Drews C, Partridge EE. A case-study of endometrial cancer in relation to cigarette smoking, serum estrogen levels and alcohol use. *Am J Obstet Gynecol.* 1993;169:1086–1091.
20. Franks AL, Kendrick JS, Tyler CW Jr. Postmenopausal smoking, estrogen replacement therapy and the risk of endometrial cancer. *Am J Obstet Gynecol.* 1987;156:20–23.
21. Doherty JA, Cushing-Haugen KL, Saltzman BS, et al. Long-term use of postmenopausal estrogen and progestin hormone therapies and the risk of endometrial cancer. *Am J Obstet Gynecol.* 2007;197:139.e1–139.e7.
22. Ingle JN. Tamoxifen and endometrial cancer: new challenges for an "old" drug. *Gynecol Oncol.* 1994;55:161–163.
23. Powles T. Prevention of breast cancer by newer SERMS in the future. *Recent Results Cancer Res.* 2011;188:141–145.
24. Pinkerton JV, Goldstein SR. Endometrial safety: a key hurdle for selective estrogen receptor modulators in development. *Menopause.* 2010;17:642–653.
25. Renehan AG, Tyson M, Egger M, et al. Body-mass index and incidence of cancer: a systematic review and meta-analysis of prospective observational studies. *Lancet.* 2008;371:569–578.
26. Parazzini F, Franceschi S, La Vecchi C, et al. The epidemiology of female genital tract cancers. *Int J Gynecol Cancer.* 1997;7:169–181.

27. Papanas N, Giatromanolaki A, Galazios G, et al. Endometrial carcinoma and diabetes revisited. *Eur J Gynaecol Oncol.* 2006;27:505–508.
28. Nicolucci A. Epidemiological aspects of neoplasms in diabetes. *Acta Diabetol.* 2010;47:87–95.
29. Creutzberg CL, van Putten WL, Koper PC, et al. Surgery and postoperative radiotherapy versus surgery alone for patients with stage-1 endometrial carcinoma: multicentre randomised trial. PORTEC Study Group. Post Operative Radiation Therapy in Endometrial Carcinoma. *Lancet.* 2000;355:1404–1411.
30. Scholten AN, van Putten WL, Beerman H, et al. Postoperative radiotherapy for stage 1 endometrial carcinoma: long-term outcome of the randomized PORTEC trial with central pathology review. *Int J Radiat Oncol Biol Phys.* 2005;63:834–838.
31. Ramirez PT, Frumovitz M, Bodurka DC, et al. Hormonal therapy for the management of grade 1 endometrial adenocarcinoma: a literature review. *Gynecol Oncol.* 2004;95:133–138.
32. Ushijima K, Yahata H, Yoshikawa H, et al. Multicenter phase II study of fertility-sparing treatment with medroxyprogesterone acetate for endometrial carcinoma and atypical hyperplasia in young women. *J Clin Oncol.* 2007;25:2798–2803.
33. Lee TS, Jung JY, Kim JW, et al. Feasibility of ovarian preservation in patients with early stage endometrial carcinoma. *Gynecol Oncol.* 2007;104:52–57.
34. Grigsby PW, Kuske RR, Perez CA, et al. Medically inoperable stage I adenocarcinoma of the endometrium treated with radiotherapy alone. *Int J Radiat Oncol Biol Phys.* 1987;13:483–488.
35. Creasman WT, Kohler MF, Odicino F, et al. Prognosis of papillary serous carcinoma, clear cell carcinoma and grade 3 stage I carcinoma of the endometrium. *Gynecol Oncol.* 2004;95:593–596.
36. Mountzios G, Barnias A, Voulgaris Z, et al. Prognostic factors in patients treated with taxane-based chemotherapy for recurrent or metastatic endometrial cancer: proposal for a new prognostic model. *Gynecol Oncol.* 2008;108:130–135.
37. McCluggage WG, Hirschowitz L, Wilson GE, et al. Significant variation in the assessment of cervical involvement in endometrial carcinoma: an interobserver variation study. *Am J Surg Pathol.* 2011;35:289–294.
38. Dietl J. Is lymphadenectomy justified in endometrial cancer? *Int J Gynecol Cancer.* 2011;21:507–510.
39. Soliman PT, Frumovitz M, Spannuth W, et al. Lymphadenectomy during endometrial cancer staging: practice patterns among gynaecological oncologists. *Gynecol Oncol.* 2010;119:291–294.
40. Chi DS, Barakat RR, Palayekar MJ, et al. The incidence of pelvic lymph node metastasis by FIGO staging for patients with adequately surgically staged endometrial adenocarcinoma of endometrioid histology. *Int J Gynecol Cancer.* 2008;18:269–273.
41. Kaneda S, Fujii S, Fukunaga T, et al. Myometrial invasion by endometrial carcinoma: evaluation with 3.0T MR imaging. *Abdom Imaging.* 2011;36:612–618.
42. Kinkel K, Forstnet R, Danza FM, et al. Staging of endometrial carcinoma with MRI: guidelines of the European Society of Urogenital Imaging. *Eur Radiol.* 2009;19:1565–1574.
43. Furukawa N, Takekuma M, Takahashi N, et al. Intraoperative evaluation of myometrial invasion and histological type and grade in endometrial cancer: diagnostic value of frozen section. *Arch Gynecol Obstet.* 2010;281:913–917.
44. Benedetti Panici P, Basile S, Maneschi F, et al. Systemic pelvic lymphadenectomy vs no lymphadenectomy in early-stage endometrial carcinoma: randomized clinical trial. *J Natl Cancer Inst.* 2008;100:1707–1716.
45. Chan JK, Cheung MK, Huh WK, et al. Therapeutic role of lymph node resection in endometrioid corpus cancer: a study of 12,333 patients. *Cancer.* 2006;107:1823–1830.
46. Todo Y, Kato H, Kaneuchi M, et al. Survival Effect of Para-aortic Lymphadenopathy in Endometrial Cancer (SEPAL study): a retrospective cohort analysis. *Lancet.* 2010;375:1165–1172.
47. Johnson N, Cornes P. Survival and recurrent disease after postoperative radiotherapy for early endometrial cancer: systematic review and meta-analysis. *BJOG.* 2007;114:1313–1320.

48. Susumu N, Sagae S, Udagawa Y, et al. Randomized phase III trial of pelvic radiotherapy versus cisplatin-based combined chemotherapy in patients with intermediate and high risk endometrial cancer: a Japanese Gynecologic Oncology Group study. *Gynecol Oncol.* 2008;108:226–233.
49. Fleming GF. Systemic chemotherapy for uterine carcinoma: metastatic and adjuvant. *J Clin Oncol.* 2007;25:2983–2990.
50. Fleming GF, Brunetto VL, Cella D, et al. Phase III trial of doxorubicin plus cisplatin with or without paclitaxel plus filgrastim in advanced endometrial carcinoma: a Gynecologic Oncology Group study. *J Clin Oncol.* 2004;22:2159–2166.
51. Mountzios G, Pectasides D, Bournakis E, et al. Developments in the systemic treatment of endometrial cancer. *Crit Rev Oncol Hematol.* 2011;79:278–292.
52. Holland C. Unresolved issues in the management of endometrial cancer. *Exp Rev Anticancer Ther.* 2011;11:57–69.
53. McKenney JK, Longacre TA. Low-grade endometrial adenocarcinoma: a diagnostic algorithm for distinguishing atypical endometrial hyperplasia and other benign (and malignant) mimics. *Adv Anat Pathol.* 2009;16:1–22.
54. Suh-Burgmann E, Hung YY, Armstrong MA. Complex atypical hyperplasia: the risk of unrecognized adenocarcinoma and value of preoperative dilation and curettage. *Obstet Gynecol.* 2009;114:523–529.
55. McCluggage WG. Miscellaneous disorders involving endometrium. *Semin Diagn Pathol.* 2010;27:287–310.
56. Allison KH, Reed SD, Voight LF, et al. Diagnosing endometrial hyperplasia: why is it so difficult to agree? *Am J Surg Pathol.* 2008;32:691–698.
57. Clarke BA, Gilks CB. Endometrial carcinoma: controversies in histopathological assessment of grade and tumour cell type. *J Clin Pathol.* 2010;63:410–415.

SECTION II

Histopathology

- **CHAPTER 3:** Preneoplastic Conditions of the Endometrium: Endometrial Hyperplasia, the Emergent Concept of Endometrial Intraepithelial Neoplasia, and Others
- **CHAPTER 4:** Endometrial Carcinoma

Preneoplastic Conditions of the Endometrium: Endometrial Hyperplasia, the Emergent Concept of Endometrial Intraepithelial Neoplasia, and Others

3

Anais Malpica, MD

In this chapter, the preneoplastic conditions of the endometrium are reviewed. The traditional approach to the preneoplastic condition of endometrioid adenocarcinoma, which is known as endometrial hyperplasia, and the more recently proposed approach, which is designated as endometrial intraepithelial neoplasia, are included. In addition, conditions that are commonly associated with endometrial hyperplasia, the metaplasias, are presented.

ENDOMETRIAL HYPERPLASIA

Endometrial hyperplasia has been the term traditionally used to designate an endometrial proliferation where there is a predominance of endometrial glands over endometrial stroma. This is the most widely accepted approach to the endometrial, endometrioid type of preneoplastic condition. Table 3-1 summarizes the World Health Organization (WHO) classification[1] of endometrial hyperplasia.

The WHO classification is based entirely on histologic features as follows: (1) a shift in the gland-to-stroma ratio with architectural alteration and (2) the presence or absence of cytologic atypia in the epithelium lining the proliferating glands. It is important to bear in mind that although the hyperplastic endometrium is usually increased in volume, in some cases, the hyperplasia is just a focal finding in an otherwise nonhyperplastic endometrium.[2]

Table 3-1	World Health Organization (WHO) Classification of Endometrial Hyperplasia
Simple endometrial hyperplasia	
Without atypia	
With atypia	
Complex endometrial hyperplasia	
Without atypia	
With atypia	

From Silverberg SG, Kurman RJ, Nogales F, et al. Tumors of the uterine corpus. Epithelial tumors and related lesions. In: Tavassoli FA, Devilee P, eds. *World Health Organization Classification of Tumours: Tumours of the Breast and Female Genital Organs.* Lyon, France: IARC Press; 2003:221–232, with permission.

Shift of the Gland-to-Stroma Ratio with Architectural Alteration

Although the WHO classification does not provide a threshold to determine what constitutes a shift in the gland-to-stroma ratio, in our practice, we follow the recommendation provided by Hendrickson et al.[3] Essentially, endometrial hyperplasia is diagnosed when the glandular proliferation is sufficient to shift the gland-to-stroma ratio from 2:1 to 3:1 (i.e., the endometrial stroma representing less than one-half to one-third of the cross-sectional area of the proliferation) (Fig. 3-1). Both glands and villoglandular structures are included in the glandular component. The hyperplastic glands usually have proliferative features (i.e., pseudostratification and mitotic activity) (Fig. 3-2), except in the uncommon cases of hyperplasia with secretory changes (Fig. 3-3).

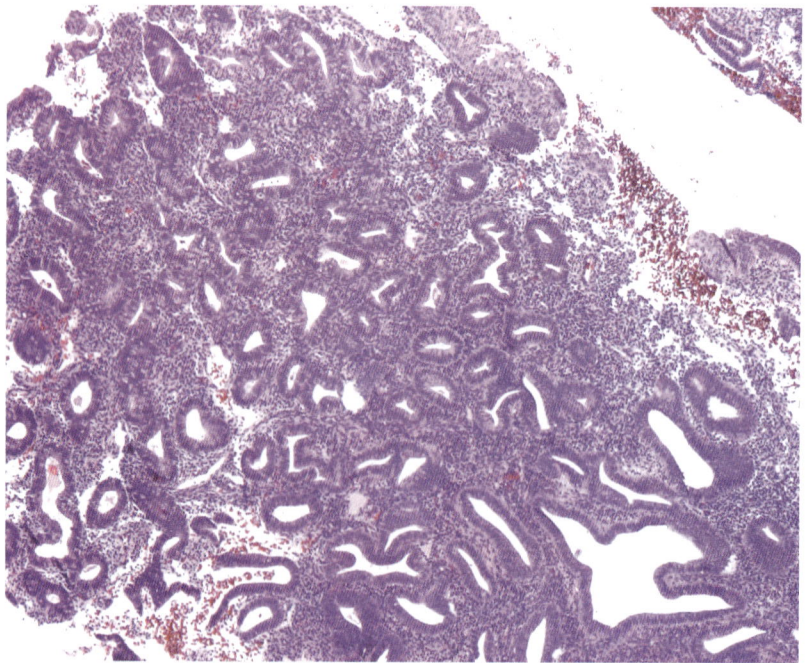

FIGURE 3-1: Endometrial hyperplasia. The glandular proliferation has shifted the gland-to-stroma ratio from 2:1 to 3:1 (the endometrial stroma represents less than one-half to one-third of the cross-sectional area of the proliferation).

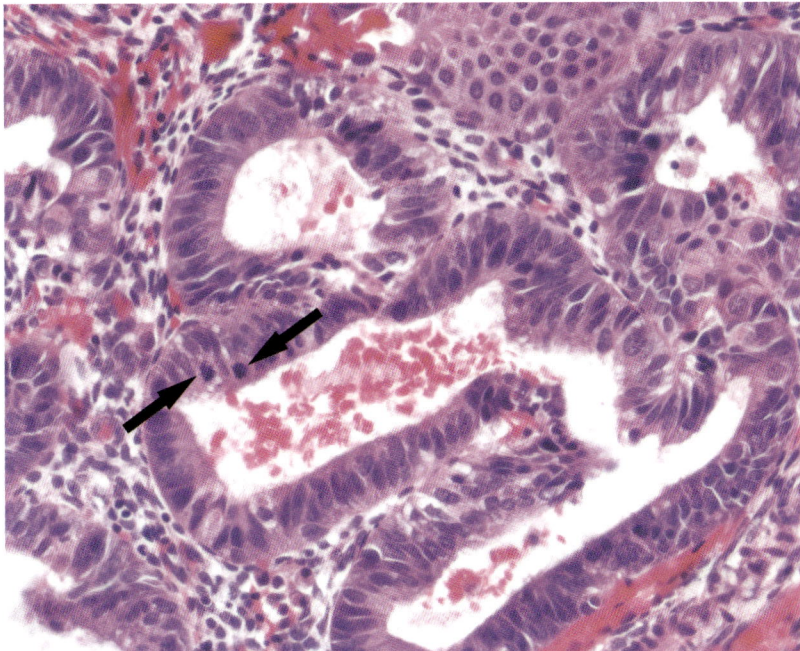

FIGURE 3-2: Endometrial epithelium usually demonstrates proliferative features such as pseudostratification and mitoses (*arrows*).

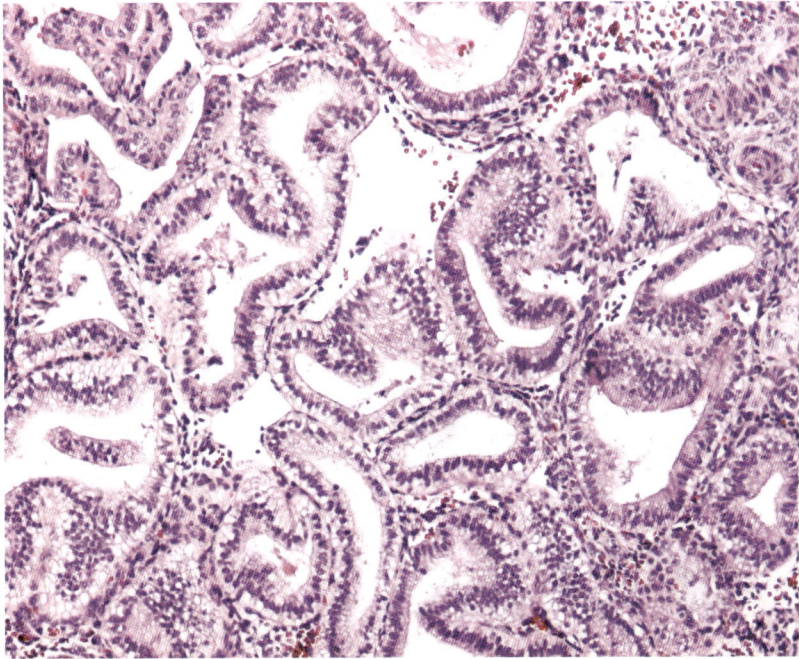

FIGURE 3-3: Secretory changes in endometrial hyperplasia.

Simple versus Complex Endometrial Hyperplasia

Simple endometrial hyperplasia is characterized by a proliferation of dilated endometrial glands of variable size, with no or slight outpouchings (Fig. 3-4), whereas in complex endometrial hyperplasia, the endometrial glands are markedly irregular in size and shape with numerous outpouchings (Fig. 3-5).

Diagnosis of Atypia

Atypia of the endometrial epithelium lining the proliferating glands is characterized by nuclear enlargement, round rather than oval nuclei, irregular distribution of the chromatin, and a variable presence of conspicuous nucleoli[4] (Figs. 3-6 and 3-7). While assessing the presence of atypia, several issues should be considered.

Artifactual Changes Secondary to Variations in Tissue Fixation and Processing

Variations in tissue fixation and processing can induce changes in the appearance of the nuclei, including alterations in the chromatin distribution and the presence of nucleoli. To prevent any misinterpretation while trying to determine whether cytologic atypia is present, it is necessary to obtain a reference point for each case by examining the nuclear features of the endometrial glands in areas without hyperplasia.

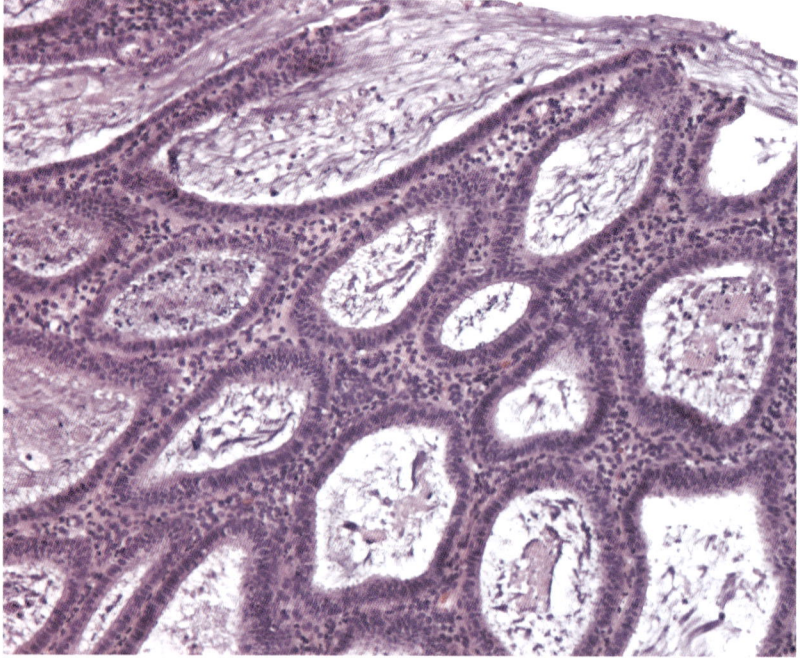

FIGURE 3-4: Simple hyperplasia. Note the proliferation of dilated endometrial glands with no or slight outpouchings.

Chapter 3 • Endometrial Hyperplasia

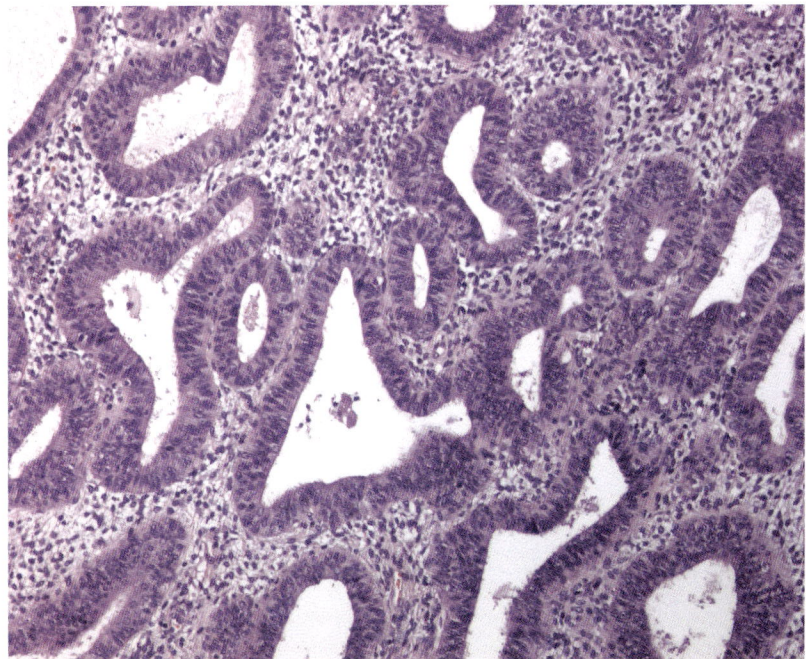

FIGURE 3-5: Complex hyperplasia. Note the proliferation of endometrial glands of variable size and shape with outpouchings.

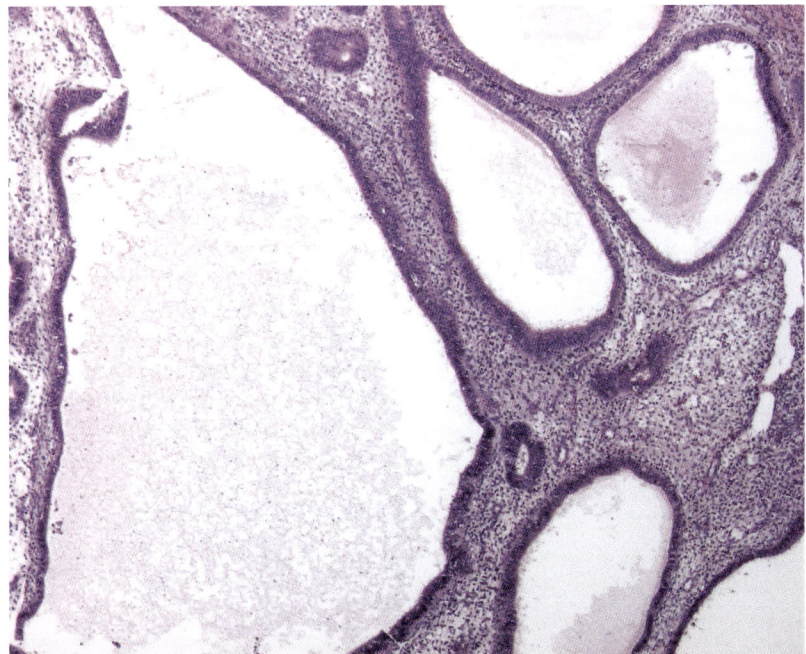

FIGURE 3-6: Simple hyperplasia with atypia (A). Note the nuclear enlargement, round nuclei, irregular distribution of the chromatin, and variable presence of nucleoli (B and C). *(continued)*

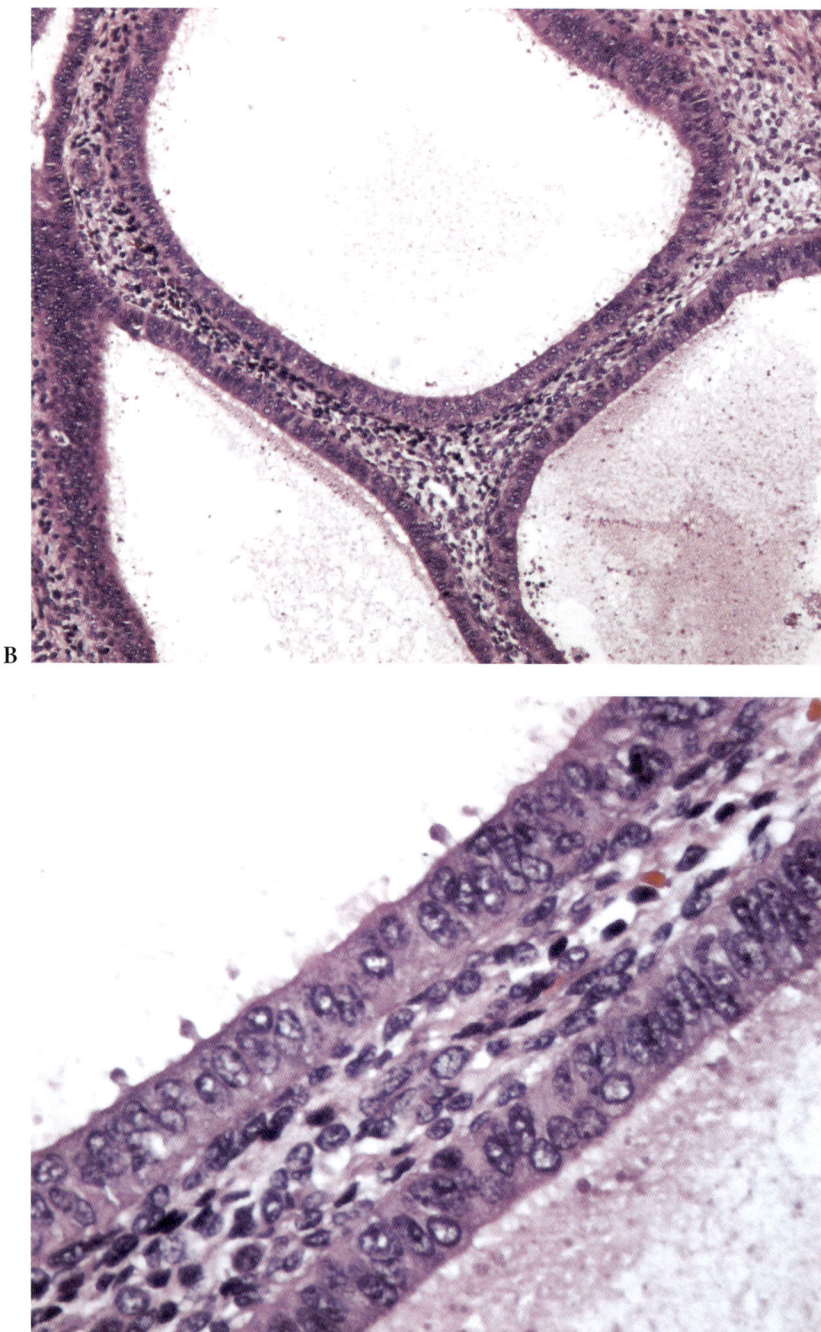

FIGURE 3-6: *(continued)*

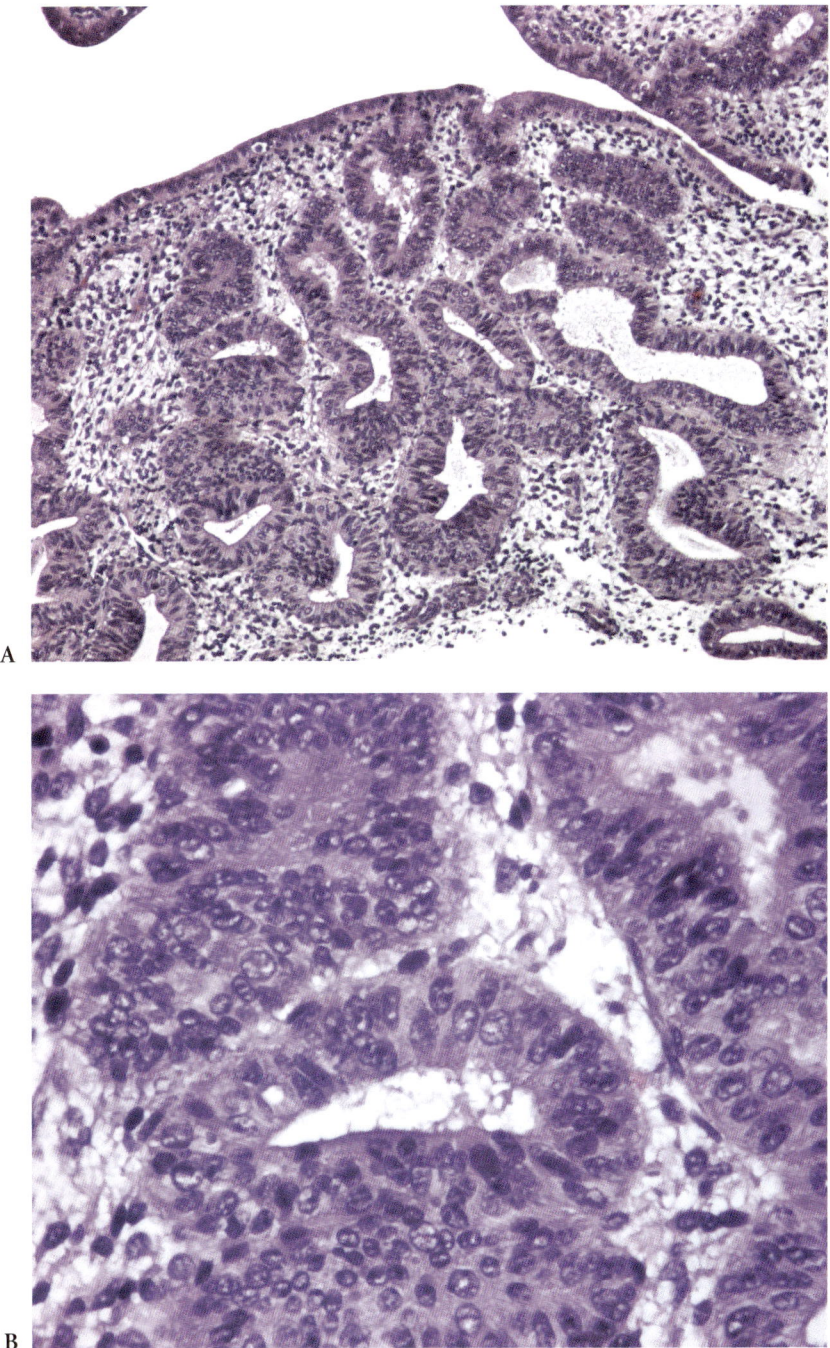

FIGURE 3-7: Complex hyperplasia with atypia (**A**). Note the nuclear enlargement, round nuclei, irregular distribution of the chromatin, and variable presence of nucleoli (**B**).

Metaplastic Changes

Nuclear changes typically seen in the endometrial glands undergoing metaplastic changes can be misinterpreted as atypia. For example, in ciliated or eosinophilic cell metaplasia, the nuclei can be enlarged and rounded; however, the chromatin distribution is uniform, and the nuclear contour is regular.

Extent and Degree of Atypia: What Is Relevant?

Hyperplastic endometrial glands with atypia may be admixed with those displaying no atypia. The minimum threshold for the diagnosis of focal atypia has not been established; however, focal atypia should be readily found without the need for an intense search (i.e., clearly atypical nuclei seen in most of the cells of several glands) in order to be considered a significant finding. Surface endometrial epithelium should be avoided for the assessment of atypia. In addition, grading the atypia (e.g., mild, moderate, severe) should be avoided because of the lack of reproducibility.[5]

DIFFERENTIAL DIAGNOSIS

Endometrial Atrophy with Cystic Change

In the atrophic endometrium with cystic changes, there is an apparent shift of the gland-to-stroma ratio that could be misinterpreted as endometrial hyperplasia. However, the endometrial epithelium in atrophy is either low columnar, cuboidal, or flattened with rare or no mitotic figures (Fig. 3-8). This epithelium contrasts with the columnar, stratified, mitotically active epithelium seen in hyperplastic endometrium.

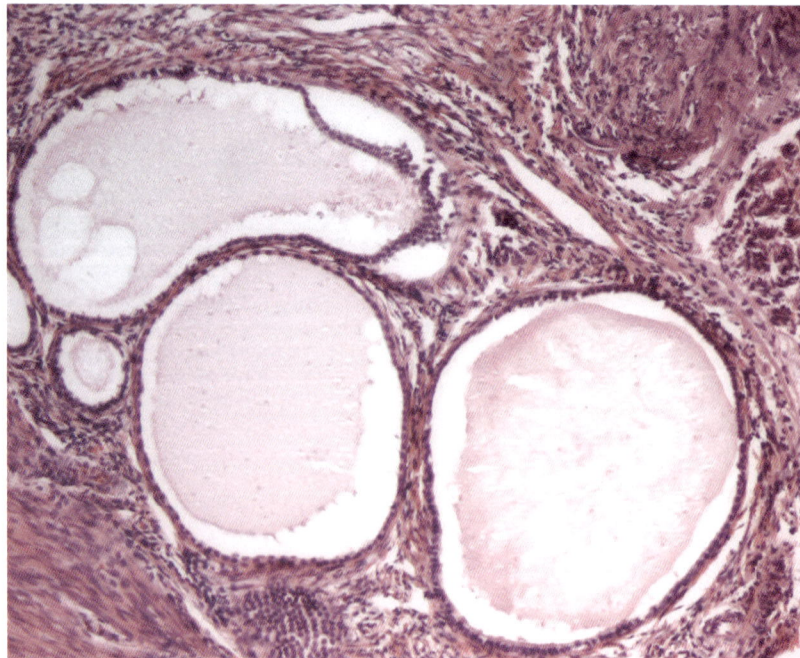

FIGURE 3-8: Cystic atrophy. The glands are dilated, but the epithelium is low columnar, cuboidal, or flattened.

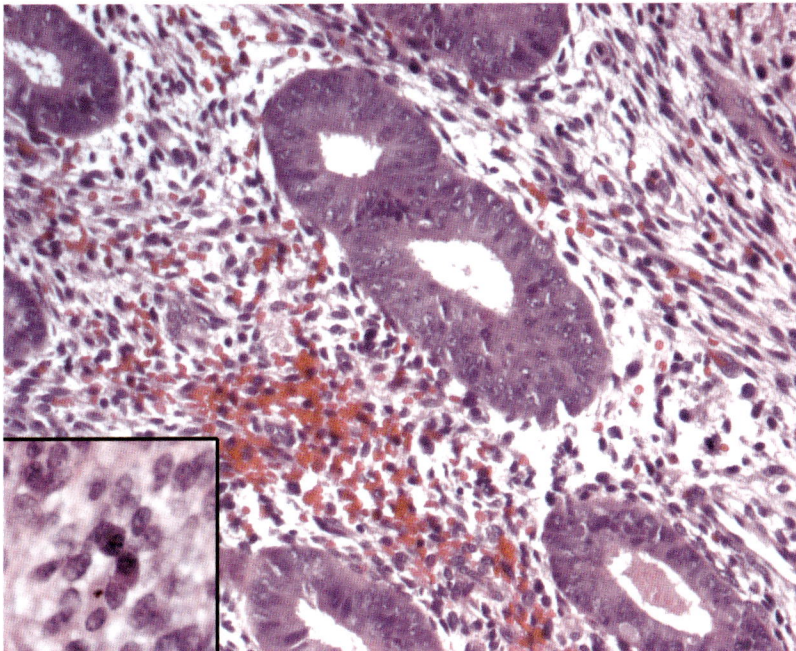

FIGURE 3-9: Reactive atypia of the glandular epithelium in endometritis. Note the presence of plasma cells in the stroma (*inset*).

Endometritis

In endometritis, especially in cases with severe inflammation, the glands may be irregularly distributed, thus mimicking endometrial hyperplasia. In addition, nuclear enlargement, a reactive change in these cases (Fig. 3-9), should not be misinterpreted as atypia. The recognition of plasma cells (Fig. 3-9, *inset*) and usually the presence of a reactive-looking stroma with spindle cells will allow the correct diagnosis.

Endometrial Polyp

An endometrial polyp can display irregularly shaped and crowded glands, thus representing a hyperplastic polyp or a polyp with areas of hyperplasia. This does not pose a problem when the classical histologic features of an endometrial polyp can be recognized in the tissue sampled (i.e., polypoid shape, thick-walled vessels, fibrous or dense stroma). However, when these features are not identified (often due to the small size of the tissue obtained), hysteroscopy and curettage may be required to ensure a correct diagnosis.[2]

Disordered Proliferative Endometrium

Disordered proliferative endometrium is usually an estrogen-related condition associated with anovulatory cycles. It is characterized by a proliferation of endometrial glands of variable size and shape, without a shift of the normal gland-to-stroma ratio (i.e., from 2:1 to 3:1; in other words, the endometrial stroma does not represent less than one-half to one-third of the cross-sectional area of the proliferation). The glands are lined by proliferative epithelium, with some of the glands becoming enlarged or cystic. Some of the glands can have an irregular contour (Fig. 3-10).[3]

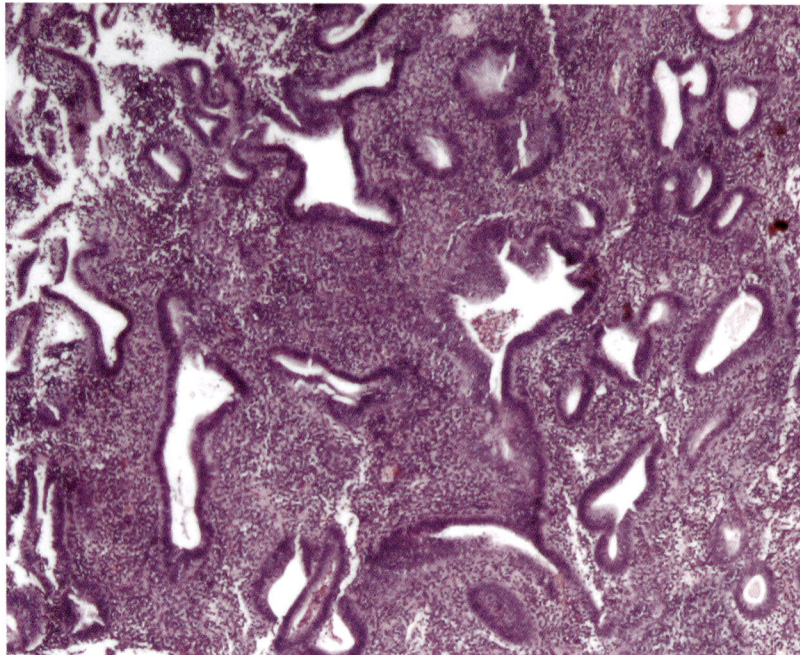

FIGURE 3-10: Disordered proliferative endometrium. Note the glands of variable size and shape. There is no shift of the normal glandular-to-stroma ratio.

Endometrioid Adenocarcinoma, International Federation of Gynecology and Obstetrics Grade 1 (Well-Differentiated Endometrioid Adenocarcinoma)

The diagnosis of endometrial, endometrioid adenocarcinoma, International Federation of Gynecology and Obstetrics (FIGO) grade 1, is made on one of the following criteria: (1) a confluent glandular growth occupying an area of at least 2 × 2 mm, (2) an extensive papillary pattern, or (3) an irregular infiltration of glands associated with a desmoplastic response.[6]

Secretory Endometrium

Secretory endometrium can have an abnormal appearance due to artifactual crowding, fragmentation, or poor orientation of the tissue sample. A proper orientation (i.e., evaluating the glands in relation to the surface epithelium) and the recognition of an organized, regular glandular pattern, mimicking a "stack of coins," in contrast to a disorganized glandular pattern, will allow the distinction of secretory endometrium with artifactual distortion from complex hyperplasia with extensive secretory changes.

Serous Carcinoma

The glandular variant of serous carcinoma can be mistaken for endometrial hyperplasia with atypia. Attention to the degree of cytologic atypia is of utmost importance to make the correct diagnosis. The presence of cells with marked variation in nuclear size and shape, an increased nuclear-to-cytoplasmic ratio, and loss of nuclear polarity lining the endometrial glands (Fig. 3-11) should raise the possibility of serous carcinoma, glandular variant. The use

Chapter 3 • Endometrial Hyperplasia

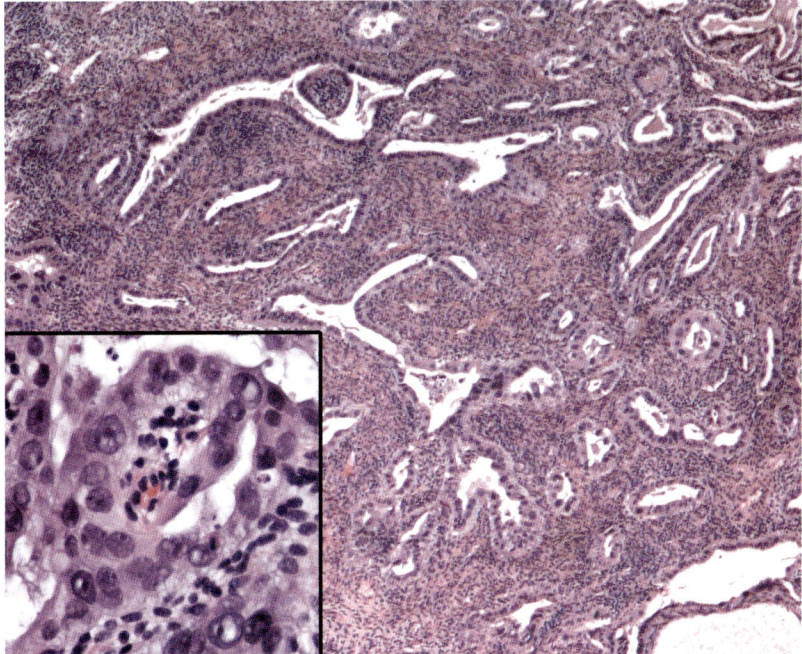

FIGURE 3-11: Glandular variant of serous carcinoma. The endometrium shows an increased number of glands with variable size and shape; note the marked cytologic atypia and loss of nuclear polarity in the epithelium (*inset*).

of immunohistochemical studies, such as Ki-67, demonstrating a high proliferative index and a strong and diffuse p53 expression confirm the diagnosis of serous carcinoma.[5,7,8]

Hyperplastic Papillary Proliferation of the Endometrium

Hyperplastic papillary proliferation of the endometrium is an uncommon lesion that is characterized by a papillary proliferation of cuboidal to low columnar bland epithelium with scanty or no mitoses. The papillary structures may or may not have a fibrovascular core. This process can have a simple or complex architecture. The former type usually involves a polyp. The simple pattern consists of small foci of papillary formations, which can be restricted to a dilated endometrial gland (Fig. 3-12). In contrast, the complex pattern is exuberant with many endometrial glands involved (Fig. 3-13). Some investigators have considered this process a form of hyperplasia associated with metaplasia and have proposed polypectomy and/or curettage as treatment.[9] However, in our opinion, patients with a complex hyperplastic papillary proliferation of the endometrium who are treated conservatively should be followed, with procurement of additional tissue if uterine bleeding persists or recurs due to the rare association with endometrial adenocarcinoma (unpublished observations). At the present time, there is no consensus regarding the most appropriate term for this entity (i.e., simple or complex hyperplastic papillary proliferation, papillary proliferation, or benign papillary change). In our practice, we use the term "complex hyperplastic papillary proliferation" for those cases displaying a complex architectural pattern. In addition, we include a comment in the report indicating that this process represents a form of complex endometrial hyperplasia with metaplastic changes. In contrast, we use the term "papillary proliferation" for those cases displaying a simple architectural pattern.[3,5,9]

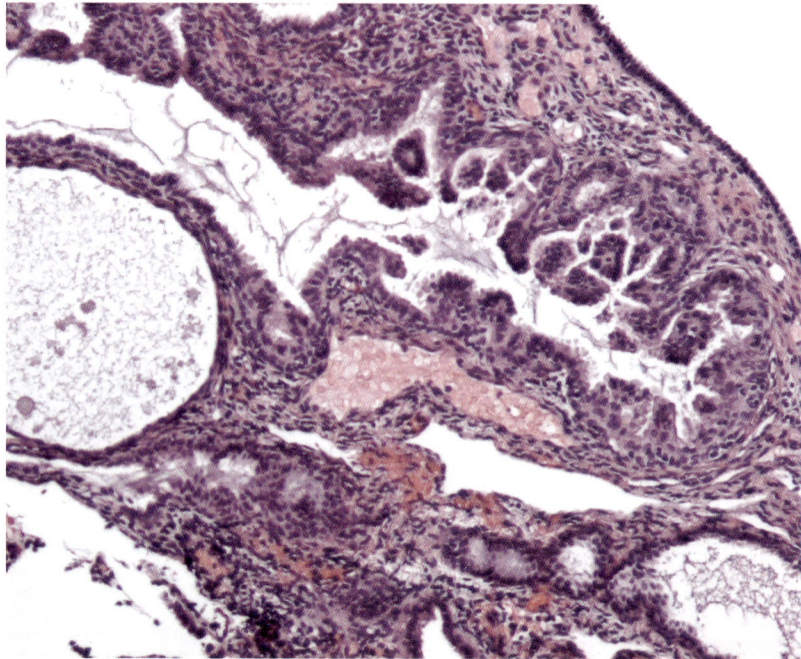

FIGURE 3-12: Simple hyperplastic papillary proliferation of the endometrium in an endometrial polyp.

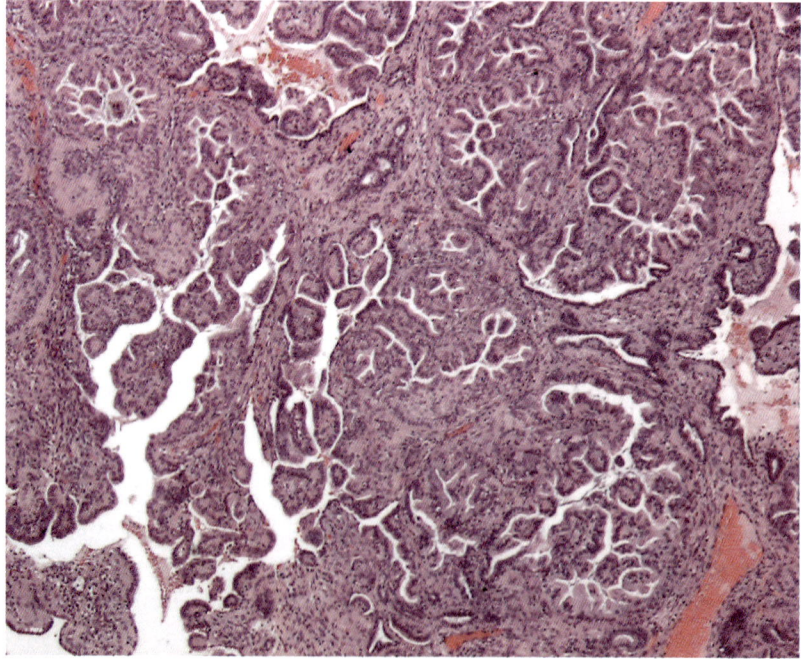

FIGURE 3-13: Complex hyperplastic papillary proliferation of the endometrium.

Artifacts and Contaminants

Artifactual distortion of the endometrial tissue or the presence of contaminants can cause the misdiagnosis of endometrial hyperplasia. The following artifacts can result in diagnostic difficulties:

1. Marked fragmentation of the tissue with subsequent dissociation of the endometrial glands from the stroma can produce the false impression of glandular crowding. This fragmentation can be secondary to mechanical disruption of the tissue during the biopsy or curettage due to artifactual glandular/stromal "breakdown" and crowding.
2. Overlapping glands or disruption of the stroma due to suboptimal histologic technique, such as improper fixation or processing and thick sectioning.
3. Poor orientation of the tissue can result in misinterpretation of irregularly shaped endometrial glands of the basalis or tangentially cut tortuous endometrial glands as endometrial hyperplasia (Fig. 3-14).
4. Telescoping is the intussusception of glands within glands due to mechanical disruption from curettage or biopsy. It can be seen in proliferative or secretory endometrium (Fig. 3-15).
5. The presence of numerous endocervical tissue fragments in an endometrial sample, especially if displaying hyperplastic changes (Fig. 3-16), can add complexity to the architecture seen at low magnification. This can be misinterpreted as endometrial hyperplasia with metaplastic changes.

ENDOMETRIAL HYPERPLASIA: CLINICAL IMPLICATIONS

The classification adopted by the WHO is linked to a reported difference in the progression to carcinoma. In one study that analyzed untreated hyperplasia, 80% of the cases of endometrial hyperplasia, simple or complex, without atypia regressed. In contrast, 69% of the cases

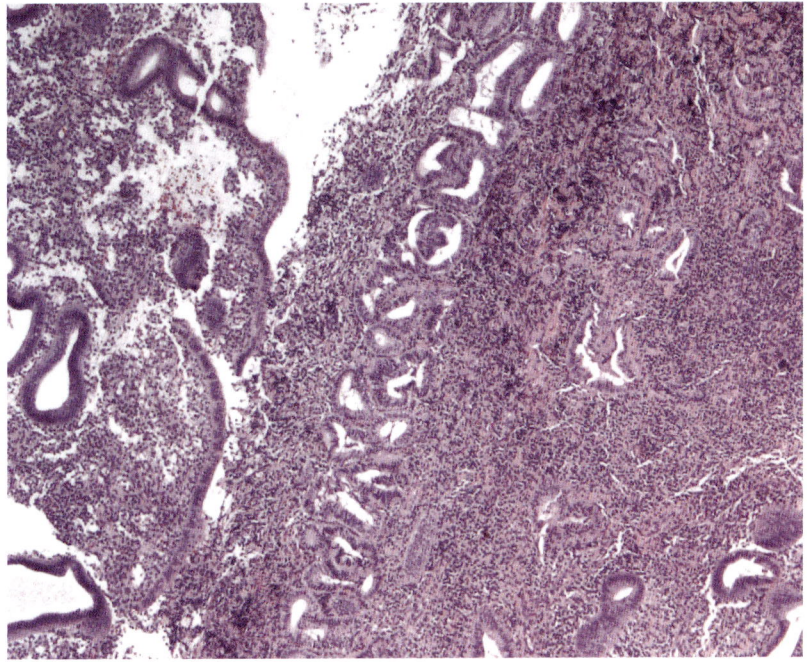

FIGURE 3-14: Tangentially cut basalis not to be mistaken for hyperplasia.

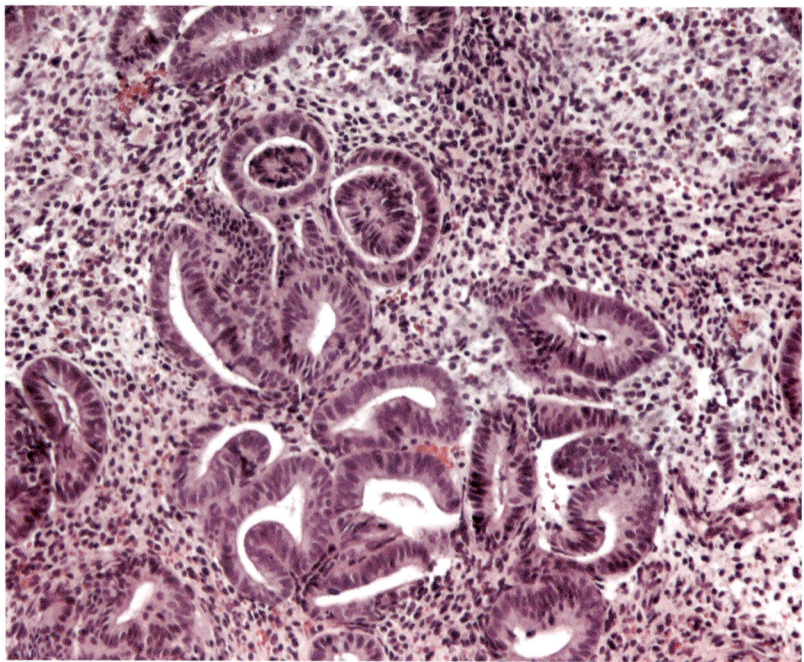

FIGURE 3-15: "Telescoping" in proliferative endometrium.

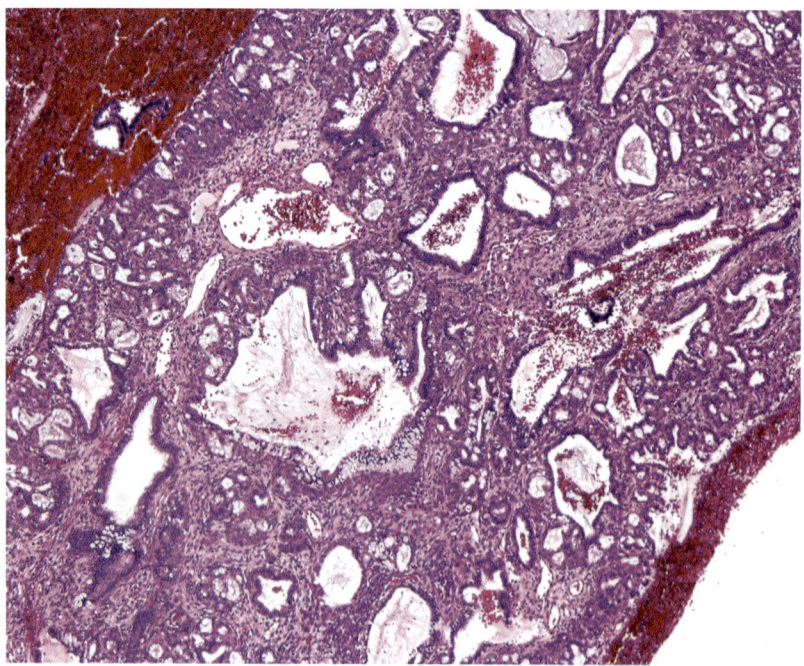

FIGURE 3-16: Fragment of endocervical tissue with microglandular hyperplasia as a contaminant in an endometrial biopsy not to be confused with endometrial hyperplasia.

of simple endometrial hyperplasia with atypia and 57% of the cases of complex endometrial hyperplasia with atypia regressed. In patients with complex endometrial hyperplasia with atypia, persistence of the lesion or progression to adenocarcinoma was seen in 14% and 29% of patients, respectively. In patients with simple hyperplasia with atypia, persistence of the lesion or progression to adenocarcinoma was seen in 23% and 8% of patients, respectively. In patients with simple endometrial hyperplasia without atypia, persistence of the lesion or progression to adenocarcinoma occurred in 19% and 1% of patients, respectively. In patients with complex endometrial hyperplasia without atypia, persistence of the lesion or progression to adenocarcinoma was seen in 17% and 3% of patients, respectively.[4] Other investigators have also reported the highest risk of progression to carcinoma in the atypical hyperplasia group, as well as the highest risk of persistence despite hormonal therapy.[10,11] One of these studies[11] found that the long-term risk of developing adenocarcinoma among women with atypical hyperplasia, either simple or complex, was approximately 30%. In addition to this risk of progression to carcinoma, it is important to bear in mind that complex endometrial hyperplasia with atypia is frequently seen in the background of low-grade endometrial, endometrioid adenocarcinoma, as demonstrated in a Gynecological Oncology Group study where 39% of the hysterectomies performed on patients diagnosed with complex endometrial hyperplasia with atypia on a biopsy or curettage contained adenocarcinoma and 33% of these were myoinvasive.[12]

Patients with complex endometrial hyperplasia with atypia, and even patients with FIGO grade 1 endometrial, endometrioid adenocarcinoma, can be managed conservatively with progestational agents or gonadotropin-releasing hormone agonists.[13] Follow-up with endometrial sampling every 3 to 6 months is required to monitor the response to treatment.[14] Patients with complex endometrial hyperplasia with atypia who are postmenopausal or premenopausal and do not wish to preserve their fertility are treated surgically. A rare case of complex endometrial hyperplasia with atypia managed with progestins progressed to FIGO grade 2 endometrial, endometrioid adenocarcinoma with lymph node metastasis in a 2.5-year period.[15]

PROBLEMS WITH THE WHO CLASSIFICATION OF ENDOMETRIAL HYPERPLASIA

Despite the clinical relevance of the WHO classification for endometrial hyperplasia, this classification has had problems with its reproducibility. Different studies evaluating the diagnostic reproducibility of the currently used WHO scheme for endometrial hyperplasia have shown κ values for overall interobserver agreement ranging from 0.2 to 0.7.[16–20] Of interest, complex endometrial hyperplasia with atypia has represented the least reproducible category, with κ values ranging from 0.28 to 0.65. This poor reproducibility underscores the lack of strict definitions for the diagnostic features used in the WHO classification (i.e., lack of strict definitions to determine what constitutes a "shift in the gland-to-stroma ratio in favor of the glands," "architectural changes," and "cytologic atypia").

ENDOMETRIAL INTRAEPITHELIAL NEOPLASIA: AN EMERGING CONCEPT

A group of investigators has proposed a new nomenclature to designate the preneoplastic endometrioid lesions of the endometrium with the intention to provide a classification system with better reproducibility and prediction of biologic behavior than the commonly used

Table 3-2	WHO and EIN Nomenclature Systems: Functional and Management Categories			
WHO Nomenclature	**EIN Nomenclature**	**Topography**	**Functional Category**	**Management**
Simple or complex hyperplasia without atypia	Endometrial hyperplasia	Diffuse	Prolonged estrogen effect	Hormonal therapy, symptomatic
Simple or complex hyperplasia with atypia	EIN	Focal progressing to diffuse	Precancerous	Hormonal therapy or surgery

EIN, endometrial intraepithelial neoplasia; WHO, World Health Organization.
Modified from Mutter GL, Zaino RJ, Baak JP, et al. Benign endometrial hyperplasia sequence and endometrial intraepithelial neoplasia. *Int J Gynecol Pathol.* 2007;26:103–114, with permission.

WHO classification.[18] In Table 3-2, this new system is shown, together with its functional categories and the clinical management.

Briefly, endometrial intraepithelial neoplasia (EIN) is considered to be the histopathologic manifestation of a monoclonal preinvasive glandular proliferation, and its diagnosis requires the following three criteria:

1. Architectural alteration: Crowded glands are present (i.e., the area of glands, combining epithelium and luminal spaces, is greater than that of the stroma that contains them; the stroma represents <50% of the tissue). The glands may vary in shape and branch slightly.
2. Cytologic alterations: Nuclear and cytoplasmic features of the epithelium in the glands with abnormal architecture differ from those in the background endometrium. Classic cytologic atypia, although often present, is not required for EIN diagnosis.
3. Size: Maximum linear dimension exceeds 1 mm.

In addition, it is necessary to exclude the following:

1. Benign mimickers: disordered proliferative endometrium, basalis, secretory endometrium, endometrial polyp, or repair
2. Carcinoma: maze-like glands, solid areas, or a significant cribriform pattern

The supporters of the concept of EIN have found this system to be superior to the WHO classification in discriminating lesions with the highest risk for progression to adenocarcinoma.[21] However, in a more recent study, women observed for at least 1 year after a biopsy-based diagnosis of endometrial hyperplasia, EIN, and atypical hyperplasia were found to have similarly increased risks of progression to adenocarcinoma. Thus, both systems identified women whose endometrial biopsies reflect a nearly 10-fold higher risk of progressing to adenocarcinoma.[22] Another interesting aspect of EIN is its relationship with the inactivation of the *PTEN* tumor suppressor *gene*, which is seen in 63% of cases (Fig. 3-17). However, the routine application of this marker for diagnosis of EIN is limited

Chapter 3 • Endometrial Hyperplasia

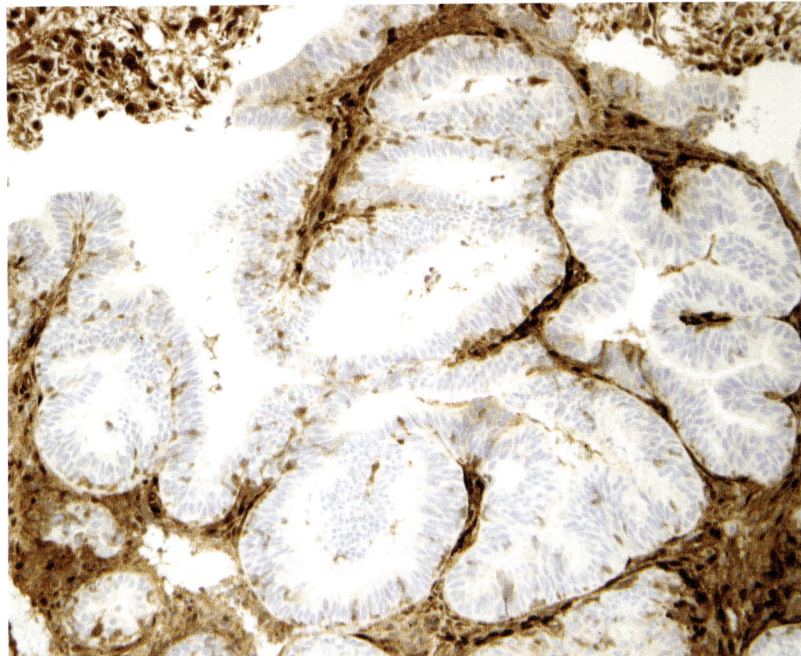

FIGURE 3-17: *PTEN* loss in an area with endometrial intraepithelial neoplasia.

because intact *PTEN* function is seen in one-third of cases; this makes *PTEN* a relatively insensitive marker for the diagnosis of this lesion. However, somatic inactivation of *PTEN* may be seen in scattered histologically unremarkable glands in 43% of otherwise healthy endometrial glands.[23]

ENDOMETRIAL METAPLASIAS

Metaplasia is the term used to describe the changes in differentiation or appearance of the regular endometrial epithelium. It is important to recognize the different types of metaplasia and distinguish them from more significant lesions.

Squamous Metaplasia

Squamous metaplasia can range from a highly keratinized form with cells capable of producing keratin debris to an immature form characterized by masses of round or spindle cells with eosinophilic or amphophilic cytoplasm and indistinct cytoplasmic borders and without obvious cytoplasmic keratinization (morules). Occasionally, squamous morules have central keratinization or necrosis (Fig. 3-18).[24] Nuclear features can be bland or obviously atypical. The former can be seen in association with normal endometrium, hyperplasia, or carcinoma, whereas the latter is usually seen in high-grade endometrioid adenocarcinoma or in the rare cases of squamous carcinoma arising in the endometrium.

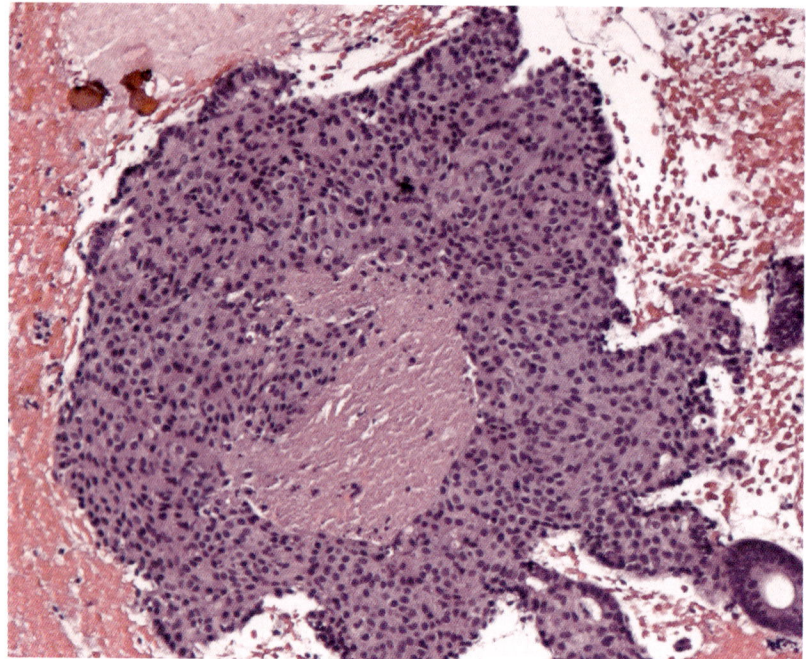

FIGURE 3-18: Squamous metaplasia.

Ciliated (Tubal) Metaplasia

Ciliated cells can be normally seen in the surface epithelium of the endometrium, especially during the proliferative phase.[25] However, ciliated cells also can be noted within glands in endometrium stimulated by unopposed estrogen[5] or in inactive endometrium (unpublished personal observation). Ciliated cells may have eosinophilic, basophilic, or pale cytoplasm. The nuclei are stratified, oval, or round, with even distribution of the chromatin and small nucleoli (Fig. 3-19). The round nuclei with nucleoli in ciliated metaplasia should not be mistaken for the atypia of hyperplasia.

Eosinophilic Metaplasia

This type of metaplasia shows columnar, cuboidal, or slightly round cells with abundant eosinophilic cytoplasm and nuclei that tend to be round, rather than oval, with evenly distributed chromatin (Fig. 3-20). These cells can be intermixed with cells containing a small amount of cytoplasmic mucin.[5] Eosinophilic metaplasia can be seen in atrophic, proliferative, or hyperplastic endometrium and in endometrioid adenocarcinoma.

Papillary Syncytial Metaplasia

Although commonly listed as a metaplastic change, papillary syncytial metaplasia is commonly associated with breakdown and bleeding, which indicates that it is most likely related to degeneration and regeneration.[26] This process can involve the surface endometrium or the endometrial glands, and it shows a syncytial growth of bland eosinophilic cells that may be arranged in small papillae without a fibroconnective tissue core

Chapter 3 • Endometrial Hyperplasia

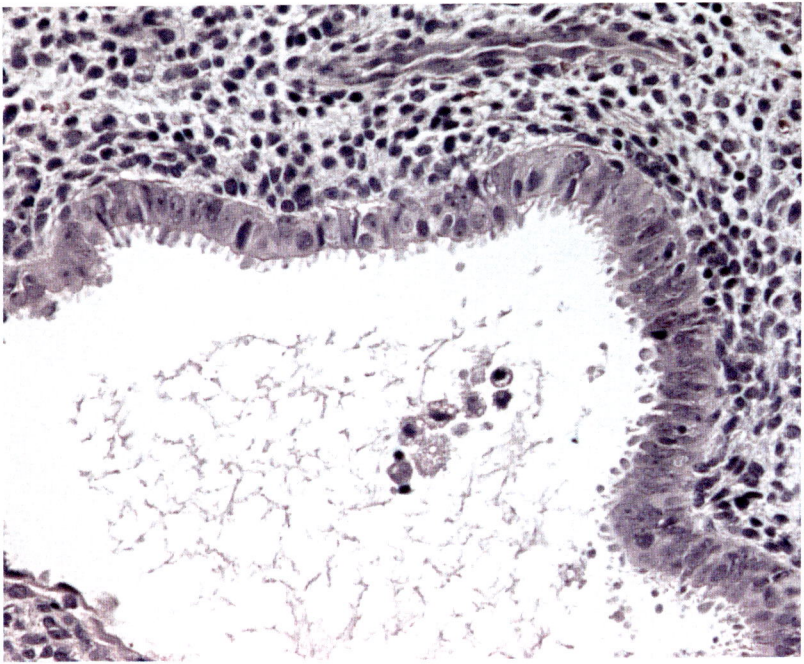

FIGURE 3-19: Ciliated metaplasia.

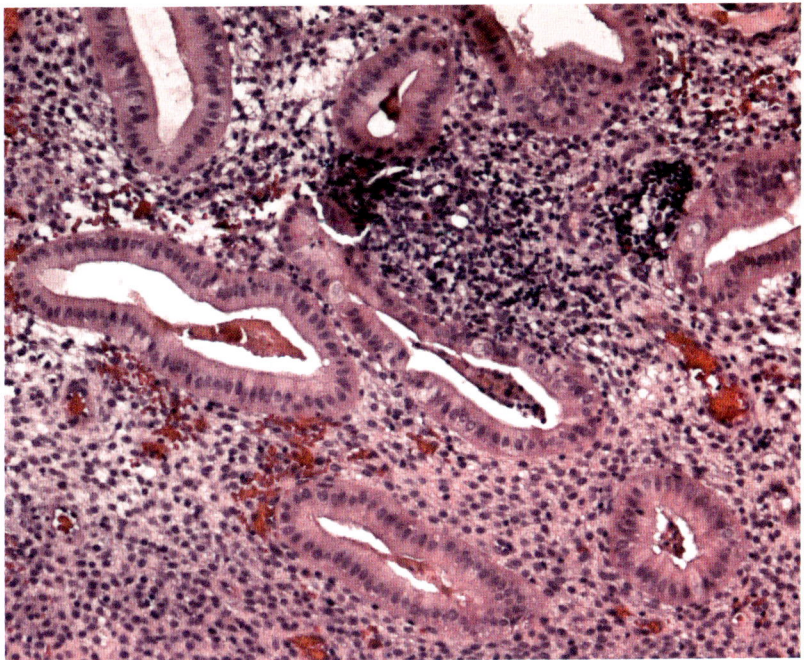

FIGURE 3-20: Eosinophilic metaplasia.

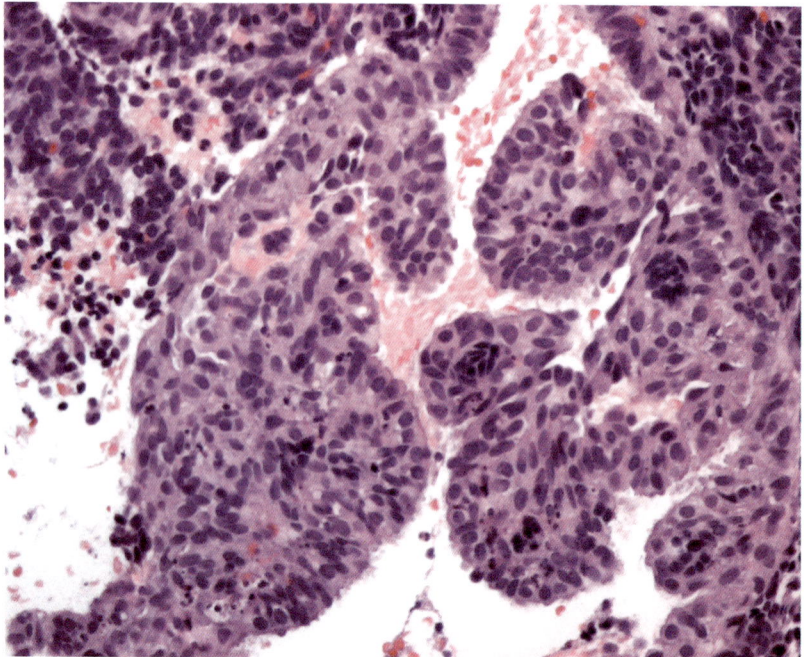

FIGURE 3-21: Papillary syncytial metaplasia.

(Fig. 3-21). Some of the nuclei can be pyknotic or show degenerative changes. Usually, it is associated with an infiltrate of polymorphonuclear leukocytes. Mitoses are rare or absent.

Mucinous Metaplasia

Mucinous metaplasia is characterized by the presence of abundant intracytoplasmic mucin in the endometrial cells (Fig. 3-22). The appearance of the endometrium with this type of change is quite variable, including endometrium without an increased number of glands (usually postmenopausal or associated with hormone replacement therapy) to hyperplasia with architectural complexity and/or cytologic atypia. Conspicuous cytologic atypia and/or a complex architectural pattern, either as small pseudoglands with rigid punched-out stroma and no supporting stroma or a filiform pattern, are seen in complex endometrial hyperplasia and adenocarcinoma.[27]

Hobnail Metaplasia

Occasionally, the endometrium is lined by nonstratified cells with a hobnail appearance (Fig. 3-23).

Clear Cell Metaplasia

Clear cell metaplasia is an uncommon finding characterized by clearing of the cytoplasm without demonstrable mucin or glycogen by histochemical methods.[24]

Chapter 3 • Endometrial Hyperplasia

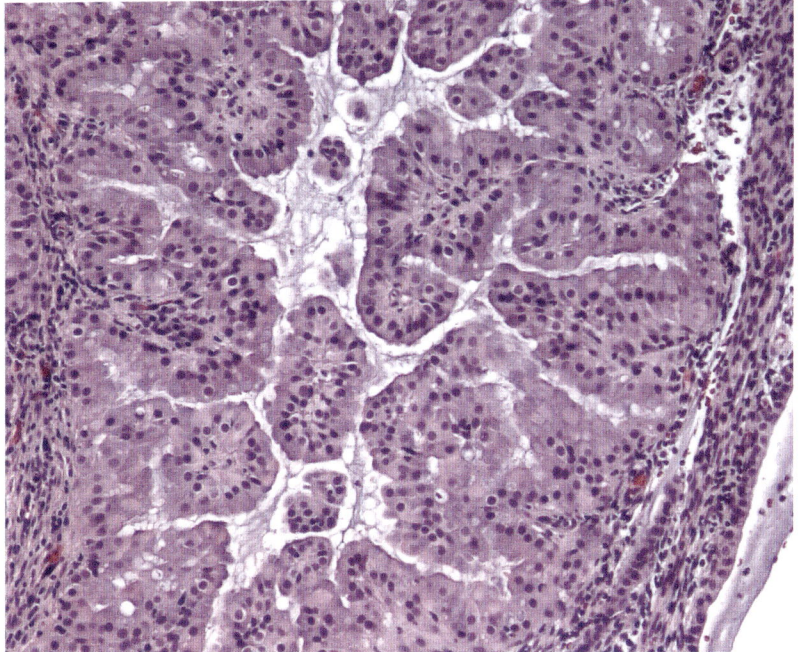

FIGURE 3-22: Mucinous metaplasia.

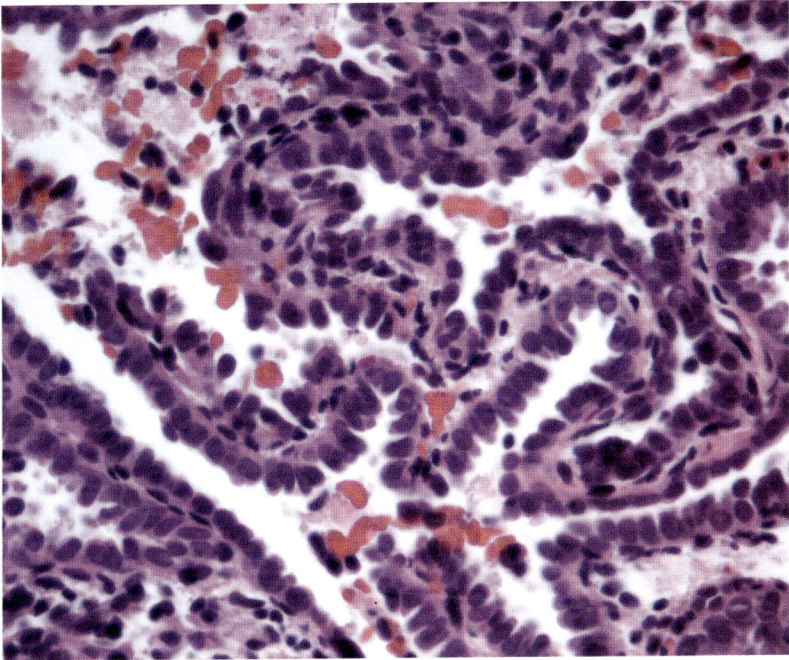

FIGURE 3-23: Hobnail metaplasia.

References

1. Silverberg SG, Kurman RJ, Nogales F, et al. Tumors of the uterine corpus. Epithelial tumors and related lesions. In: Tavassoli FA, Devilee P, eds. *World Health Organization Classification of Tumours: Tumours of the Breast and Female Genital Organs*. Lyon, France: IARC Press; 2003:221–232.
2. Mazur MT. Endometrial hyperplasia/adenocarcinoma. A conventional approach. *Ann Diagn Pathol*. 2005;9:174–181.
3. Hendrickson MR, Longacre TA, Kempson RL. The uterine corpus. In: Mills SE, Carter D, Greenson JK, et al., eds. *Sternberg's Diagnostic Surgical Pathology*. Philadelphia: Lippincott Williams & Wilkins; 2004:2435–2542.
4. Kurman RJ, Kaminski PF, Norris HJ. The behavior of endometrial hyperplasia. A long-term study of "untreated" hyperplasia in 170 patients. *Cancer*. 1985;56:403–412.
5. Mazur MT, Kurman RJ. Endometrial hyperplasia, endometrial intraepithelial carcinoma, and epithelial cytoplasmic change. In: Mazur MT, Kurman RJ, eds. *Diagnosis of Endometrial Biopsies and Curettings: A Practical Approach*. New York: Springer-Verlag; 2005:178–207.
6. Kurman RJ, Norris HJ. Evaluation of criteria for distinguishing atypical endometrial hyperplasia from well-differentiated carcinoma. *Cancer*. 1982;49:2547–2559.
7. Wheeler DR, Bell KA, Kurman RJ, et al. Minimal uterine serous carcinoma: diagnosis and clinicopathologic correlation. *Am J Surg Pathol*. 2000;24:797–806.
8. Zheng W, Khurana R, Farahmand S, et al. p53 immunostaining as a significant adjunct diagnostic method for uterine surface carcinoma: precursor of uterine papillary serous carcinoma. *Am J Surg Pathol*. 1998;22:1463–1473.
9. Lehman MB, Hart WR. Simple and complex hyperplastic papillary proliferations of the endometrium: a clinicopathologic study of nine cases of apparently localized papillary lesions with fibrovascular stromal cores and epithelial metaplasia. *Am J Surg Pathol*. 2001;25:1347–1354.
10. Horn LC, Neinel A, Handzel R, et al. Histopathology of endometrial hyperplasia and endometrial carcinoma: an update. *Ann Diagn Pathol*. 2007;11:297–311.
11. Lacey JV, Ioffe OB, Ronnett BM, et al. Endometrial carcinoma risk among women diagnosed with endometrial hyperplasia: the 34-year experience in a large health plan. *Br J Cancer*. 2008;98:45–53.
12. Trimble CL, Kauderer J, Zaino R, et al. Concurrent endometrial carcinoma in women with a biopsy diagnosis of atypical endometrial hyperplasia: a Gynecologic Oncology Group study. *Cancer*. 2006;106:812–819.
13. Ramirez PT, Frumovitz M, Bodurka DC, et al. Hormonal therapy for the management of grade 1 endometrial adenocarcinoma: a literature review. *Gynecol Oncol*. 2004;95:133–138.
14. Montgomery BE, Daum GS, Dunton CJ. Endometrial hyperplasia: a review. *Obstet Gynecol Surv*. 2004;59:368–378.
15. Rubatt JM, Slomovitz BM, Burke TW, et al. Development of metastatic endometrial endometrioid adenocarcinoma while on progestin therapy for endometrial hyperplasia. *Gynecol Oncol*. 2005;99:472–476.
16. Skov BG, Broholm H, Engel U, et al. Comparison of the reproducibility of the WHO classifications of 1975 and 1994 of endometrial hyperplasia. *Int J Gynecol Pathol*. 1997;16:33–37.
17. Kendell BS, Ronnett BM, Isacson C, et al. Reproducibility of the diagnosis of endometrial hyperplasia, atypical hyperplasia, and well-differentiated carcinoma. *Am J Surg Pathol*. 1998;22:1012–1219.
18. Bergeron C, Nogales FF, Masseroli M, et al. A multicentric European study testing the reproducibility of the WHO classification of endometrial hyperplasia with proposal of a simplified working classification for biopsy and curettage specimens. *Am J Surg Pathol*. 1999;23:11012–11018.
19. Allison KH, Reed SD, Voigt LF, et al. Diagnosing endometrial hyperplasia. Why is it so difficult to agree? *Am J Surg Pathol*. 2008;32:691–698.

20. Zaino RJ, Kauderer J, Trimble CL, et al. Reproducibility of the diagnosis of atypical endometrial hyperplasia: a Gynecologic Oncology Group study. *Cancer.* 2006;106:804–811.
21. Baak JP, Mutter GL, Robboy S, et al. The molecular genetics and morphometry-based endometrial intraepithelial neoplasia classification system predicts disease progression in endometrial hyperplasia more accurately than the 1994 World Health Organization classification system. *Cancer.* 2005;103:2304–2312.
22. Lacey JV, Mutter GL, Nucci MR, et al. Risk of subsequent endometrial carcinoma associated with endometrial intraepithelial neoplasia classification of endometrial biopsies. *Cancer.* 2008;113:2073–2081.
23. Mutter GL, Zaino RJ, Baak JP, et al. Benign endometrial hyperplasia sequence and endometrial intraepithelial neoplasia. *Int J Gynecol Pathol.* 2007;26:103–114.
24. Hendrickson MR, Kempson RL. Endometrial epithelial metaplasias: proliferations frequently misdiagnosed as adenocarcinoma. Report of 89 cases and proposed classifications. *Am J Surg Pathol.* 1980;4:525–542.
25. Masterson R, Armstrong EM, More IAR. The cyclical variation in the percentage of ciliated cells in the normal human endometrium. *J Reprod Fertil.* 1975;42:537–540.
26. Zaman SS, Mazur MT. Endometrial papillary syncytial change. A nonspecific alteration associated with active breakdown. *Am J Clin Pathol.* 1993;99:741–745.
27. Nucci MR, Prasad CJ, Crum CP, et al. Mucinous endometrial epithelial proliferations: a morphologic spectrum of changes with diverse clinical significance. *Mod Pathol.* 1999;12:1137–1142.

Endometrial Carcinoma

4

▶ Anais Malpica, MD

In this chapter, a brief overview of the current classifications of endometrial carcinoma is presented, with a more detailed review of the histopathology of endometrial carcinoma and an emphasis on features that are clinically relevant.

PATHOGENETIC CLASSIFICATION OF ENDOMETRIAL CARCINOMA

From a pathogenetic standpoint, sporadic endometrial carcinoma has been classified into two categories: type I and type II.[1] These two categories differ in their pathologic, molecular, and clinical findings, as summarized in Table 4-1.[1-4] Some cases of endometrial carcinoma may have overlapping features of these two categories, underscoring the existence of exceptions to this dualistic model of endometrial tumorigenesis (author's unpublished observations).[2]

HISTOLOGIC CLASSIFICATION OF ENDOMETRIAL CARCINOMA

The current World Health Organization (WHO) histologic classification of endometrial carcinoma is shown in Table 4-2.[5] In this chapter, we review the histologic subtypes and variants included in this classification, as well as other variants not included in it.

Endometrioid Adenocarcinoma

Endometrioid adenocarcinoma is the most common type of endometrial carcinoma, accounting for 80% of cases.[3] This tumor is composed of glands that resemble those seen in the normal endometrium. The variably sized glands seen in this type of tumor are usually oval or round, although they can be angulated or branched. They are lined by columnar cells with stratified or pseudostratified nuclei. The degree of nuclear atypia is usually mild to moderate. The cytoplasm is either basophilic, amphophilic, or slightly eosinophilic (Fig. 4-1). Intraluminal mucin can be seen, and in some cases, this becomes a prominent finding. Intracellular mucin, usually focal and less frequently diffuse, may also be noted (Fig. 4-2).[6,7] Ciliated cells, necrosis of the glands or within luminal spaces (Fig. 4-3), foamy stromal cells, signet ring cells (Fig. 4-4), and infrequently, intestinal differentiation, including goblet cells and argentaffin cells, can be seen.[7-11] In addition, psammoma bodies and focal, bland-looking heterologous elements (fat, cartilage, osteoid) are occasionally found (Fig. 4-5).[12,13]

Table 4-1 Pathogenetic Classification of Sporadic Endometrial Carcinoma

	Type I	Type II
Age	Premenopausal and perimenopausal	Postmenopausal
Unopposed estrogen stimulation	Present	Absent
Background endometrium	Hyperplasia	Atrophy
Histologic type	Endometrioid Mucinous	Serous Clear cell
Estrogen/progesterone receptors expression	Present	Absent or weakly positive
Behavior	Favorable	Aggressive
Molecular alterations	*PTEN* inactivation Microsatellite instability Mutations of K-ras and β-catenin	p53 mutation Loss of heterozygosity at different loci Inactivation of p16 and E-cadherin Amplification of HER2/neu

Table 4-2 World Health Organization (WHO) Classification of Endometrial Carcinoma

Endometrioid adenocarcinoma
    Variants
        With squamous differentiation
    Villoglandular
        Secretory
        Ciliated cell
Mucinous adenocarcinoma
Serous carcinoma
Clear cell carcinoma
Mixed carcinoma
Squamous carcinoma
Transitional cell carcinoma
Small-cell carcinoma
Undifferentiated carcinoma
Others

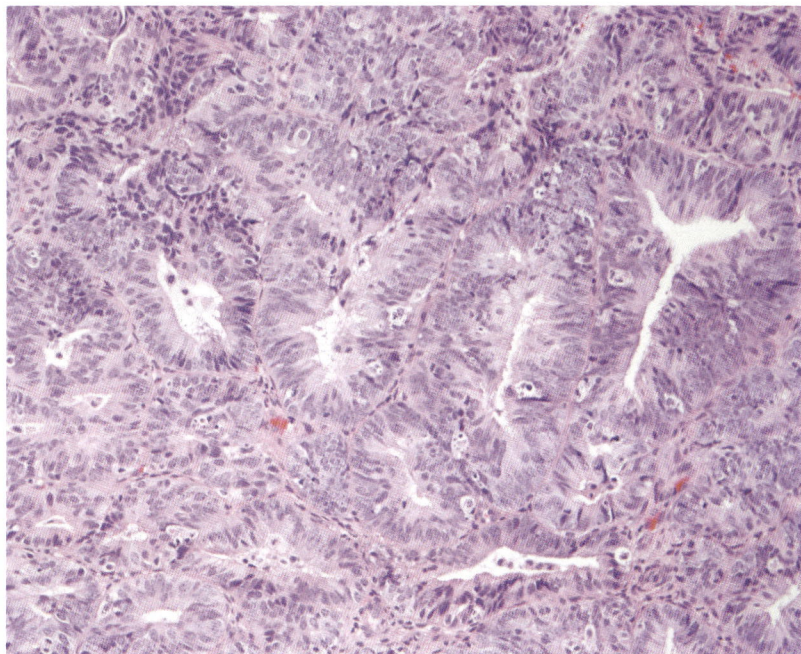

FIGURE 4-1: Endometrioid adenocarcinoma; glands are lined by columnar cells with stratified nuclei. The luminal contour of the glands is smooth.

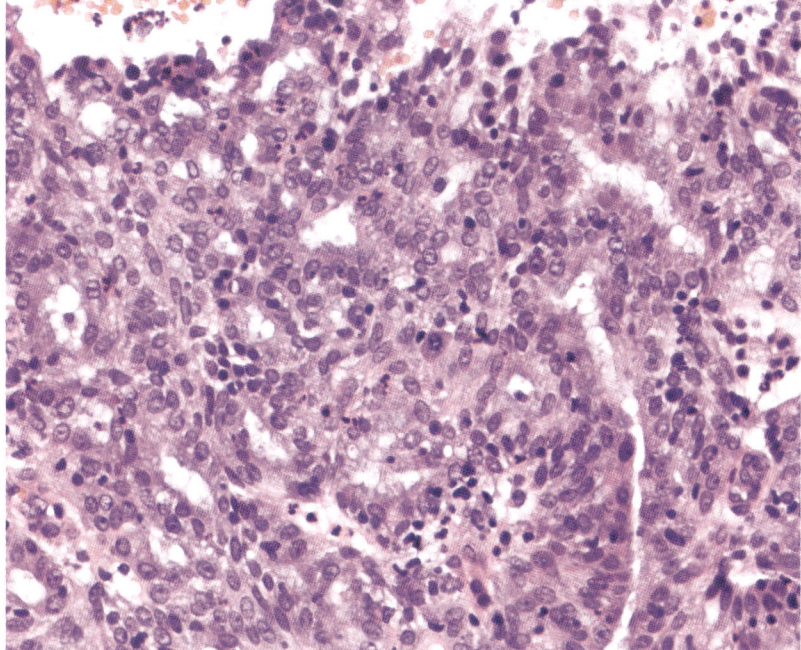

FIGURE 4-2: Endometrioid adenocarcinoma with intracellular (intracytoplasmic) mucin.

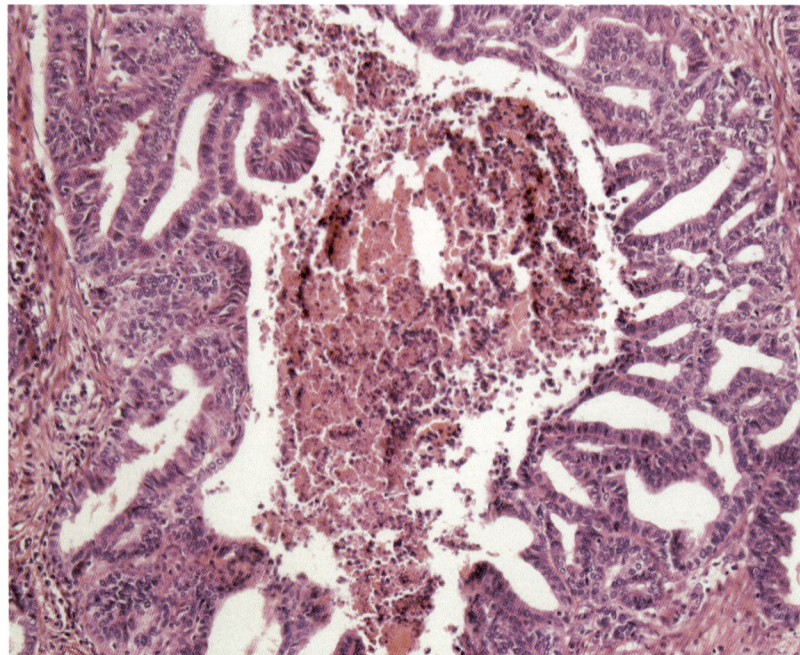

FIGURE 4-3: Endometrioid adenocarcinoma with dirty necrosis within glandular luminal spaces.

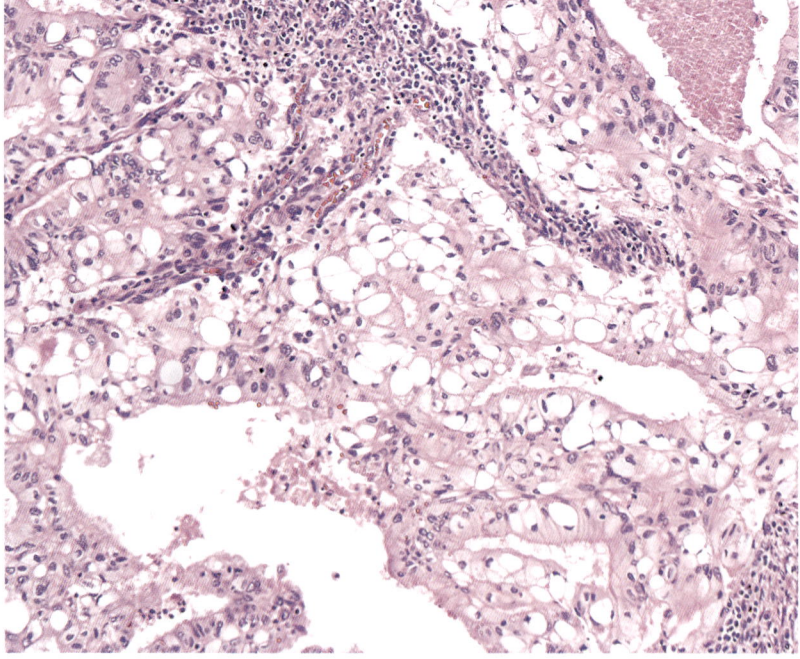

FIGURE 4-4: Endometrioid adenocarcinoma with signet ring-like cells.

Chapter 4 • Endometrial Carcinoma

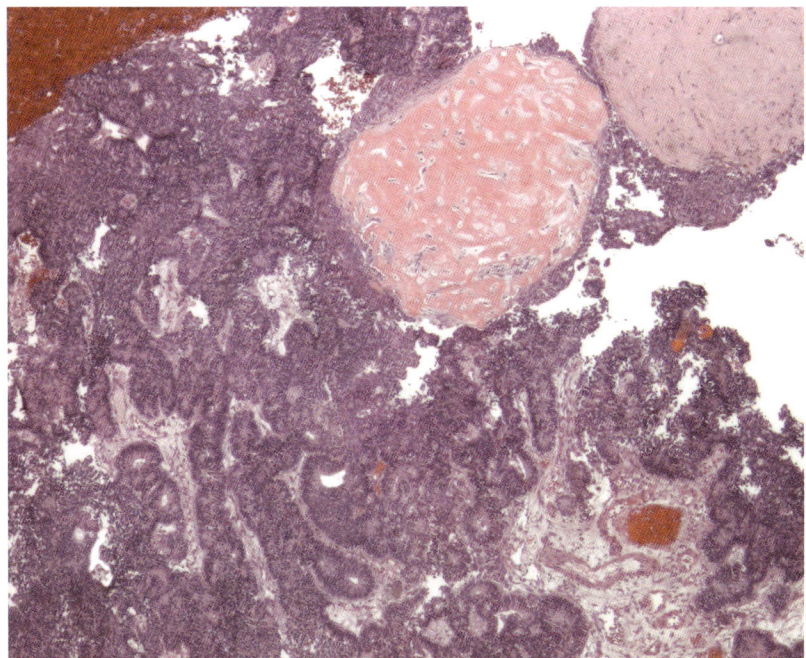

FIGURE 4-5: Endometrioid adenocarcinoma with osseous metaplasia.

Variants of Endometrioid Adenocarcinoma

Variant with Squamous Differentiation
Squamous differentiation in endometrioid adenocarcinoma can have a variable appearance: (1) morular (rounded intraluminal masses of bland-looking eosinophilic or amphophilic cells), (2) nests or sheets of tumor cells resembling keratinized squamous carcinoma, (3) nests or sheets of squamous cells rich in glycogen, (4) sheets of spindled cells with minimal evidence of squamous differentiation, and (5) papillae with associated mucinous metaplasia and neutrophils (Fig. 4-6). The previously used terms "adenoacanthoma" and "adenosquamous carcinoma" are considered obsolete and should not be used.[5]

Villoglandular Variant
This variant is characterized by the presence of slender, finger-like papillae lined by columnar cells with low-grade cytologic atypia. The nuclei of the neoplastic cells preserve their polarity in relation to the basement membrane of the epithelium, and the contour of the papillae is smooth (Fig. 4-7). The presence of this variant within the myoinvasive component of an endometrial adenocarcinoma has been found to be associated with higher incidences of vascular/lymphatic invasion and lymph node metastasis.[14]

Secretory Variant
This rare variant of endometrioid adenocarcinoma is usually seen in postmenopausal patients, although it can also occur in premenopausal patients, with or without a history of endogenous or exogenous progestational effect. Its histologic hallmark is the presence of intracytoplasmic vacuoles in most of the neoplastic cells. These vacuoles can be supranuclear, subnuclear, or both (Fig. 4-8).[15,16]

Ciliated Variant
This uncommon variant of endometrial adenocarcinoma shows neoplastic glands lined predominantly by ciliated cells (Fig. 4-9).[8,17]

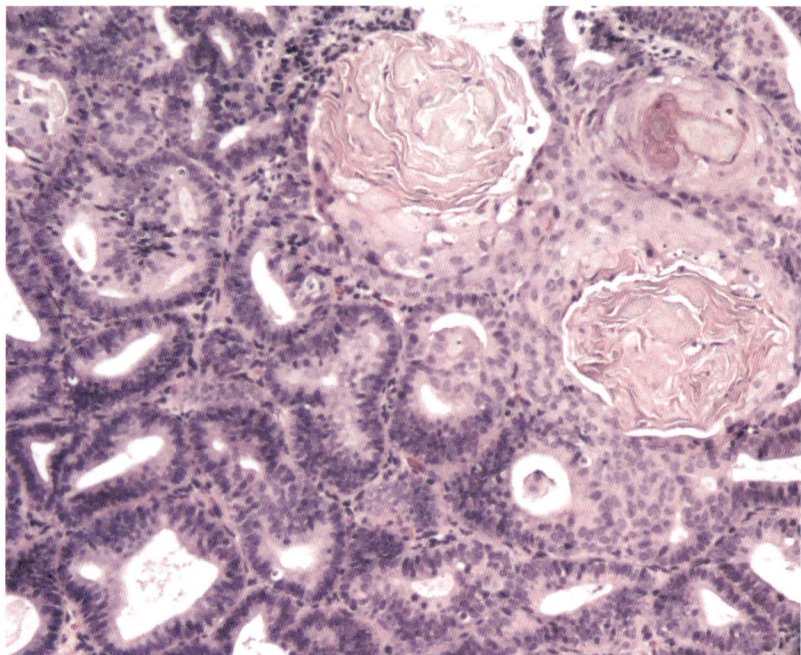

FIGURE 4-6: Endometrioid adenocarcinoma with squamous differentiation.

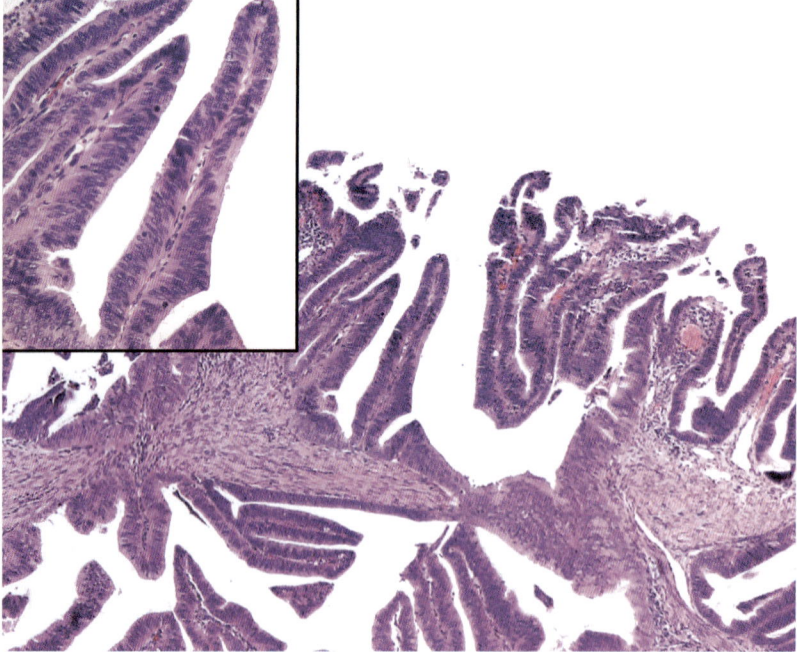

FIGURE 4-7: Endometrioid adenocarcinoma with a villoglandular pattern. Finger-like papillae with fibroconnective tissue cores, lined by cells with nuclei that have preserved their polarity. Note the smooth outer contour of the papillae (*inset*).

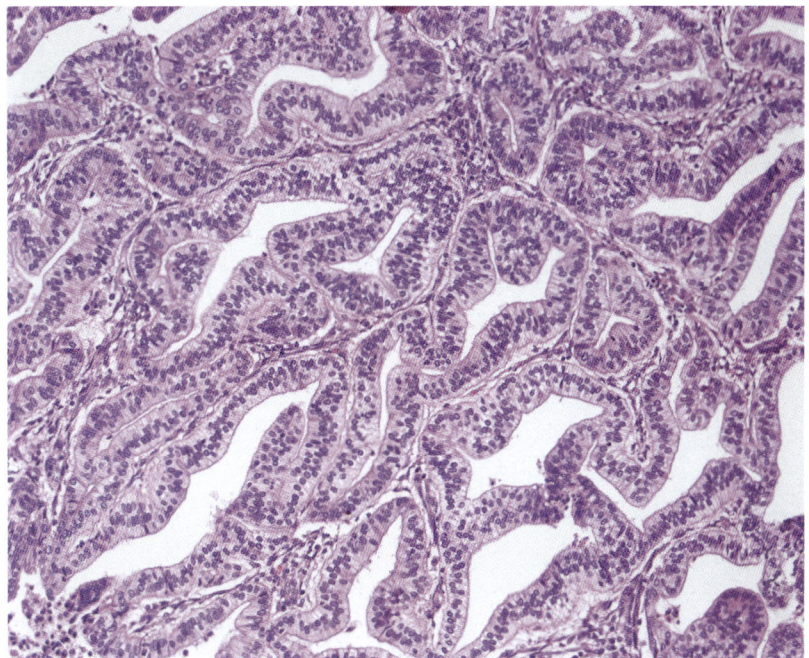

FIGURE 4-8: Endometrioid adenocarcinoma, secretory variant.

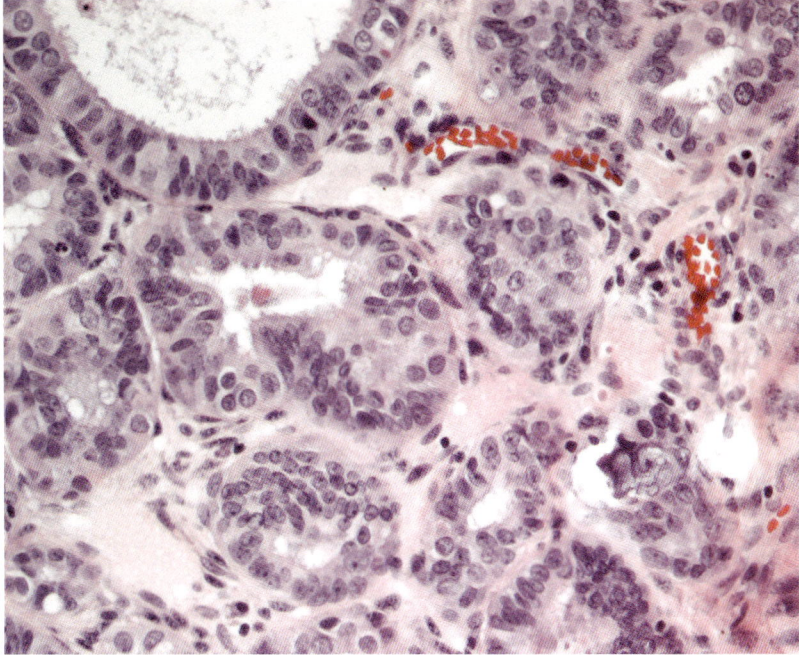

FIGURE 4-9: Endometrioid adenocarcinoma, ciliated cell variant.

Other Changes

SARCOMATOID (SPINDLE CELL) FEATURES

Sarcomatoid (spindle cell) features also can be seen in endometrioid adenocarcinoma. This is usually a focal finding, and the recognition of the area where the spindle cells merge with the glandular component of the tumor is crucial to avoid the misinterpretation of the spindle

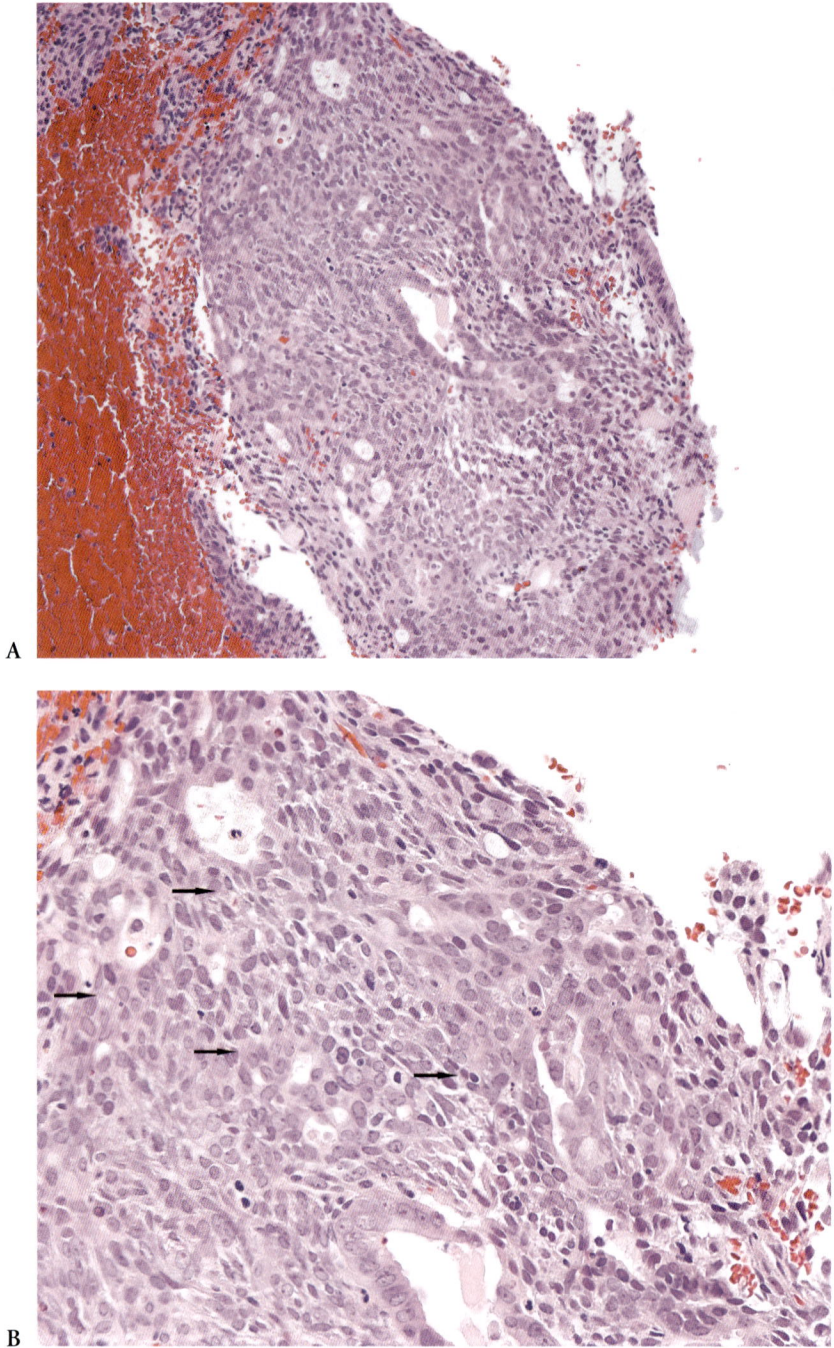

FIGURE 4-10: **A.** Endometrioid adenocarcinoma with spindle cell features. **B.** Note how the cells lining the neoplastic endometrial glands merge with the spindle cells (*arrows*).

cells as a true sarcoma (Fig. 4-10A–B). The use of a keratin cocktail and epithelial membrane antigen (EMA) may assist in making the correct diagnosis; however, these immunostains can be only focally positive.

CLEAR CELL CHANGES

The cytoplasm of the neoplastic cells in endometrioid adenocarcinoma can be focally clear. The specific cause of this finding is usually unknown, although it may be related to the presence of intracytoplasmic lipid.[18]

MICROGLANDULAR HYPERPLASIA-LIKE PATTERN

Endometrioid adenocarcinoma with a prominent microglandular hyperplasia-like pattern is uncommon and usually seen in postmenopausal women with a history of exogenous hormone use (i.e., medroxyprogesterone acetate, estradiol, or a combination of both).[19] This type of neoplasm shows a proliferation of small glands lined by one or more layers of cuboidal, columnar, or flattened cells, with a variable amount of amphophilic or mucin-rich cytoplasm. In certain areas, the glands can be large or cystic or the neoplastic cells can be arranged in solid nests. The degree of cytologic atypia is variable, from none to moderate, and the mitotic index is also variable, ranging from one mitosis per 10 high-power fields (HPFs) to frequent mitoses per 10 HPFs (Fig. 4-11). Abnormal mitotic figures can be seen. The luminal spaces contain mucin, and there are numerous neutrophils. In addition, lymphocytes and plasma can be found. Immunohistochemically, this type of neoplasm stains variably with carcinoembryonic antigen (CEA), vimentin, and Ki-67.[20–23] Recently, some investigators have found p16 immunostaining to be positive in endometrial adenocarcinoma with a microglandular hyperplasia-like pattern and negative in microglandular hyperplasia of the uterine cervix.[24] Because experience with p16 immunostaining is limited, the definitive diagnosis of this type of tumor requires the recognition of continuity between the tumor and endometrium.

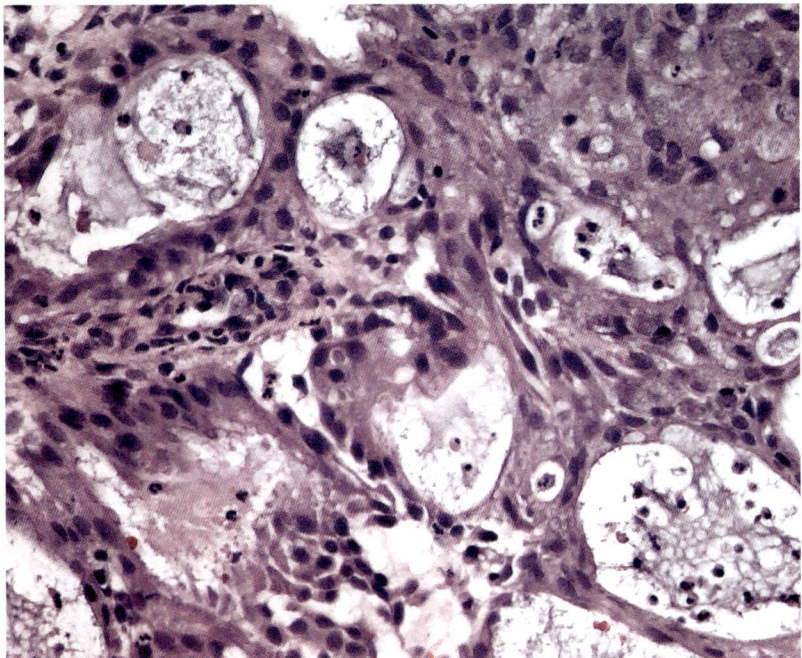

FIGURE 4-11: Endometrioid adenocarcinoma, microglandular hyperplasia-like.

SMALL NONVILLOUS PAPILLAE

This pattern consists of small, simple or complex papillae protruding with the glandular component of an otherwise typical International Federation of Gynecology and Obstetrics (FIGO) grade 1 or 2 endometrioid adenocarcinoma or from the finger-like papillae of a villoglandular adenocarcinoma. The neoplastic cells have eosinophilic cytoplasm and low-grade nuclear features (Fig. 4-12).[25]

SERTOLIFORM PATTERN

The presence of a sertoliform pattern in endometrioid adenocarcinoma arising in the endometrium is rare. This pattern is characterized by tubules, cords, and nests of columnar cells with eosinophilic or clear apical cytoplasm mimicking a Sertoli cell tumor. This pattern can be focal or diffuse. Immunohistochemically, the tumor cells are positive for EMA and vimentin and positive or negative for keratin. A rare case has also expressed α-inhibin, calretinin, WT-1, and Melan-A, indicating true sex cord differentiation.[26] Smooth muscle markers such as desmin, smooth muscle actin (SMA), and HHF35 are negative.[26–28]

SEX CORD-LIKE PATTERN AND HYALINIZATION

This rare pattern of endometrioid adenocarcinoma shows cords or clusters of epithelioid and/or spindle cells that are intermixed and usually merge with typical endometrioid adenocarcinoma. Usually, the neoplastic cells are embedded in a hyalinized matrix. The degree of hyalinization can be so pronounced that it can resemble osteoid material. Squamous differentiation is common (Fig. 4-13). Immunohistochemically, the tumor cells have a variable expression of keratin and EMA, ranging from no staining to diffuse staining; however, the expression is typically seen in less than 50% of the cells. Although this pattern could be mistaken for a malignant mixed müllerian tumor, attention to the cytologic features and mitotic activity (this pattern displays less cytologic atypia and less mitotic activity than a malignant mixed müllerian tumor) is necessary to make the correct diagnosis.[29]

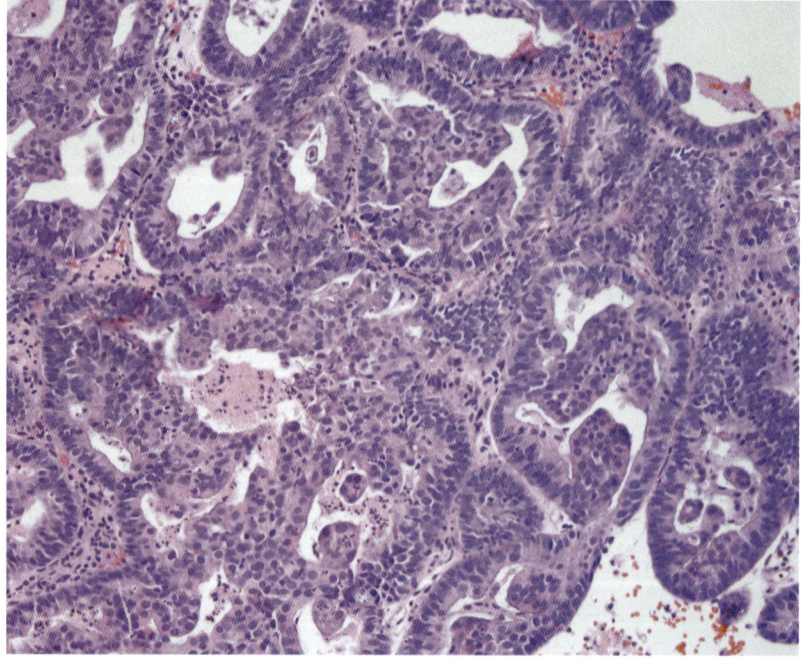

FIGURE 4-12: Endometrioid adenocarcinoma with small nonvillous papillae.

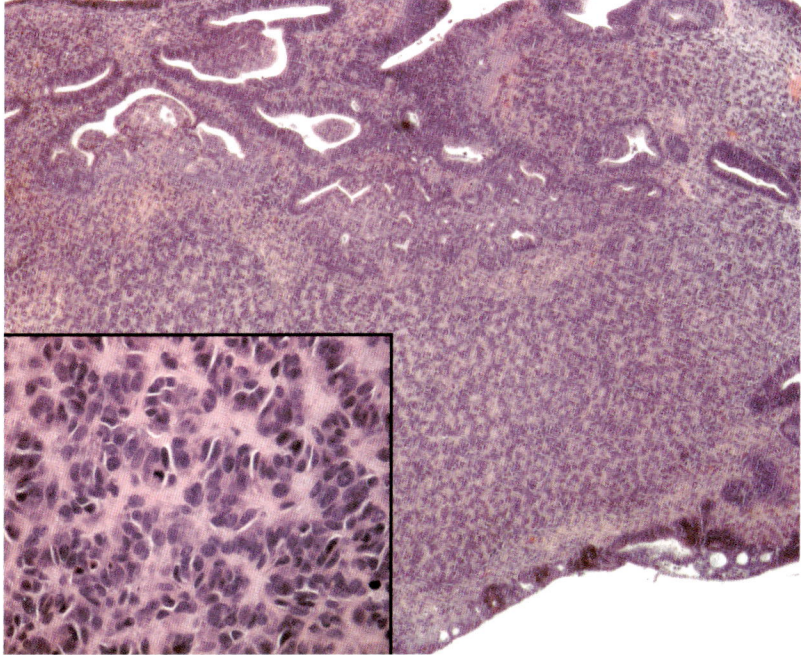

FIGURE 4-13: Endometrioid adenocarcinoma with sex cord-like pattern (*inset*).

OXYPHILIC (ONCOCYTIC) CHANGES

This rare pattern of endometrioid adenocarcinoma is seen mostly in postmenopausal patients. Tumors with this pattern display, either predominantly or entirely, large oxyphilic cells (Fig. 4-14). Some cases have been found to be rich in mitochondria.[30–32]

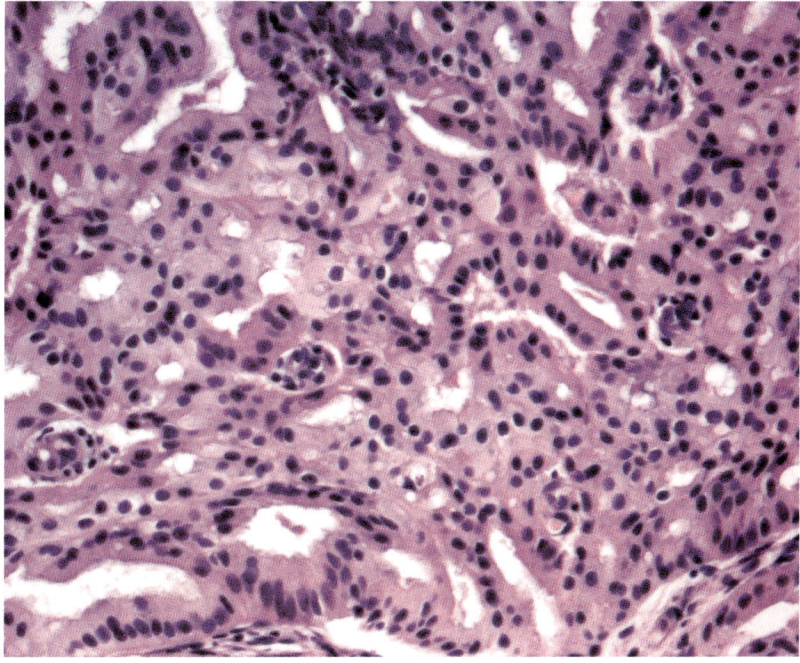

FIGURE 4-14: Endometrioid adenocarcinoma, oxyphilic variant.

Differential Diagnosis

Endometrioid Adenocarcinoma versus Complex Endometrial Hyperplasia with or without Atypia
One of the three following criteria is required for the diagnosis of endometrioid adenocarcinoma:

1. Back-to-back endometrial glandular proliferation occupying an area of at least 2 × 2 mm (Fig. 4-15)
2. An extensive papillary pattern (Fig. 4-16)
3. A desmoplastic or fibroblastic stroma infiltrated by irregular glands (Fig. 4-17)

The last criterion mentioned earlier must be used with caution because the stromal reaction secondary to a recent endometrial curettage and the fibroblastic stroma of an endometrial polyp with torsion may mimic this feature.

Endometrioid Adenocarcinoma with a Villoglandular Pattern versus Papillary Endometrial Adenocarcinoma of Intermediate Grade versus Serous Carcinoma
The papillae seen in the villoglandular pattern are slender and finger-like and lined by neoplastic cells with low-grade cytologic features and nuclei that preserve their polarity. In addition, the outer surface of the papillae is smooth. In contrast, the papillae seen in papillary endometrial adenocarcinoma of intermediate grade are long or short and lined by cells with moderate cytologic atypia and nuclei that have partially lost their polarity. The outer surface of the papillae is somehow irregular (Figs. 4-18A–B and 4-19A–B). Serous carcinoma can have either long or blunt papillae, with or without fibroconnective cores, lined by markedly atypical cells usually showing conspicuous mitotic activity. Immunohistochemically, villoglandular adenocarcinoma and intermediate-grade papillary endometrial adenocarcinoma are usually either negative or focally positive for p53 (author's unpublished observations), whereas serous carcinoma is usually positive for this immunomarker.[33,34]

Endometrioid Adenocarcinoma versus Glandular Variant of Serous Carcinoma
The presence of marked cytologic atypia in an endometrioid-looking tumor composed mostly of glands should raise the diagnostic possibility of serous carcinoma, glandular variant (Fig. 4-20). The use of an immunohistochemical panel that includes p53, progesterone receptor (PR), and *PTEN* will assist in making the correct diagnosis. The combination of lack of p53 expression, positive PR expression, and loss of *PTEN* is in keeping with the diagnosis of endometrioid adenocarcinoma.[34]

Endometrioid Adenocarcinoma with Glycogenated Squamous Differentiation versus Clear Cell Carcinoma
Attention to histologic features is of utmost importance in making the correct diagnosis. In cases of endometrioid adenocarcinoma with glycogenated squamous differentiation (Fig. 4-21), there are areas with overt squamous differentiation in the vicinity. In contrast, clear cell carcinoma usually demonstrates a combination of architectural patterns: solid, tubuloglandular, and papillary.

Endometrioid Adenocarcinoma with Sarcomatoid (Spindle Cell) Features or with Sex Cord-Like Pattern/Hyalinization versus Malignant Mixed Müllerian Tumor
Careful attention to histologic features will allow the correct diagnosis of these neoplasms. As mentioned earlier, endometrioid adenocarcinoma with sarcomatoid (spindle cell) features demonstrates areas where the spindle cell component merges with the glandular component,

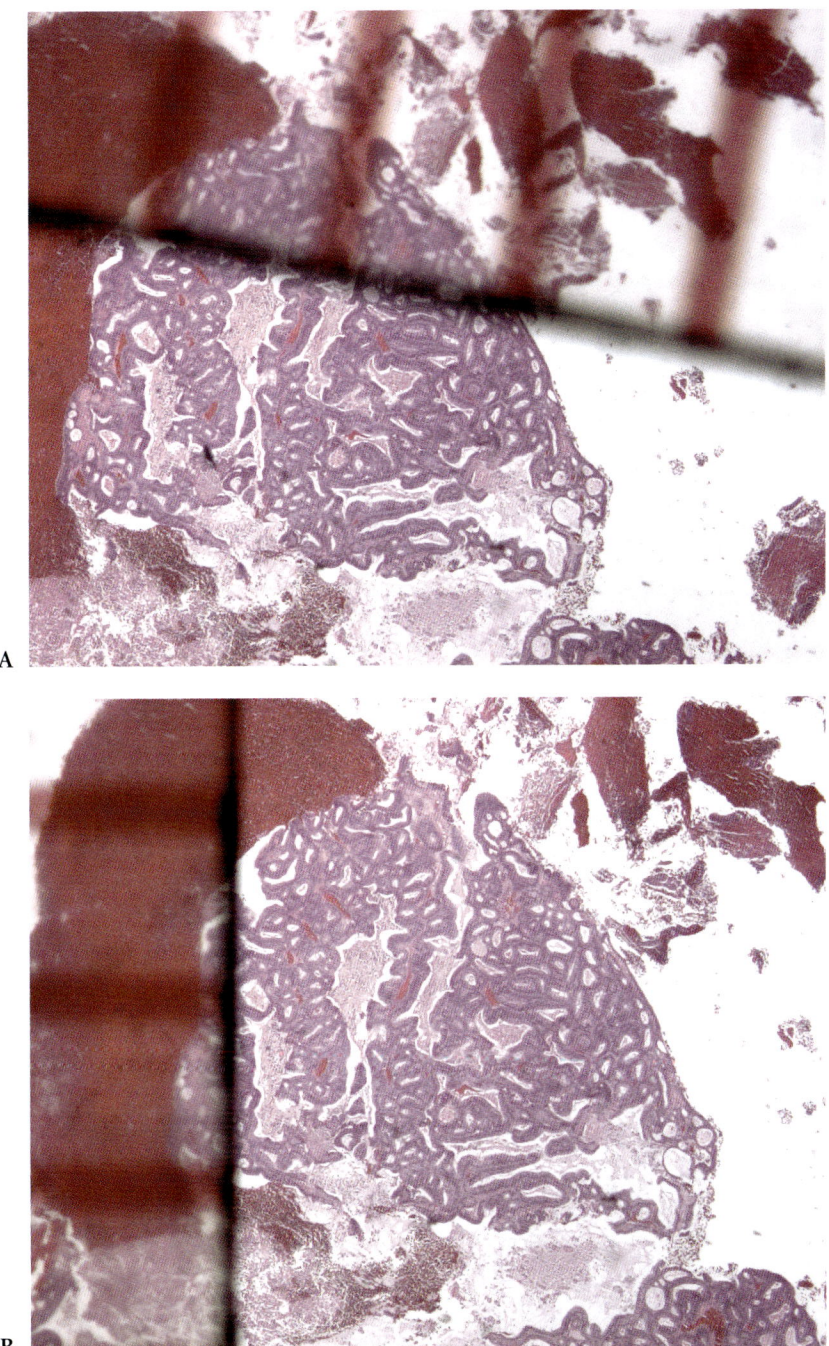

FIGURE 4-15: Endometrioid adenocarcinoma; the diagnosis is based on a back-to-back glandular proliferation occupying an area measuring 2 × 2 mm (**A and B**).

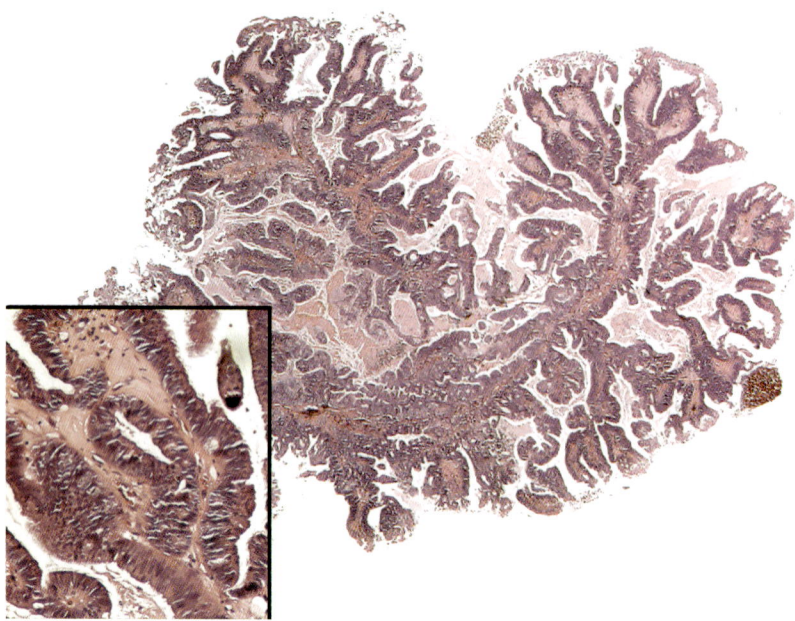

FIGURE 4-16: Endometrioid adenocarcinoma; the diagnosis is based on the presence of an extensive papillary pattern. Note the absence of marked cytologic atypia in the cells lining the papillae (*inset*).

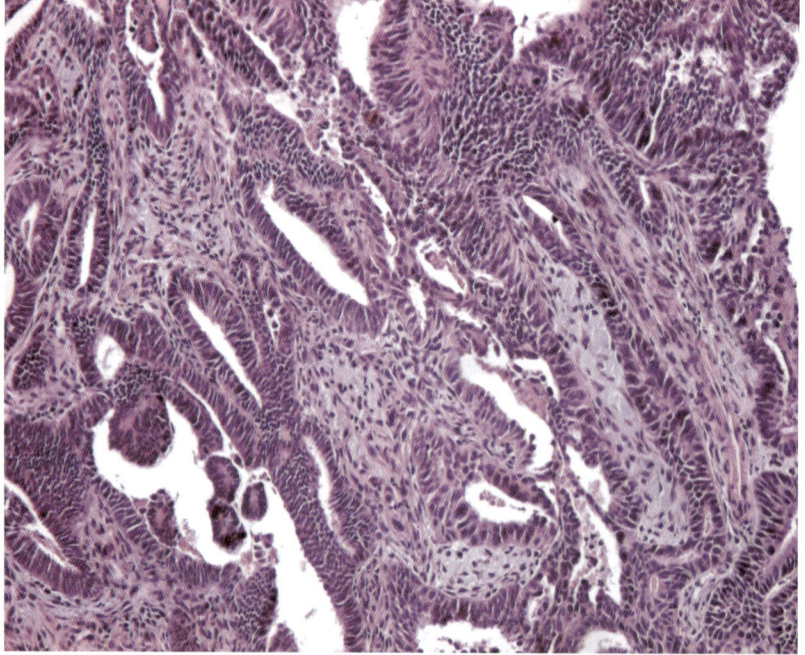

FIGURE 4-17: Endometrioid adenocarcinoma; the diagnosis is based on the presence of irregular glands embedded in a desmoplastic stroma.

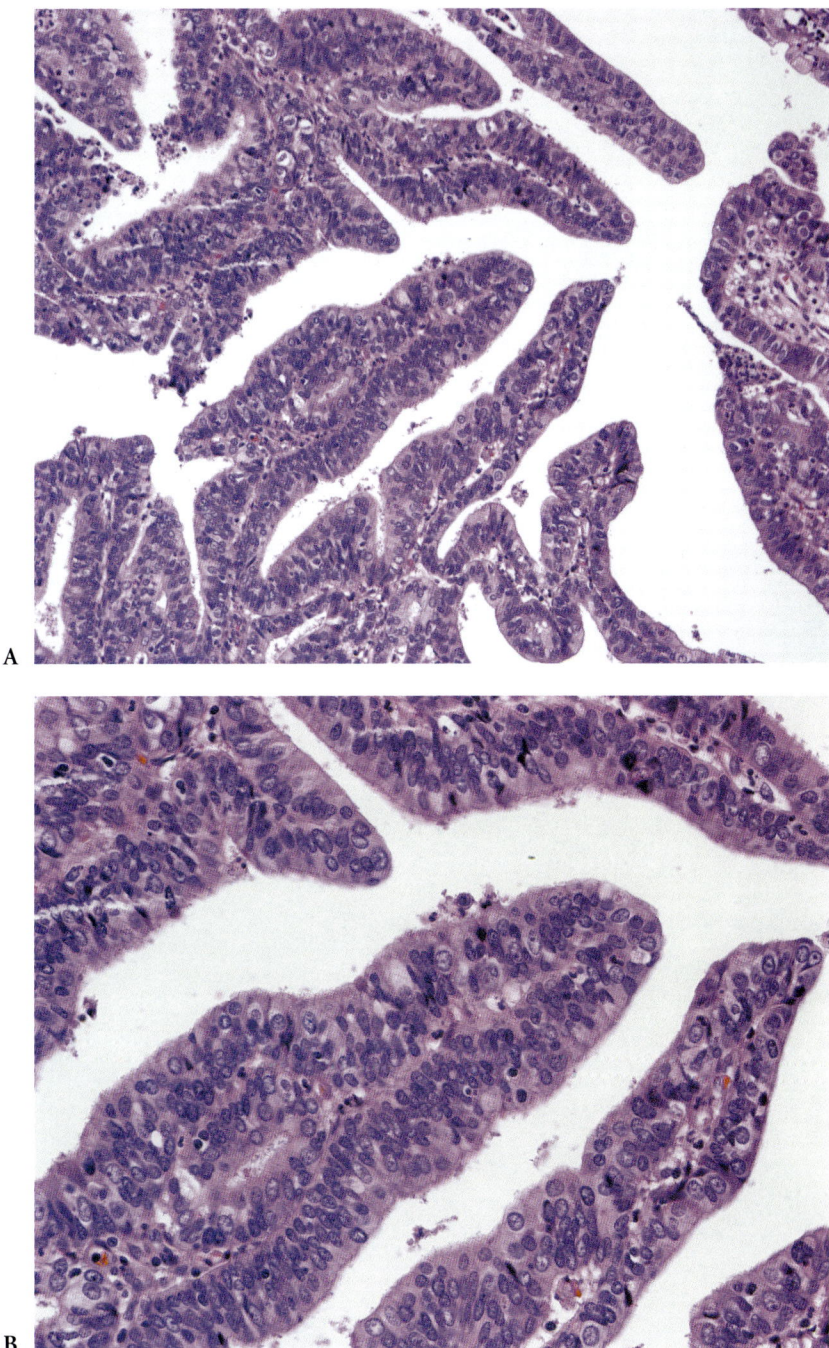

FIGURE 4-18: Papillary endometrial adenocarcinoma of intermediate-grade, papillary structures (**A**), lined by cells that have lost the polarity of their nuclei (**B**).

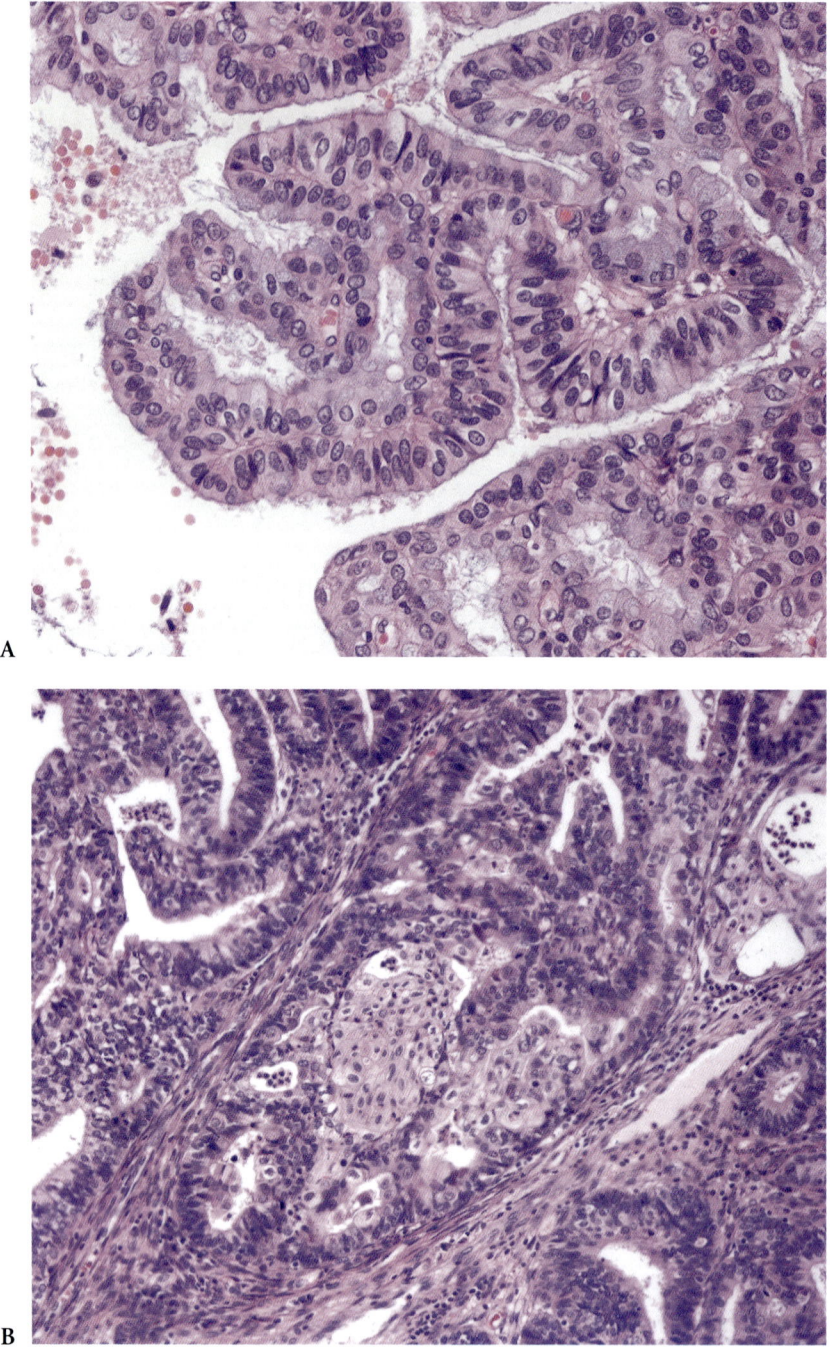

FIGURE 4-19: Papillary endometrial adenocarcinoma of intermediate grade. Frequently seen features include mucinous metaplasia (**A**) and squamous differentiation (**B**).

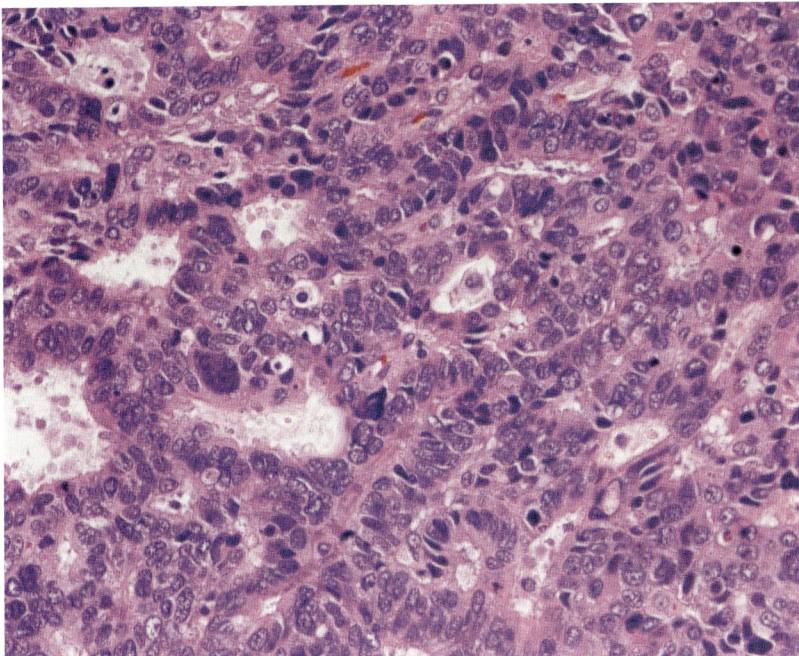

FIGURE 4-20: Serous carcinoma, not to be mistaken for endometrioid adenocarcinoma. Note the presence of marked cytologic atypia, including the loss of polarity of the nuclei of the cells lining the neoplastic glands.

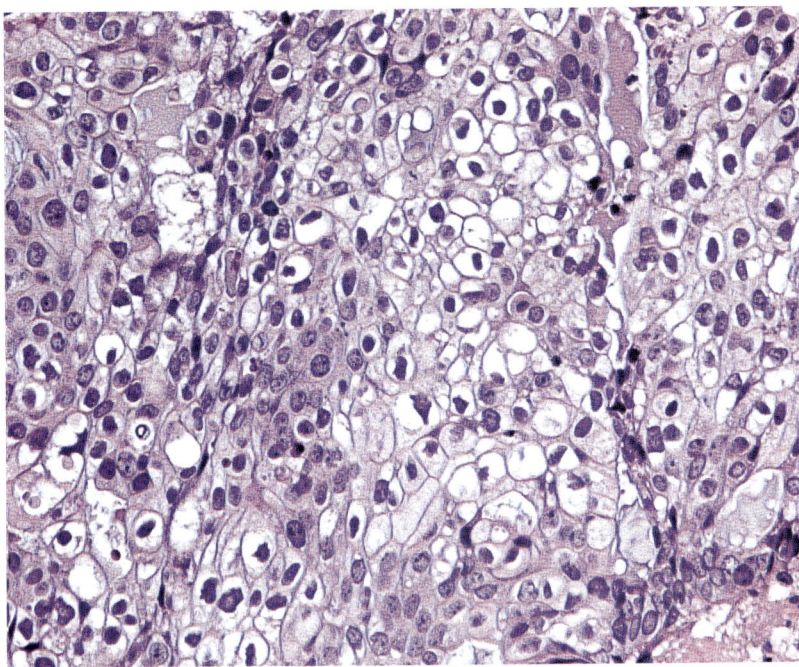

FIGURE 4-21: Endometrioid adenocarcinoma with glycogenated squamous differentiation.

whereas endometrioid adenocarcinoma with sex cord-like pattern and hyalinization shows a constellation of typical features such as the formation of cords and clusters of spindle and epithelioid cells in a background of hyalinized material usually associated with squamous differentiation. The value of immunohistochemical studies, such as EMA and keratin, to enhance the epithelial nature of the spindle cells is limited because they can be negative or only focally positive in these neoplasms.[29] In addition, the sarcoma component of a malignant mixed müllerian tumor can be focally or diffusely positive for keratin and EMA.[35]

Endometrioid Adenocarcinoma Associated with Primitive Neuroectodermal Tumor versus Malignant Mixed Müllerian Tumor

Rare cases of endometrioid carcinoma associated with primitive neuroectodermal tumor (PNET) have been described (Fig. 4-22A–D). The neuroectodermal component is characterized by the presence of uniform oval, round, or slightly elongated cells with a scanty or moderate amount of cytoplasm arranged in sheets, nests, or trabeculae. The presence of perivascular rosettes, Homer Wright rosettes, ependymal-type rosettes, astrocyte-like cells in a fibrillary background, or ganglion-like cells is variable. Immunohistochemical studies show that cells with neuroectodermal differentiation are positive for neurofilament, synaptophysin, and CD99 (although some cases show nonspecific staining for the latter). These cells also are either negative or focally positive for keratin.[36,37] When molecular studies detect the rearrangement of the *EWSR1* gene, the diagnosis of peripheral PNET can be made. In contrast, cases lacking this finding should be designated as tumors with neuroectodermal differentiation or, alternatively, as central-type PNET rather than "PNET, not otherwise specified" to avoid confusion with the former. Of interest, some cases of uterine PNET are part of a malignant mixed müllerian tumor.[37] Combined endometrioid adenocarcinoma and PNET have been described in patients ranging from 47 to 71 years of age and have been associated with advanced-stage disease and a poor prognosis.[36,37]

Endometrioid Adenocarcinoma, FIGO Grade 1, with Myometrial Invasion versus Atypical Polypoid Adenomyoma

The diagnosis of atypical polypoid adenomyoma (APA) should be considered whenever a proliferation of endometrial glands is seen within a smooth muscle or fibromuscular background arranged in intersecting fascicles (Fig. 4-23). In the typical case of APA, the glandular proliferation is similar to that seen in hyperplasia and tends to have squamous morules. The glandular size and shape are variable, as is the presence of cytologic atypia.[38] The following features distinguish APA from myoinvasive endometrioid adenocarcinoma, FIGO grade 1:

1. Young age (average age, 39 years)
2. The presence of intersecting fascicles of smooth muscle or fibromuscular tissue
3. A more cellular smooth muscle than the normal myometrium seen in cases of myoinvasive endometrioid adenocarcinoma
4. The presence of endometrioid proliferation exclusively in fragments containing smooth muscle or fibromuscular tissue

Endometrioid Adenocarcinoma Arising in the Endometrium versus Endometrioid Adenocarcinoma Arising in the Uterine Cervix

Carcinomas arising in the endometrium or endocervix may have overlapping histologic features. In cases where, upon review of the hematoxylin and eosin–stained slides, the origin of the tumor (i.e., endometrium versus endocervix) cannot be determined, the

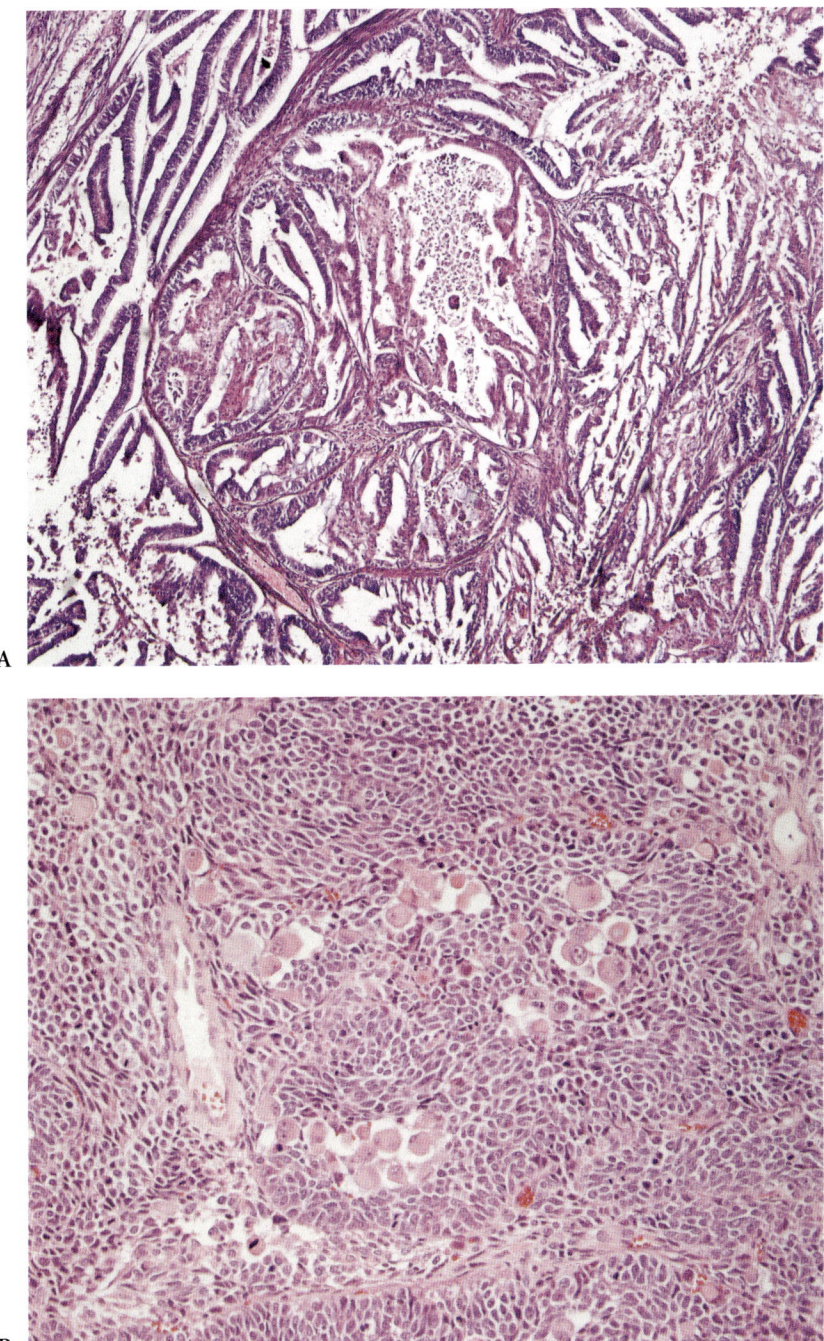

FIGURE 4-22: Endometrioid adenocarcinoma, FIGO grade 1 (**A**), associated with primitive neuroectodermal tumor. Note the ganglion cells within nests of small blue cells (**B**), synaptophysin-positive staining (**C**), and neurofilament-positive staining (**D**). *(continued)*

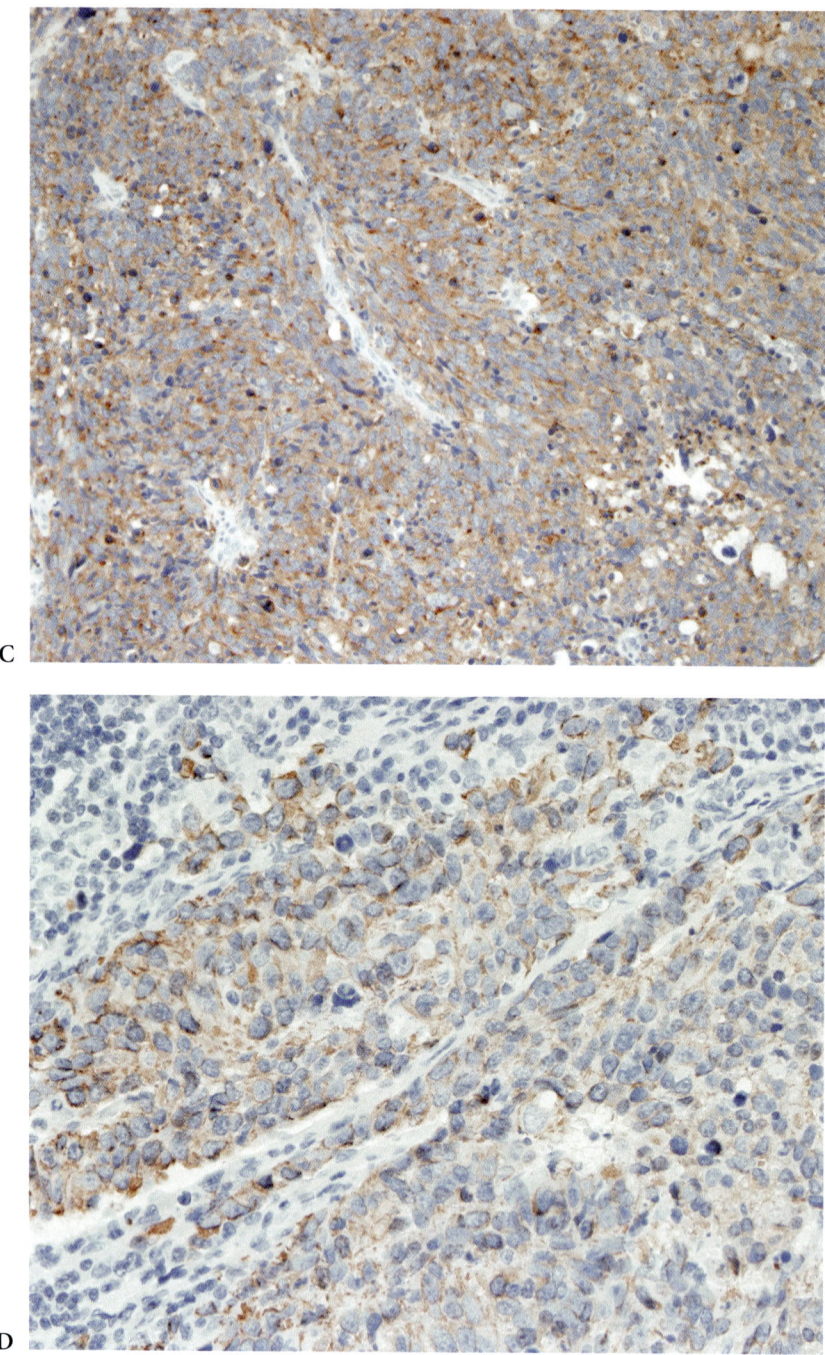

FIGURE 4-22: *(continued)*

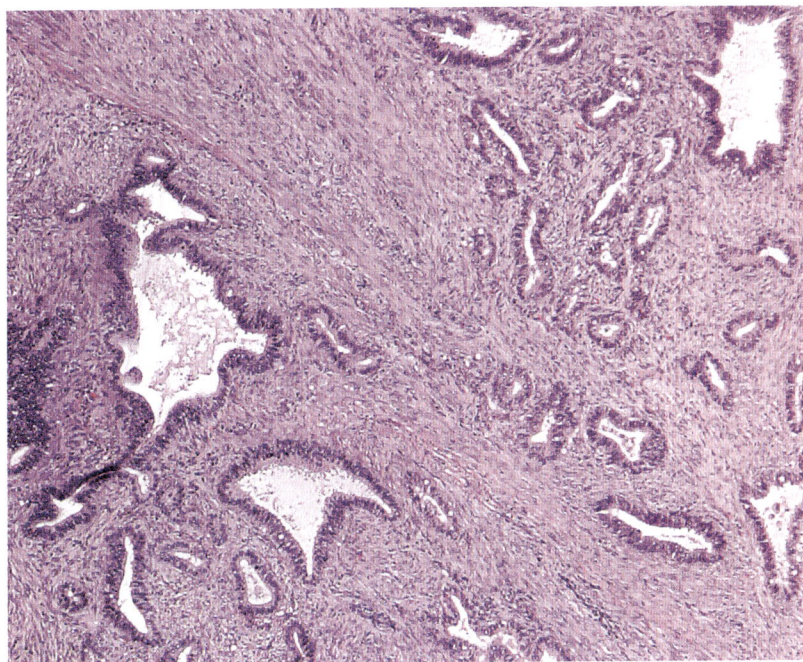

FIGURE 4-23: Atypical polypoid adenomyoma displaying a proliferation of endometrial glands embedded in a background of intersecting myometrial fascicles, not to be mistaken for endometrial adenocarcinoma with myometrial invasion.

use of immunohistochemical studies is indicated. Tumors positive for vimentin and estrogen receptor (ER) and negative for CEA are favored to have an endometrial origin (Fig. 4-24A–D), whereas tumors that are positive for CEA and negative for vimentin and ER are favored to be endocervical in origin.[39] p16 is another immunomarker recommended to assist in the distinction between these two types of tumor. It is usually diffusely expressed by adenocarcinomas of endocervical origin and has patchy expression in endometrioid endometrial adenocarcinomas[40]; however, there are two caveats to bear in mind: (1) p16 is also diffusely expressed in high-grade endometrial adenocarcinomas (serous, clear cell, and grade 3 endometrioid), and (2) in a small biopsy, a tumor with patchy expression of p16 can falsely appear to have diffuse expression of this marker. Human papillomavirus (HPV) in situ hybridization is another tool used to confirm the cervical origin of a given tumor; however, up to 30% of cases of cervical carcinoma can be negative for this test.[41] In a small subset of cases, the results of these ancillary tests are discordant, and imaging studies and/or fractioned curettage are required to determine with certainty the site of origin of the tumor.

Serous Carcinoma

Overview

Serous carcinoma accounts for 10% of all endometrial carcinomas.[42] This tumor is usually found in postmenopausal patients, although it can be seen in patients younger than age 56 years.[43] An association with breast carcinoma is noted in approximately 16% of patients; this association increases to 23% in patients younger than age 56 years.[44] In some cases, there

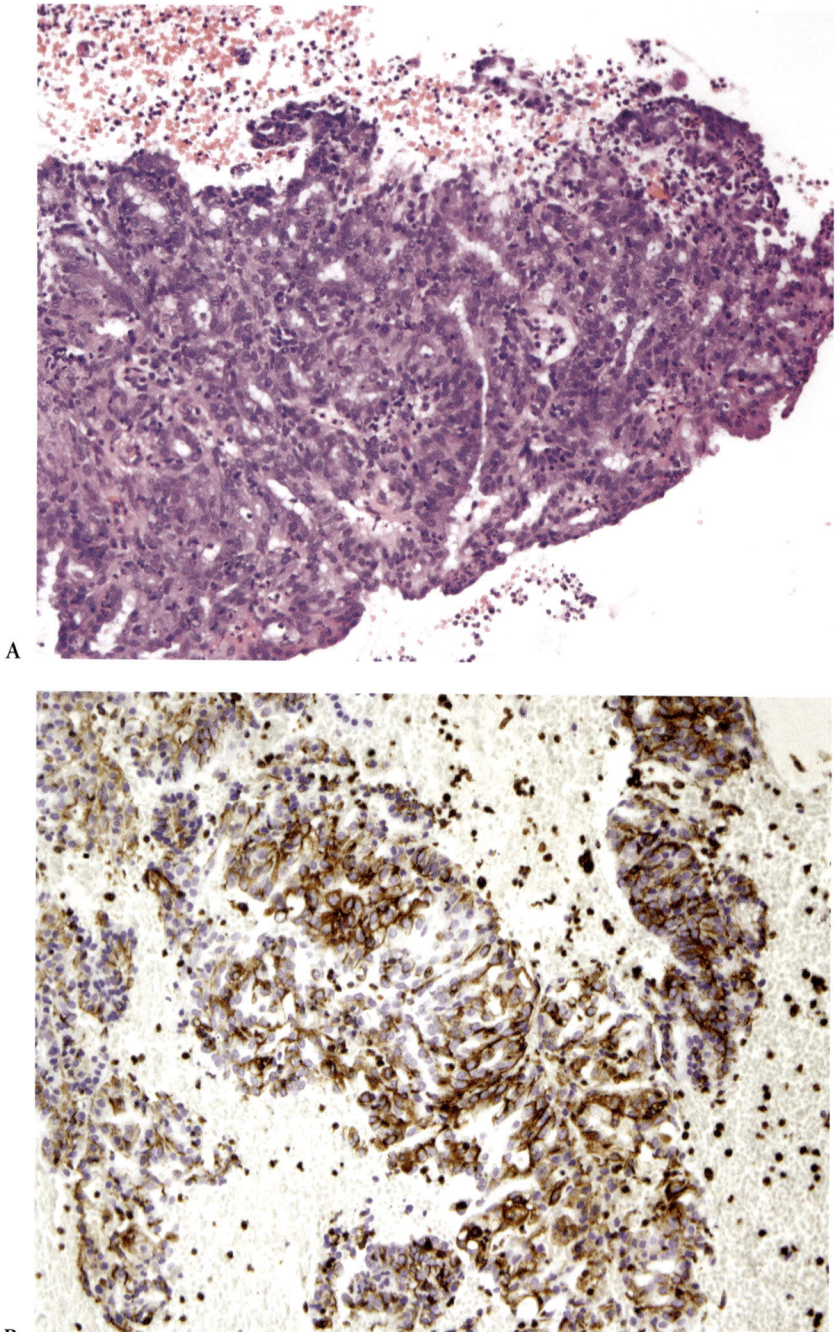

FIGURE 4-24: Endometrioid adenocarcinoma with mucinous metaplasia. Tumor difficult to differentiate from an endocervical adenocarcinoma on hematoxylin and eosin–stained slide (**A**). Immunoperoxidase studies show positive staining for vimentin (**B**) and estrogen receptor (**C**) and negative staining for carcinoembryonic antigen (CEA) (**D**). *(continued)*

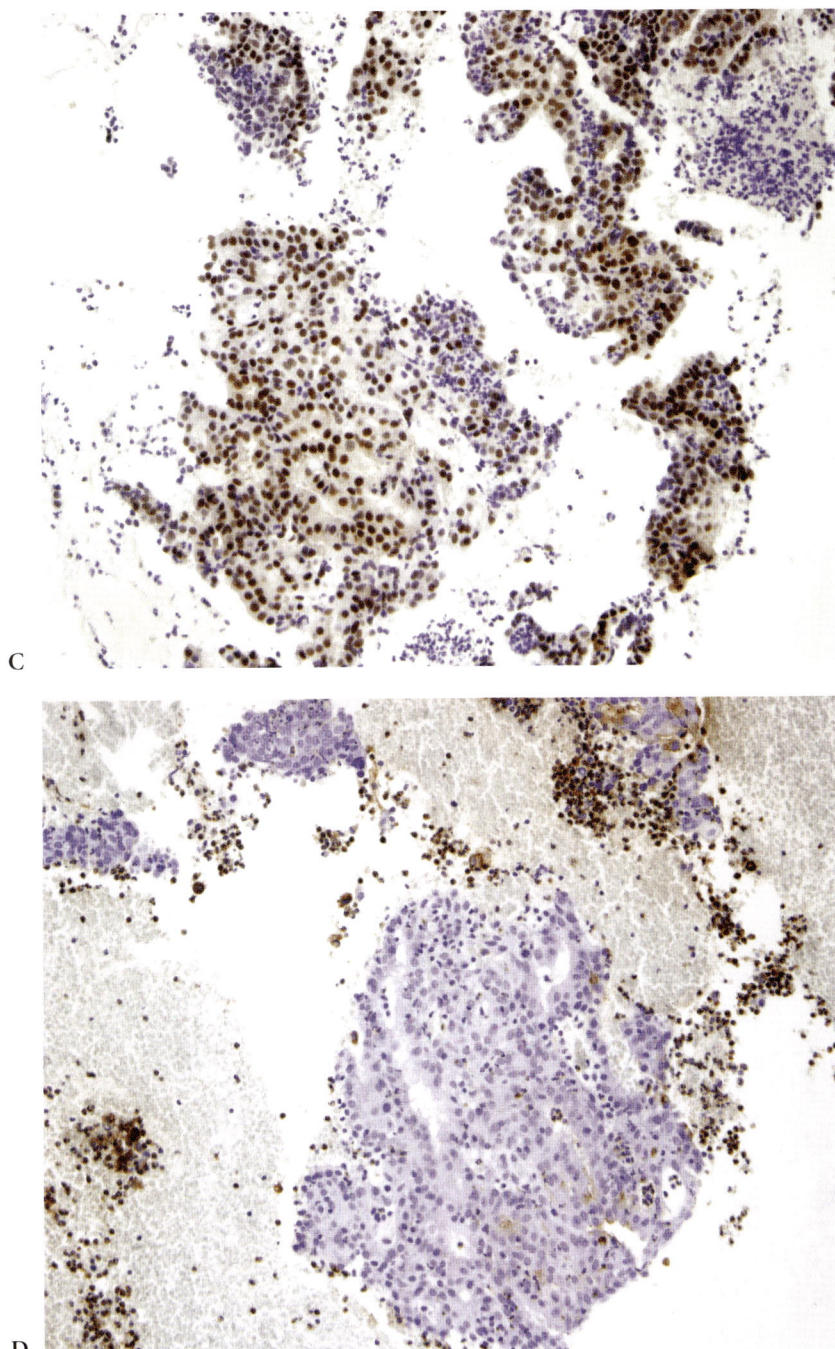

FIGURE 4-24: (continued)

is an association between serous carcinoma and pelvic irradiation, tamoxifen use, *BRCA1* mutation, cervical or axillary lymph node metastasis at presentation, paraneoplastic hypercalcemia, or high levels of serum CEA.[45–52]

Serous carcinoma is characterized by the presence of marked cytologic atypia. The neoplastic cells are arranged in papillary, glandular, or solid patterns (Fig. 4-25A–C). Usually, there is tufting with detachment of the neoplastic cells. The mitotic activity is high. Hobnail cells, tumor giant cells, abnormal mitotic figures, and psammoma bodies can also be seen.[53]

Differential Diagnosis

Serous Carcinoma versus Endometrioid Adenocarcinoma, Villoglandular Variant

In the villoglandular variant of endometrioid adenocarcinoma, the papillae are finger-like, with smooth contours, and are lined by columnar cells with preserved polarity of the nuclei and bland cytology. In serous carcinoma, there is marked cytologic atypia and no preservation of the nuclear polarity.

Serous Carcinoma versus Papillary Endometrial Adenocarcinoma of Intermediate Grade

Papillary endometrial adenocarcinoma of intermediate grade is not included in the WHO classification; however, it is recognized by some investigators.[54,55] This tumor has features that are between those of endometrioid adenocarcinoma with villoglandular features and serous carcinoma. Papillary endometrial adenocarcinoma of intermediate grade appears as papillae that are lined by cells with nuclei that are mildly or moderately disorganized, without preservation of their polarity but with less atypia than is seen in serous

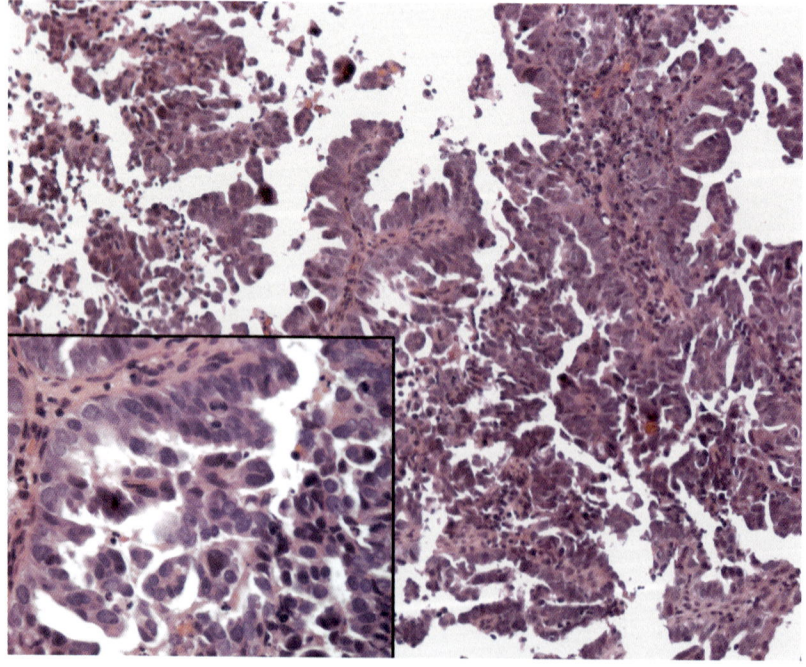

FIGURE 4-25: Serous carcinoma. Tumor characterized by the marked cytologic atypia of its neoplastic cells. Papillary pattern (**A**) (*inset*), glandular pattern (**B**), and solid pattern (**C**). *(continued)*

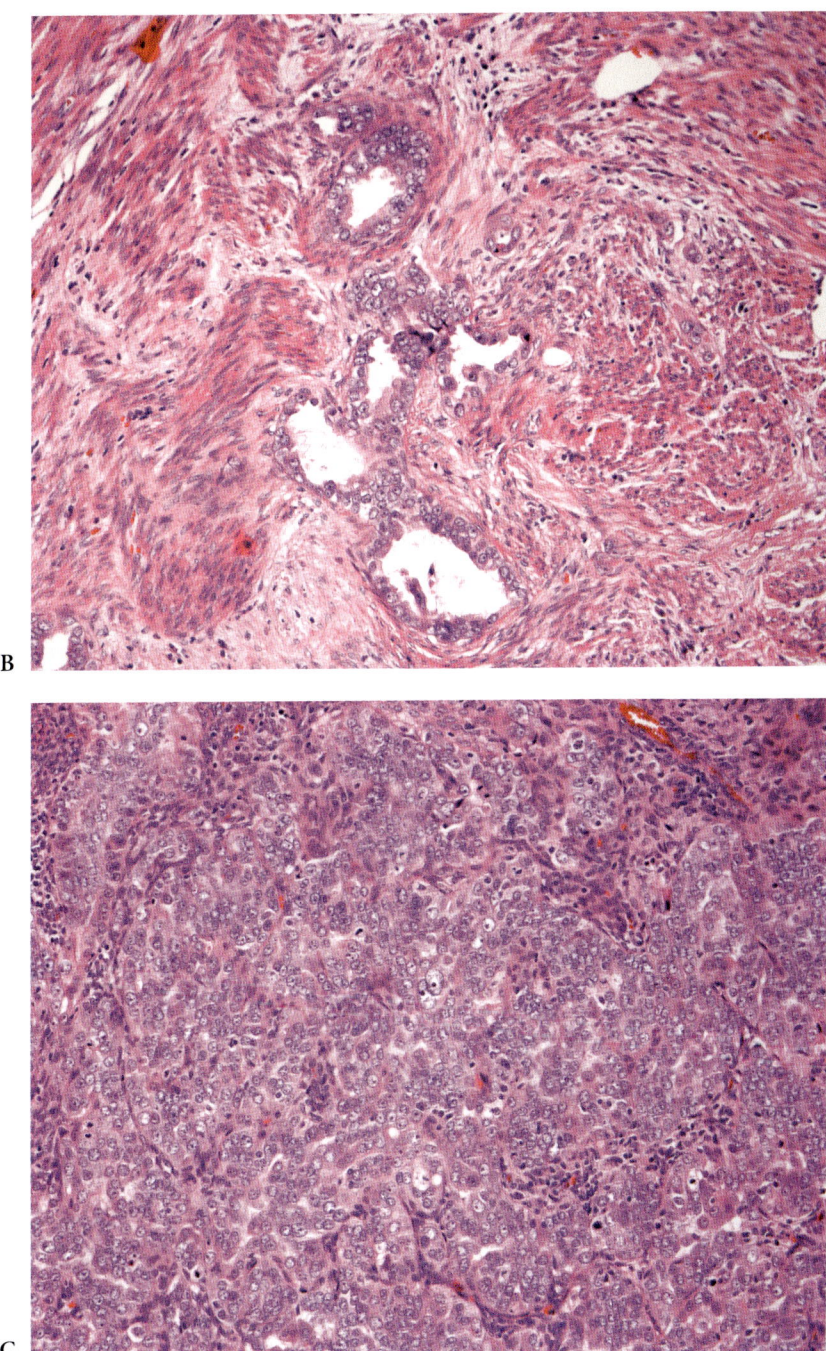

FIGURE 4-25: *(continued)*

carcinoma (Fig. 4-26). Foci of squamous and mucinous differentiation are usually seen (Fig. 4-27A–B). In addition, the pattern of invasion described as microcystic, elongated, and fragmented (MELF pattern) is commonly seen. This type of tumor is associated with a higher incidence of vascular/lymphatic invasion, advanced stage at presentation, and recurrences than a typical FIGO grade 2 endometrioid adenocarcinoma.[55]

Serous Carcinoma versus Endometrial Adenocarcinoma, FIGO Grade 1, and Complex Endometrial Hyperplasia

These two processes are characterized by a proliferation of well-formed glands lacking marked cytologic atypia. In contrast, the glandular variant of serous carcinoma shows open glands lined by cells with marked cytologic atypia (i.e., increased nuclear-to-cytoplasmic ratio, nuclear pleomorphism, and loss of nuclear polarity).

Serous Carcinoma versus Clear Cell Carcinoma

The papillae seen in clear cell carcinoma are usually lined by a single row of neoplastic cells with clear or eosinophilic cytoplasm and tend to show hyalinization of the stromal cores. In contrast, the papillae of serous carcinoma are usually more complex than the ones seen in clear cell carcinoma, and the neoplastic cells tend to have a basophilic or amphophilic cytoplasm. However, occasionally the neoplastic cells are eosinophilic or show focal clearing of the cytoplasm.

Serous Carcinoma versus Papillary Syncytial Metaplasia

This process lacks the marked cytologic atypia and the high mitotic index seen in serous carcinoma.

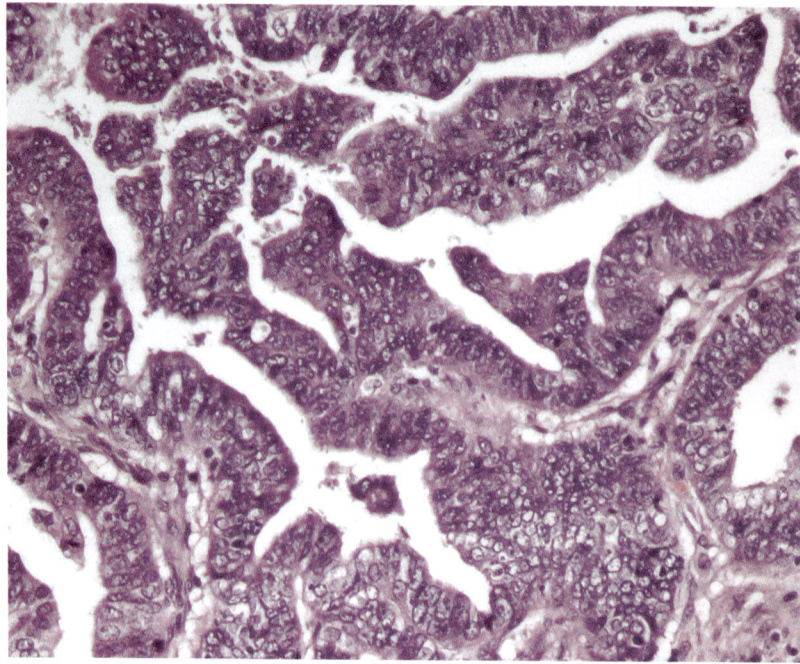

FIGURE 4-26: Papillary endometrial adenocarcinoma of intermediate grade.

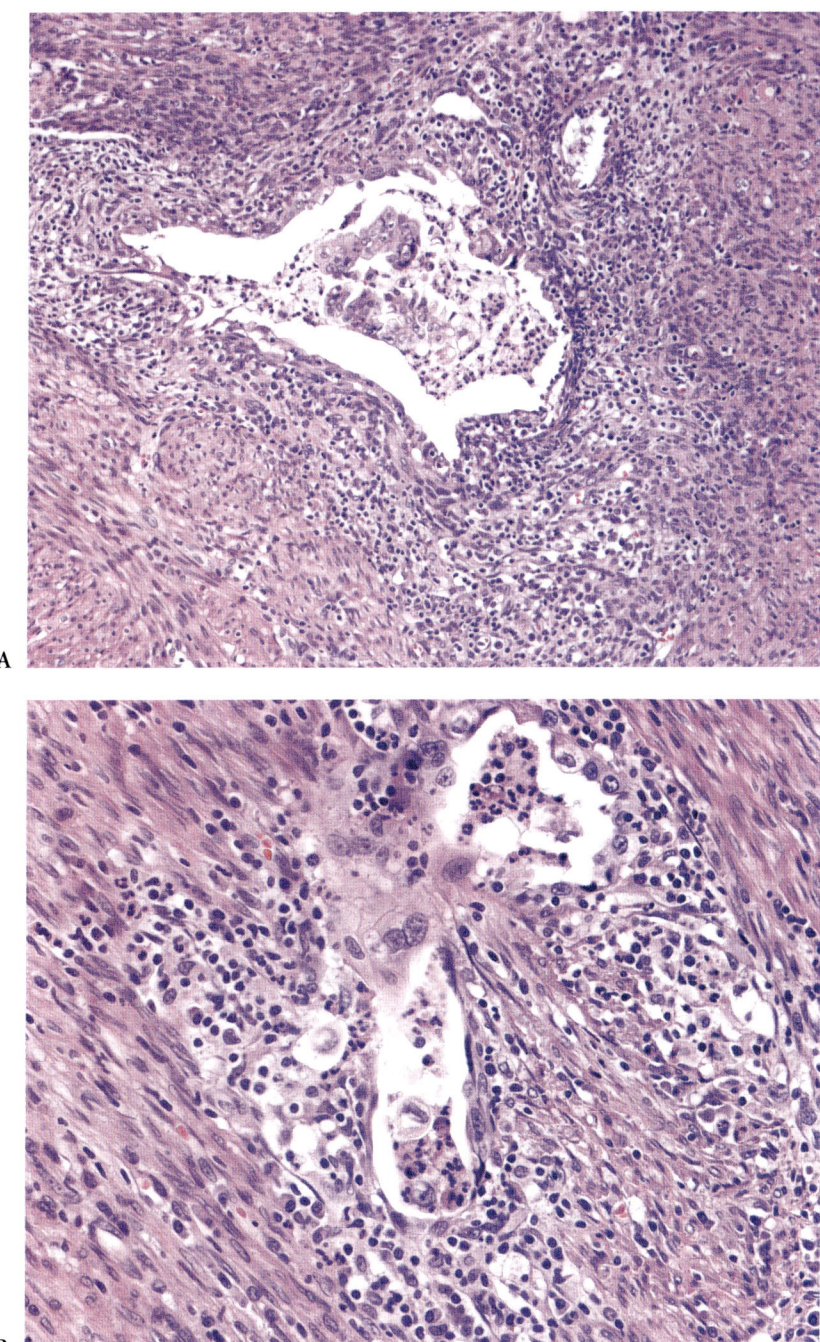

FIGURE 4-27: Papillary endometrial adenocarcinoma of intermediate grade, with typical pattern of invasion seen in this type of neoplasm. Note the incomplete glands with attenuated epithelium and prominent inflammatory infiltrate (**A and B**).

Clear Cell Carcinoma

Overview

Clear cell carcinoma represents approximately 5% of all endometrial carcinomas.[56] This tumor is composed of clear, eosinophilic (oncocytic), or hobnail cells arranged in tubulocystic, papillary, or solid patterns (Figs. 4-28A–C and 4-29). The cells can be polygonal,

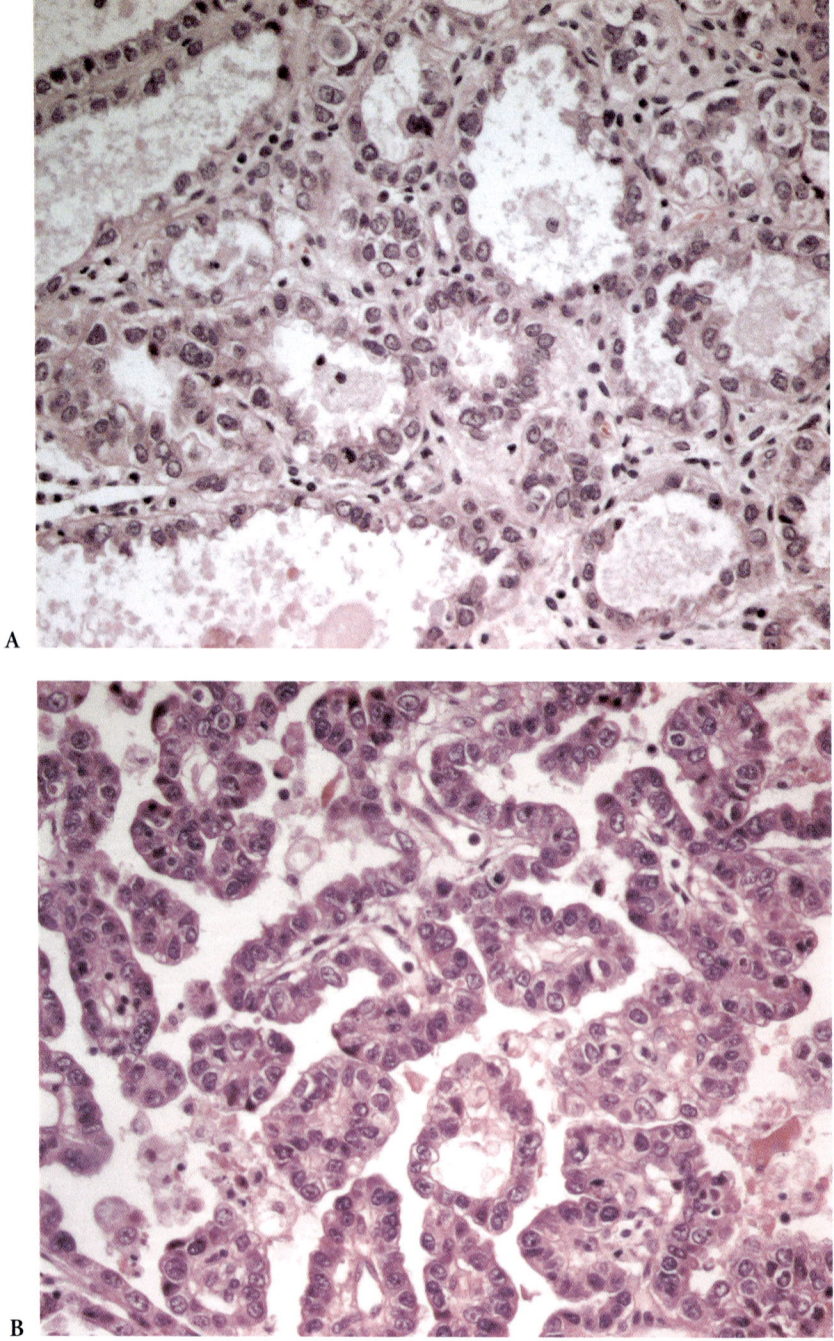

FIGURE 4-28: Clear cell carcinoma, tubulocystic pattern (**A**), papillary pattern (**B**), and solid pattern (**C**). *(continued)*

Chapter 4 • Endometrial Carcinoma

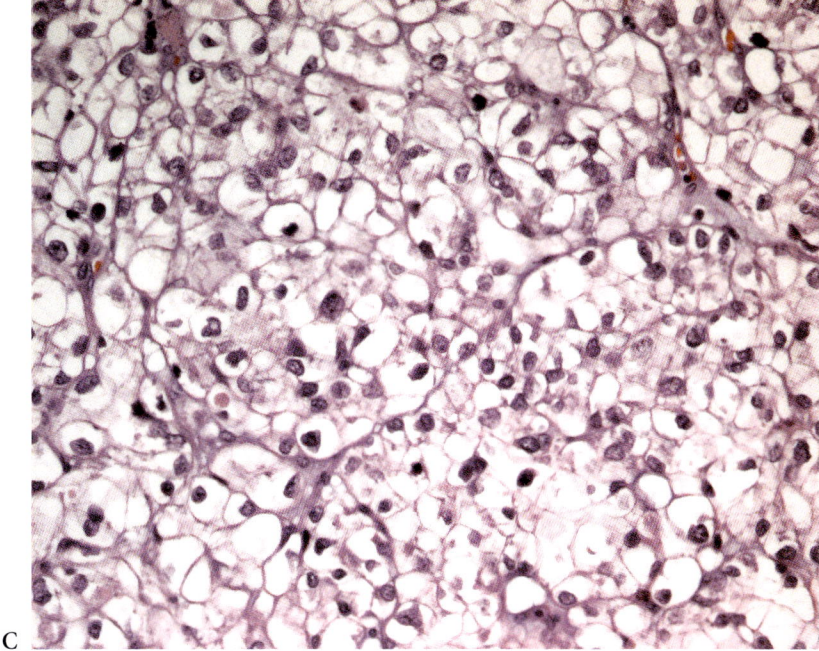

C

FIGURE 4-28: *(continued)*

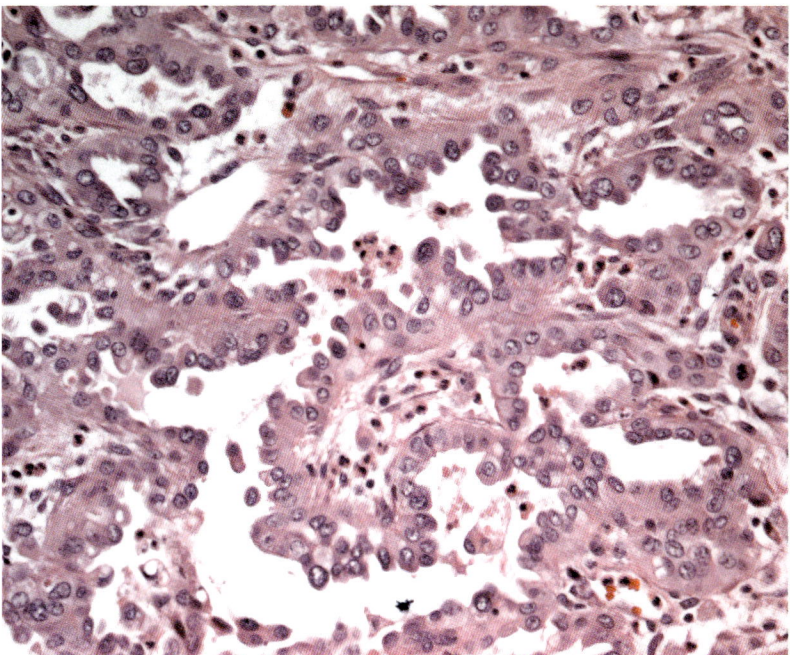

FIGURE 4-29: Clear cell carcinoma with eosinophilic cells.

cuboidal, or flattened. The degree of atypia is variable, usually marked and less frequently mild or absent. The mitotic index is also variable, ranging from 0 mitoses per 10 HPFs to greater than 10 mitoses per 10 HPFs. The stroma can be hyalinized. Epithelial hyaline bodies, eosinophilic granular or homogeneous intraluminal material, and psammoma bodies also can be seen.[57,58] Immunohistochemically, clear cell carcinoma is negative for PR and has a high Ki-67 proliferation index and variable expression of p53 and ER.[59,60] Clear cell carcinoma is usually detected in postmenopausal patients with a mean age of 65 years (range, 21 to 91 years).[56,57]

Differential Diagnosis

Clear Cell Carcinoma versus Serous Carcinoma
This distinction is discussed in the previous section.

Clear Cell Carcinoma versus Endometrioid Carcinoma with Squamous Differentiation Rich in Glycogen
Areas of typical squamous differentiation are noted in the vicinity of the areas of concern in endometrioid carcinoma with squamous differentiation. In contrast, clear cell carcinoma usually shows a combination of architectural patterns including the tubulocystic, papillary, and solid patterns.

Clear Cell Carcinoma versus Endometrioid Carcinoma with Secretory Changes
Endometrioid tumors with secretory changes have columnar cells with supra- and subnuclear glycogen vacuoles and no atypia. In contrast, clear cell carcinoma shows polygonal, cuboidal, or flattened cells with total clearing of the cytoplasm and at least focal atypia.

Clear Cell Carcinoma versus Clear Cell Changes
In an endometrioid carcinoma with clear cell changes, the clearing of the cytoplasm in the neoplastic cells is due to the accumulation of lipids or to secretory changes. The neoplastic cells do not show marked cytologic atypia. In addition, the typical architectural patterns seen in clear cell carcinoma are absent.

Clear Cell Carcinoma versus Clear Cell Metaplasia
Clear cell metaplasia is usually associated with progestin use. It tends to be focal and lacks cytologic atypia.

Clear Cell Carcinoma versus Reactive Atypia Including Hobnail Metaplasia
Reactive atypia including hobnail metaplasia is usually a focal finding secondary to inflammation, progestin therapy, infarction of a polyp, recent curettage, or intrauterine device.

Clear Cell Carcinoma versus Arias-Stella Reaction
Arias-Stella reaction is usually associated with pregnancy, although it can be seen in nonpregnant or older patients. Attention to the following features will facilitate the proper recognition of Arias-Stella reaction: (1) patient's young age, clinical history of pregnancy, or progestin use; (2) areas with decidualization of the stroma; and (3) scarce mitoses. In challenging cases, the use of immunohistochemical studies including Ki-67 and p53 has been proposed because most cases of Arias-Stella reaction are negative for these two markers, whereas the reverse is true for clear cell carcinoma.[61]

Mucinous Adenocarcinoma

Overview

Although the WHO classification system defines a mucinous adenocarcinoma of the endometrium as a tumor in which most of the neoplastic cells contain prominent intracytoplasmic mucin, this classification does not provide a percentage cutoff.[5] Two different percentage cutoffs have been proposed in the literature to render this diagnosis: >50%[6] or >70%[62] of the tumor cells showing mucinous differentiation. In our practice, we use the >50% cutoff.

Mucinous adenocarcinomas are characterized by architectural complexity, including any of the following patterns: glandular, villous, villoglandular, or solid (Fig. 4-30). The degree of cytologic atypia tends to be mild or moderate. In rare cases, marked cytologic atypia is noted. The mitotic index ranges from 0 to 8 mitoses per 10 HPFs.[6,63] Rare cases with either intestinal differentiation (i.e., goblet cells) or signet ring cells have been seen.[10,64]

The term "microglandular hyperplasia-like or endocervical-like endometrial adenocarcinoma" has been used to designate cases of well-differentiated mucinous endometrial adenocarcinoma composed of small- to medium-sized glands lined by cells with no to minimal cytologic atypia and low mitotic activity.

Differential Diagnosis

Mucinous Adenocarcinoma versus Microglandular Hyperplasia of the Uterine Cervix

The diagnosis of microglandular hyperplasia should not be rendered in an endometrial biopsy of a postmenopausal patient. When dealing with such a case, a descriptive diagnosis should be provided, and additional sampling in the form of a fractional curettage should be obtained to rule out an endometrial mucinous adenocarcinoma. The following features have been proposed as suggestive of a low-grade mucinous adenocarcinoma of

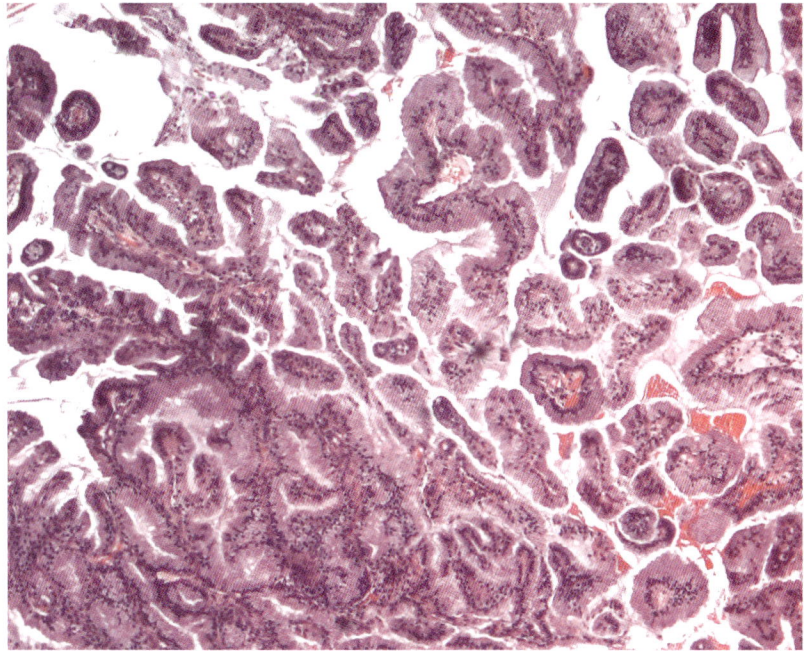

FIGURE 4-30: Mucinous adenocarcinoma.

the endometrium: (1) luminal squamous metaplasia, (2) stromal foam cells, (3) mitotic activity (>3 mitoses per 10 HPFs), (4) vimentin expression, and (5) Ki-67 expression in ≥5% of the epithelium. It is important to underscore that the expression of vimentin may be limited to the basal portion of the cells and that a negative result does not allow for the distinction of microglandular hyperplasia of the uterine cervix from a low-grade mucinous endometrial adenocarcinoma because the expression of vimentin in low-grade mucinous endometrial adenocarcinoma is variable. The use of CEA, ER, PR, or p53 has no value in distinguishing these two lesions.[63]

Mucinous Adenocarcinoma versus Metaplastic Mucinous Proliferation (Hyperplasia with Mucinous Metaplasia)

According to Nucci et al.,[65] mucinous proliferations in the endometrium can be classified as follows: type A, no more than slightly complex architecture, with or without micropapillary tufting, and mild cytologic atypia; type B, more glandular complexity than type A, microglands, and mild cytologic atypia; and type C, high degree of architectural complexity, cribriforming, branching of villous structures, and moderate-to-severe cytologic atypia. According to these investigators, the risk of carcinoma ranged from 0% to 64.5% to 100% for types A, B, and C, respectively. Other authors have found that combining types B and C into a single category yielded 100% sensitivity and 19% specificity for the diagnosis of carcinoma.[66]

Squamous Carcinoma

Overview

Squamous carcinoma is rare, accounting for fewer than 1% of the carcinomas arising in the endometrium.[67] Its diagnosis requires the following: (1) an absence of coexisting endometrial adenocarcinoma, (2) a lack of continuity with the squamous epithelium of the uterine cervix, (3) no synchronous or preexisting invasive squamous carcinoma of the uterine cervix, and (4) clear evidence of keratinization and/or intercellular bridges.[5] Most cases are seen in postmenopausal patients, and up to one-third present with FIGO stage III or IV disease. Predisposing factors include cervical stenosis, uterine prolapse, chronic pyometra, extensive squamous metaplasia of the endometrium, and a history of pelvic irradiation.[68,69] Rare cases have been positive for HPV type 31, 33, or 16.[67] Histologically, these neoplasms can range from well differentiated to poorly differentiated (Fig. 4-31). The term verrucous carcinoma is used to designate tumors that are well differentiated and have a pushing border. In rare cases, squamous carcinoma of the endometrium can have spindle cells (sarcomatoid variant).[70]

Differential Diagnosis

Squamous Carcinoma versus Endometrial Endometrioid Adenocarcinoma with Extensive Squamous Differentiation

A thorough sampling of endometrial endometrioid tumors with extensive squamous differentiation will allow the identification of the glandular component, which can be overshadowed by extensive squamous differentiation in an endometrioid adenocarcinoma.

Squamous Carcinoma versus Extension from a Cervical Squamous Carcinoma, Invasive or In Situ

Clinical correlation and a thorough sampling of the uterine cervix will allow the correct diagnosis.

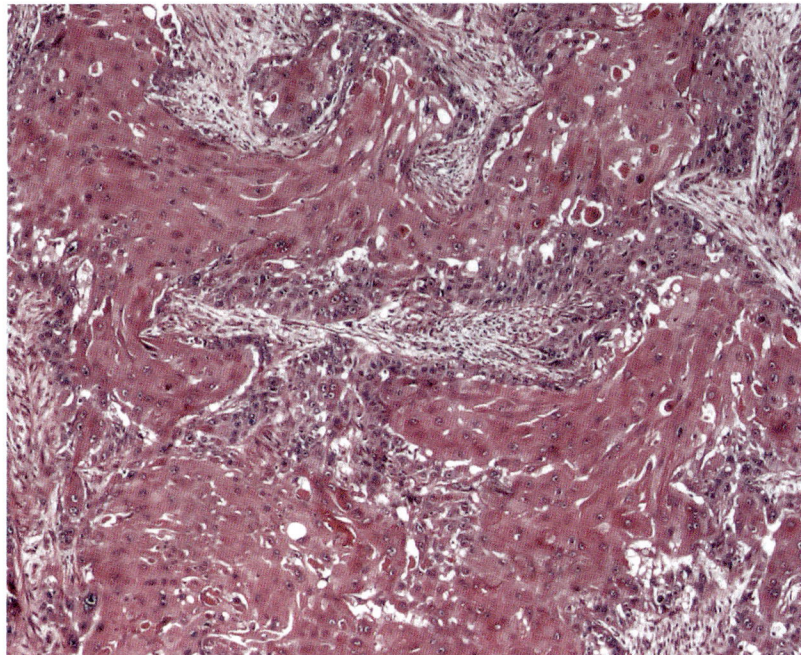

FIGURE 4-31: Squamous carcinoma.

Squamous Carcinoma versus Squamous Metaplasia

Extensive squamous metaplasia of the endometrium, also known as "ichthyosis uteri," requires the evaluation of an adequate amount of tissue for its diagnosis. Extensive squamous metaplasia of the endometrium lacks the cytologic atypia that is found in squamous carcinoma. In addition, it does not have the myometrial invasion usually seen in squamous carcinoma.

Transitional Cell Carcinoma

Overview

This uncommon tumor has the histologic features typically seen in carcinomas arising in the urinary tract (i.e., papillae with fibrovascular cores lined by transitional-like epithelium) (Fig. 4-32). Transitional cell carcinoma of the endometrium is usually detected in postmenopausal patients who present with vaginal bleeding; however, rare cases have been diagnosed in patients in their 40s. The tumor ranges in size from 0.4 to 10 cm (mean, 4.4 cm) and is usually associated with other carcinoma histotypes such as endometrioid, mucinous, or serous. A rare case has been described as part of a carcinosarcoma (malignant mixed müllerian tumor).[71] Areas of squamous differentiation, poorly formed acini, secondary "micropapillae," or condylomatous changes can be noted. Nuclear grooves are rare. The degree of cytologic atypia tends to be moderate to severe, and mitotic activity is conspicuous.[72–74]

Immunohistochemically, transitional cell carcinoma of the endometrium is usually positive for cytokeratin 7 and negative for cytokeratin 20, WT-1, and thrombomodulin.[71–73] This tumor is diffusely positive for vimentin and can be positive or negative for ER and PR.[71,73] The better differentiated areas of the tumor express p63 in the basal layer of the epithelium, whereas in the less differentiated areas, this marker is expressed in scattered cells higher in the epithelium. p16 is usually diffusely expressed, although it can be focal.[71] A few cases have been associated with HPV 16.[75] Of interest, rare cases have been associated with Brenner tumors of the ovary.[76,77]

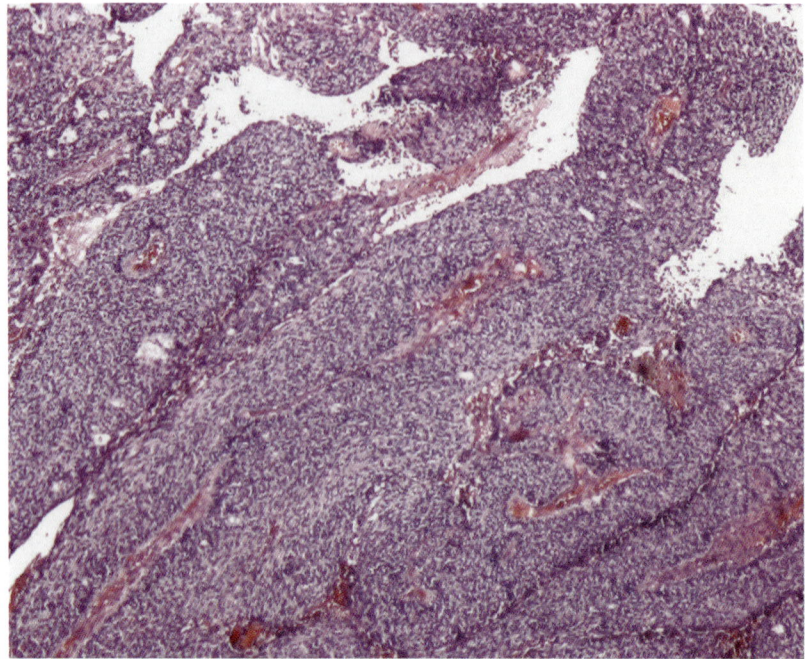

FIGURE 4-32: Transitional cell carcinoma.

Differential Diagnosis

Transitional Cell Carcinoma versus Papillary Squamous Carcinoma

In a sample with a limited amount of tissue, the distinction between transitional cell carcinoma of the endometrium and papillary squamous carcinoma of the uterine cervix can be very difficult; however, the correct diagnosis can be rendered if other histotypes of endometrial adenocarcinoma are identified.

Transitional Cell Carcinoma versus Secondary/Metastatic Transitional Cell Carcinoma of the Urinary Tract

In contrast to transitional cell carcinoma of the endometrium, transitional cell carcinoma of the urinary tract expresses cytokeratins 7 and 20.[71,73]

Small-Cell Carcinoma

Overview

This uncommon tumor is composed of small- or intermediate-sized cells arranged in sheets, nests, or cords. The cells are either round or spindled. The small cells have uniform nuclei with coarse or granular chromatin and inconspicuous nucleoli, whereas the intermediate-sized cells have pleomorphic, irregular nuclei, with or without nucleoli (Fig. 4-33). Areas of necrosis, marked mitotic activity, numerous apoptotic bodies, and vascular and myometrial invasion are usually seen.[78,79] Small-cell carcinoma of the endometrium can be associated with endometrioid or serous carcinoma or be part of a malignant mixed müllerian tumor.[78–80] Immunohistochemically, the tumor cells are usually positive for keratin, EMA, and CAM 5.2, although the staining can be focal, and for one or more of the

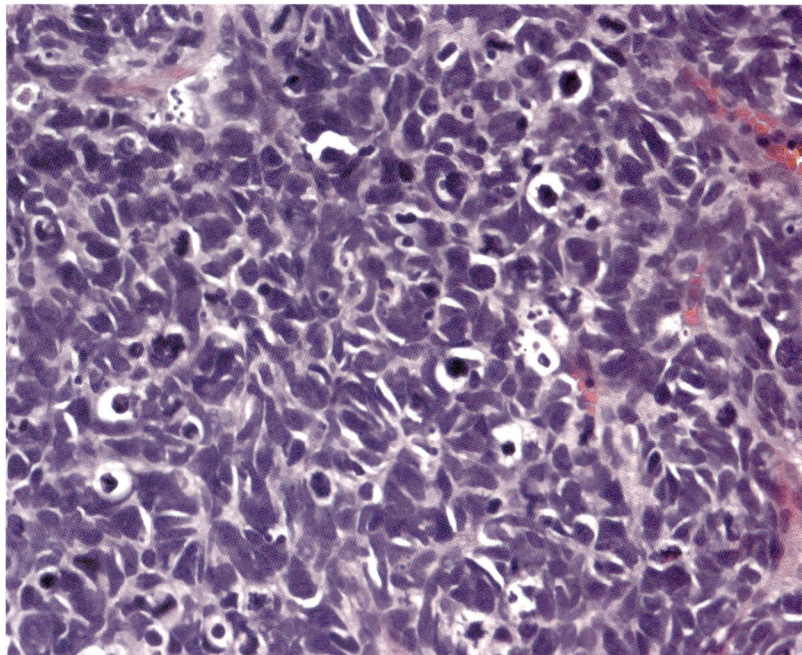

FIGURE 4-33: Small-cell carcinoma.

neuroendocrine markers, such as CD56, CD57, synaptophysin, chromogranin, neuron-specific enolase, glucagon, and calcitonin (Fig. 4-34).[78,79] Staining for p16 and S-100 has also been reported.[81] Small-cell carcinoma of the endometrium is usually detected in postmenopausal patients (age range, 23 to 78 years) who present with vaginal bleeding and advanced-stage disease.[82]

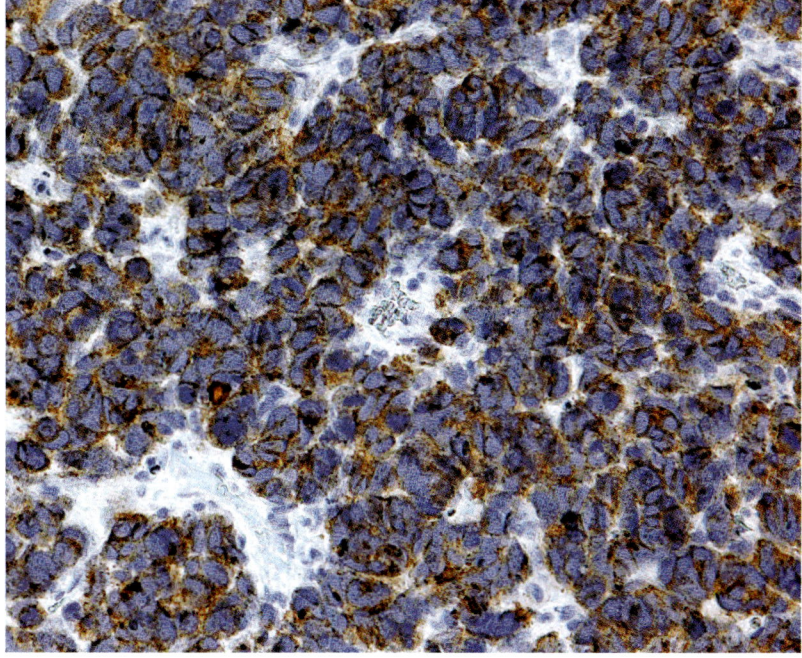

FIGURE 4-34: Small-cell carcinoma; positive staining for synaptophysin.

Differential Diagnosis

Small-Cell Carcinoma versus Small-Cell Carcinoma of the Uterine Cervix

Small-cell carcinoma of the uterine cervix is more common than its counterpart in the endometrium. Therefore, a cervical origin must be excluded clinically. The histologic examination will be able to determine the origin of the tumor only if an association with other carcinomas can be detected (i.e., squamous carcinoma or cervical adenocarcinoma, which is in keeping with a cervical origin, versus endometrioid or serous carcinoma, which is in keeping with an endometrial origin).

Small-Cell Carcinoma versus Primitive Neuroectodermal Tumor

Attention to the histologic and immunohistochemical features mentioned earlier will allow for the correct diagnosis of these two entities.

Small-Cell Carcinoma versus Malignant Mixed Müllerian Tumor

In cases where small-cell carcinoma is associated with an endometrioid adenocarcinoma, the tumor can be mistaken for a malignant mixed müllerian tumor. The expression of neuroendocrine markers will distinguish small-cell carcinoma from an undifferentiated sarcoma.

Undifferentiated Carcinoma

Overview

Undifferentiated carcinoma has been considered rare, and its WHO definition is vague (i.e., "a tumor lacking any evidence of differentiation"); however, in our experience, this neoplasm is frequently intermixed with endometrioid adenocarcinoma (detected in up to 9% of cases of endometrial carcinomas at a single institution), and it has specific histologic features that allow for its proper recognition.[83]

This type of neoplasm occurs mostly in postmenopausal patients, although it can occur in younger patients. Histologically, it is characterized by a proliferation of medium-sized, monotonous epithelial cells, usually arranged in a solid pattern. Focal trabecular or cord formations, rhabdoid-like cells, and pleomorphism can be noted. Areas of necrosis are common (Fig. 4-35). Immunohistochemically, the tumor cells are only focally positive (5% to 10% of the tumor cells) for pankeratin cocktail, although in rare cases, the expression is diffuse (>75% of the cells stain). Of interest, the expression of pankeratin is very heterogeneous in this type of tumor. Therefore, in many cases, it is necessary to perform this immunostain on at least two different tissue blocks before obtaining a positive result. Undifferentiated carcinoma of the endometrium also expresses EMA, usually focally (10% to 20% of the cells) and less frequently diffusely (>75% of the cells).[83] Neuroendocrine markers such as synaptophysin and chromogranin can be expressed focally.

Differential Diagnosis

Undifferentiated Carcinoma versus Endometrioid Adenocarcinoma

A common problem is the misclassification of a mixed carcinoma composed of endometrioid adenocarcinoma, FIGO grade 1 or 2, and undifferentiated carcinoma (dedifferentiated carcinoma) as an endometrioid adenocarcinoma of a higher grade (i.e., FIGO grade 2 or 3). This problem is due to the misinterpretation of the undifferentiated carcinoma as the solid component of an endometrioid adenocarcinoma. Attention to the histologic features listed

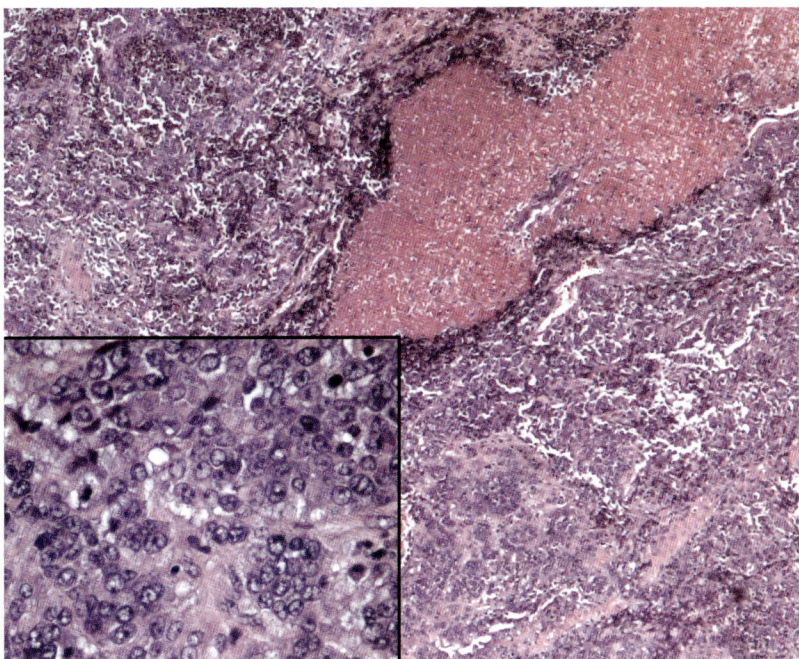

FIGURE 4-35: Undifferentiated carcinoma; note the monotonous appearance of the tumor cells (*inset*).

previously and the use of immunoperoxidase studies will facilitate the correct diagnosis. Pankeratin and EMA stain the solid component of an endometrioid adenocarcinoma diffusely; in contrast, these markers will be only focally expressed in undifferentiated carcinoma.

Undifferentiated Carcinoma versus Neuroendocrine Carcinoma
Attention to the histologic features of small- and large-cell neuroendocrine carcinoma described earlier and later, respectively, in this text and to the expression of neuroendocrine markers such as synaptophysin and chromogranin will facilitate the correct classification of a given tumor.

Undifferentiated Carcinoma versus High-Grade Sarcoma
Uterine high-grade sarcomas are seldom composed of epithelioid cells, except for epithelioid leiomyosarcoma. In these cases, the use of desmin, caldesmon, and SMA facilitates the identification of smooth muscle differentiation of these neoplasms.

Undifferentiated Carcinoma versus Malignant Mixed Müllerian Tumor
The solid pattern typically seen in undifferentiated carcinoma associated with an endometrioid adenocarcinoma can be mistaken for the sarcoma component of a malignant mixed müllerian tumor. Attention to the histologic features listed earlier and awareness of the common association of these two histotypes will allow the correct classification of the tumor.

Large-Cell Neuroendocrine Carcinoma

Overview

This uncommon tumor, detected usually in postmenopausal patients, is characterized by the presence of cells with abundant amphophilic or basophilic cytoplasm and vesicular or hyperchromatic nuclei with visible nucleoli. The tumor cells are arranged in a solid, insular,

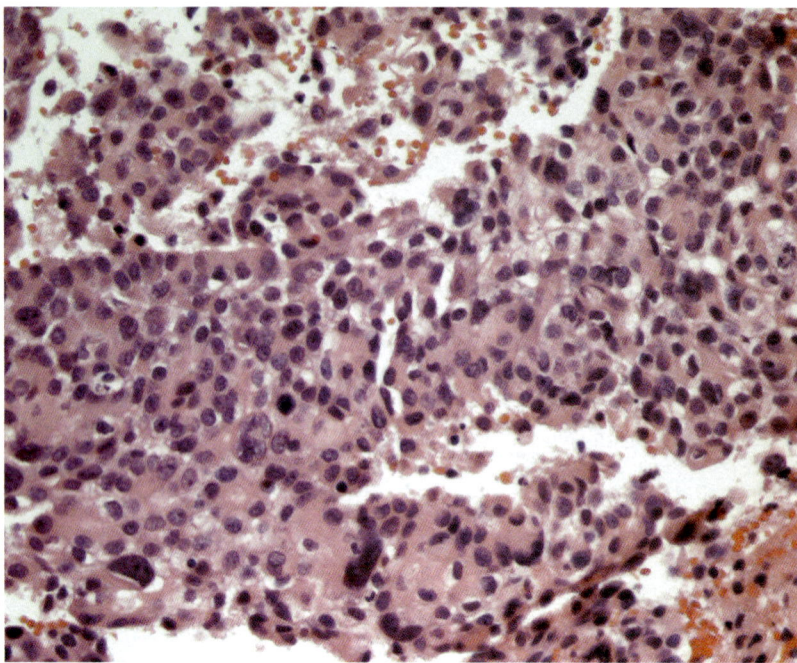

FIGURE 4-36: Large-cell neuroendocrine carcinoma.

or trabecular pattern (Fig. 4-36). Other typical features are conspicuous mitotic activity and apoptosis, as well as tumor necrosis. Large-cell neuroendocrine carcinoma might be associated with other histotypes, mostly endometrioid, and less frequently serous carcinoma.[84,85] Immunohistochemically, the neoplastic cells are positive for CAM 5.2, cytokeratin 7, AE1/AE3, CD56, p16, neuron-specific enolase (NSE), chromogranin, and synaptophysin (with variable results for the neuroendocrine markers) (Fig. 4-37A–B). CD56 and NSE lack specificity and can be expressed in endometrioid carcinoma.[84]

Differential Diagnosis

Large-Cell Neuroendocrine Carcinoma versus Small-Cell Carcinoma
Attention to the cytologic features delineated earlier will facilitate a correct diagnosis.

Large-Cell Neuroendocrine Carcinoma versus Undifferentiated Carcinoma
In contrast to large-cell neuroendocrine carcinoma, undifferentiated carcinoma is either negative or only focally positive for chromogranin and/or synaptophysin.

Lymphoepithelioma-Like Carcinoma

This tumor is rare and has been reported in postmenopausal patients only.

Lymphoepithelioma-like carcinoma is composed of sheets or groups of or individual polygonal cells with indistinct cell borders, vesicular nuclei, prominent nucleoli, and prominent inflammatory infiltrate composed of lymphocytes and plasma cells. No association with Epstein-Barr virus has been found. Immunohistochemically, the tumor cells express cytokeratin and EMA and are negative for leukocyte common antigen. The use of these immuno-

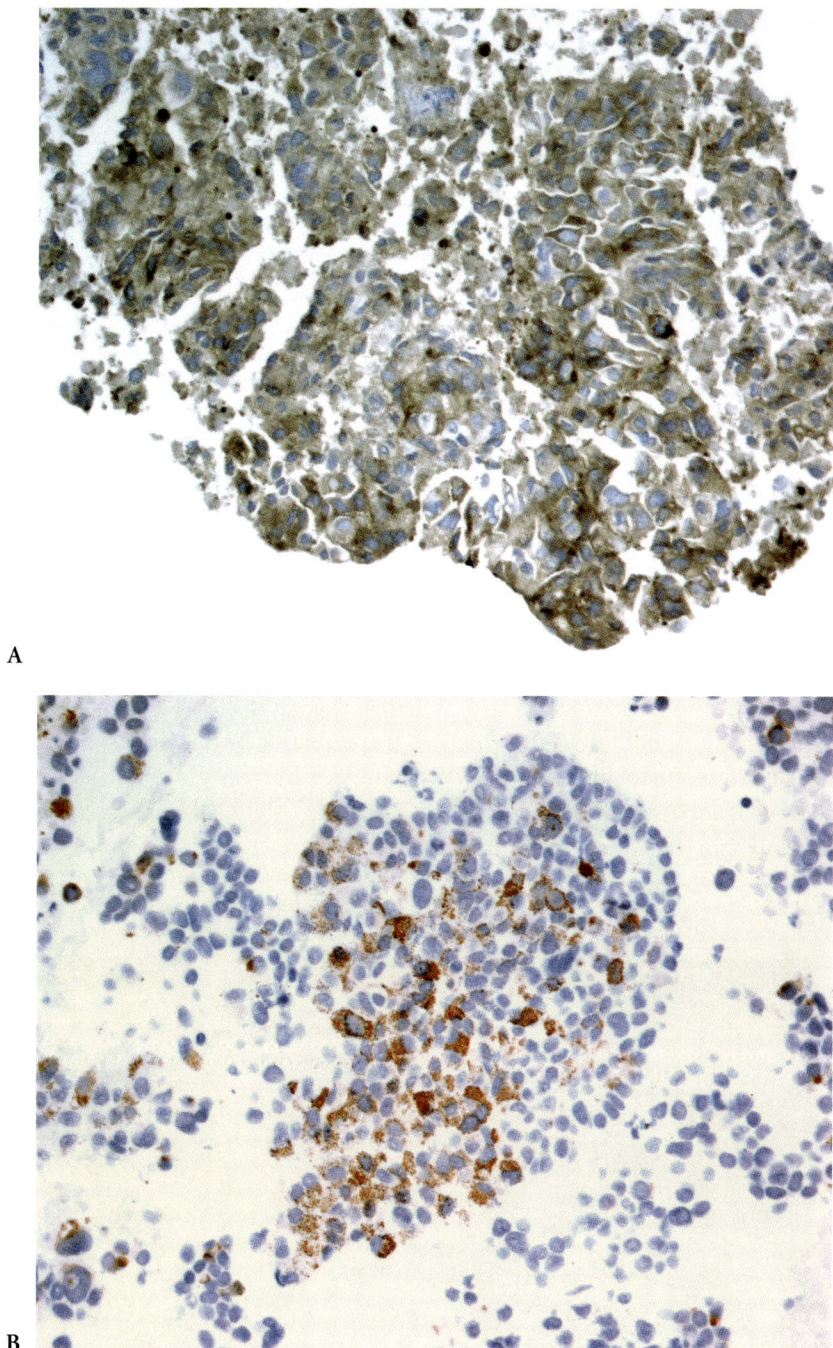

FIGURE 4-37: Large-cell neuroendocrine carcinoma; positive staining for synaptophysin (**A**) and chromogranin (**B**).

histochemical studies will allow the distinction of this type of tumor from a lymphoma-like lesion and lymphoma.[86–88]

Giant-Cell Carcinoma

Overview

This rare tumor is usually detected in postmenopausal patients. Histologically, it is characterized by numerous large, bizarre, eosinophilic, frequently multinucleated cells arranged in a solid or nested pattern. The cells can be discohesive, contain intracytoplasmic vacuoles, or be focally spindled (Fig. 4-38). A prominent infiltrate of neutrophils and eosinophils with emperipolesis can be seen. Mitoses are frequent and usually abnormal. This type of tumor is typically associated with other histotypes, usually endometrioid adenocarcinoma. The tumor cells are positive for keratin and EMA.[89]

Differential Diagnosis

Giant-Cell Carcinoma versus Trophoblastic Tumors

Placental site trophoblastic tumor (PSTT) and choriocarcinoma are tumors seen in women of reproductive age. Histologically, the former is composed of intermediate trophoblast cells, which can be multinucleated in areas, whereas the latter shows a distinct biphasic pattern in which cytotrophoblasts, intermediate trophoblasts, and syncytiotrophoblasts are recognized. Immunohistochemically, PSTT expresses human placental lactogen (hPL), MUC-4, HLA-G, and melanoma cell adhesion molecule (Mel-CAM or D146); human chorionic gonadotropin (hCG) is expressed focally. In contrast, choriocarcinoma expresses hCG

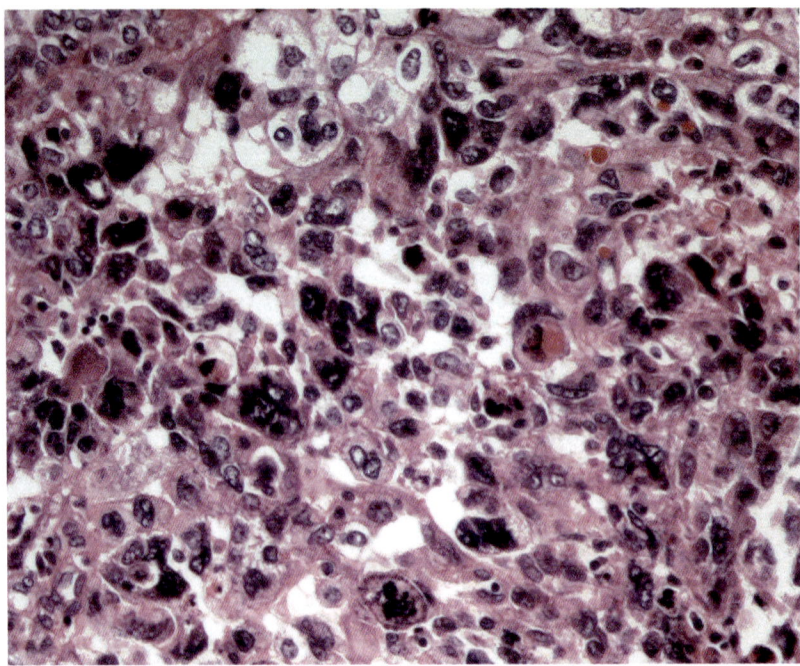

FIGURE 4-38: Giant-cell carcinoma.

in the syncytiotrophoblast; hPL, HLA-G, MUC-4, and Mel-CAM in the intermediate trophoblast; and β-*catenin* in the cytotrophoblasts.[90,91]

Giant-Cell Carcinoma versus Pleomorphic Rhabdomyosarcoma

The presence of cross-striations and the expression of markers such as desmin, myogenin, and myo-D1 will allow confirmation of the striated muscle differentiation in pleomorphic rhabdomyosarcoma, which distinguishes it from giant-cell tumors.

Giant-Cell Carcinoma versus Malignant Mixed Müllerian Tumor

Malignant mixed müllerian tumor shows definitive sarcoma differentiation, which is absent in giant-cell carcinoma.

Giant-Cell Carcinoma versus Carcinoma with Trophoblastic Differentiation

Carcinoma with trophoblastic differentiation expresses hCG immunohistochemically. This expression is absent in giant-cell carcinoma.

Hepatoid Carcinoma

This exceedingly rare tumor has been reported in postmenopausal patients who presented with vaginal bleeding and an elevated serum α-fetoprotein (AFP) level. All cases have been associated with another histotype of endometrial carcinoma, usually endometrioid type. Histologically, this tumor is composed of eosinophilic polygonal cells arranged in trabeculae, thus mimicking the appearance of hepatocellular carcinoma (Fig. 4-39). The differential diagnosis includes endometrioid carcinoma with oxyphilic metaplasia and the oxyphilic variant of clear cell carcinoma. The diagnosis of hepatoid carcinoma is confirmed with positive immunostaining for AFP (see *inset* of Fig. 4-39).[92–96]

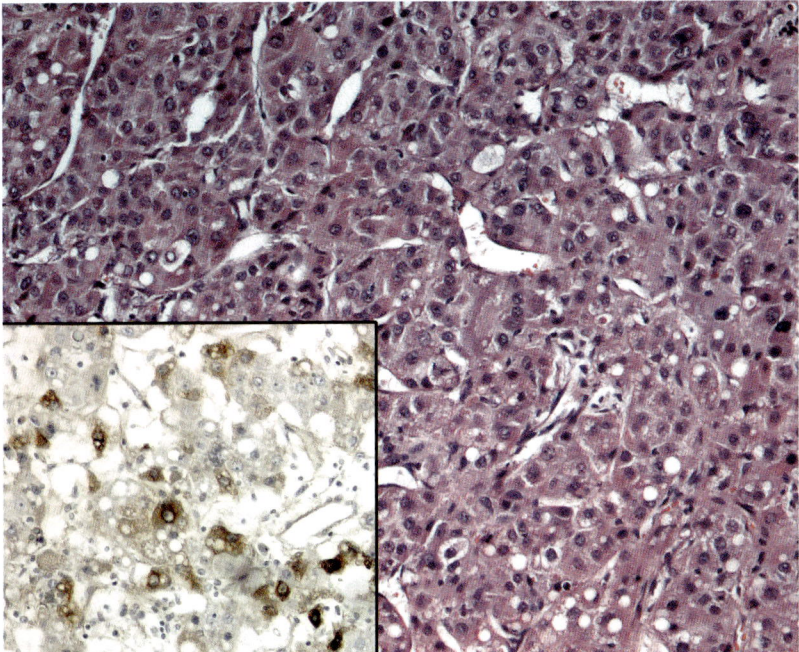

FIGURE 4-39: Hepatoid carcinoma showing eosinophilic polygonal cells, focal staining for α-fetoprotein (AFP) (*inset*).

Carcinoma with Trophoblastic Differentiation

This type of tumor is rare and usually found in postmenopausal patients with an elevated hCG level. Histologically, these tumors display areas of trophoblastic differentiation, either as isolated syncytiotrophoblastic cells or as choriocarcinoma, intermixed with adenocarcinoma, usually of the endometrioid type (Fig. 4-40A). Immunohistochemically, the trophoblastic com-

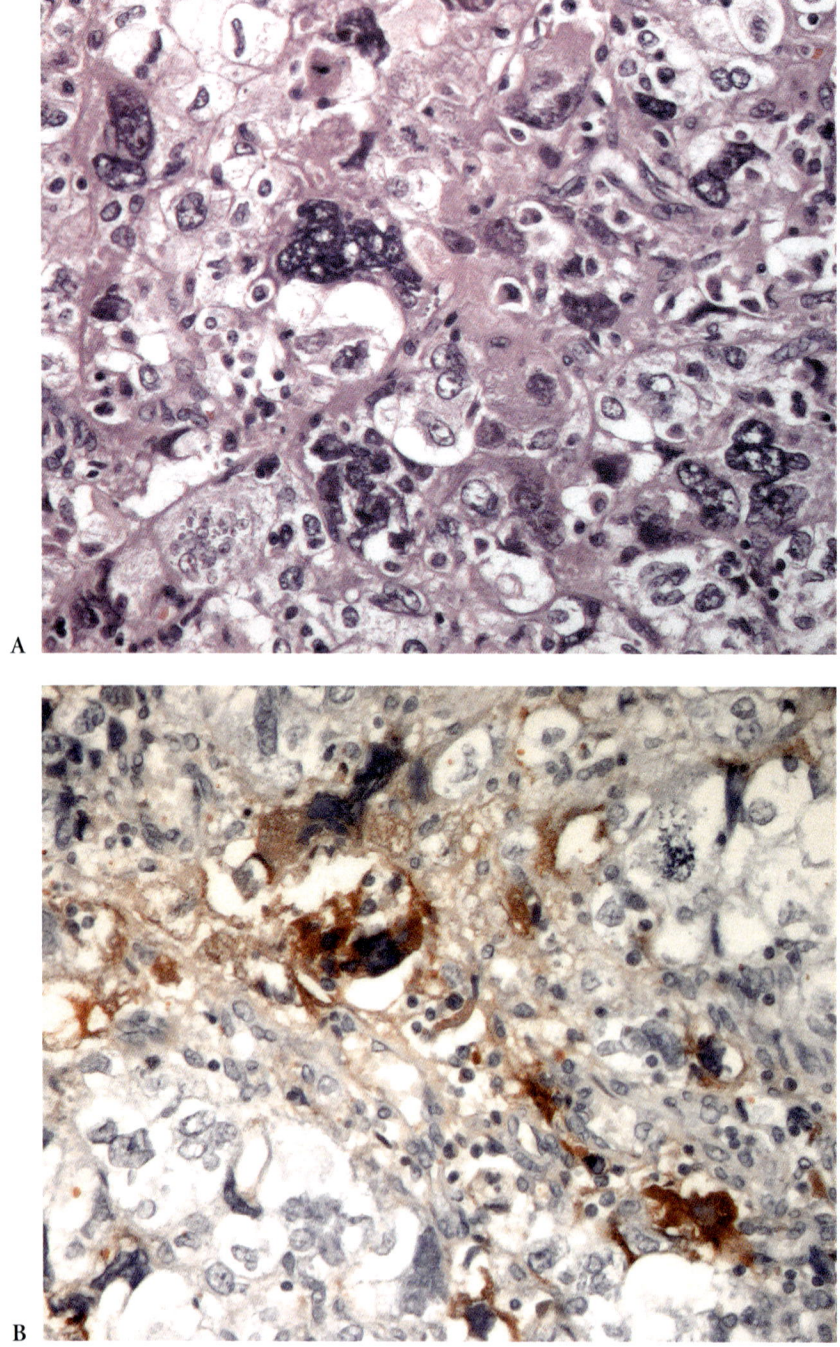

FIGURE 4-40: Carcinoma with trophoblastic differentiation; hematoxylin and eosin–stained slide (**A**) and positive staining for hCG (**B**).

ponent expresses hCG (Fig. 4-40B). The differential diagnosis includes giant-cell carcinoma and choriocarcinoma. An immunoperoxidase study for hCG facilitates distinction from the former, whereas the admixture of adenocarcinoma and the patient's age exclude choriocarcinoma.[97–100]

Metastatic Carcinoma

Metastatic carcinoma to the uterine body is uncommon, and it usually involves the myometrium followed by the endometrium. The isolated involvement of the endometrium is exceedingly rare. The most common primary sites are the breast and gastrointestinal tract, with rare cases reported of metastases from the lung, kidney, urinary bladder, pancreas, gallbladder, and thyroid. In addition, cutaneous melanomas, sarcomas, and carcinoid tumors have metastasized to the endometrium.[101,102]

Attention to the following histologic features should alert the pathologist to the possibility of metastatic carcinoma to the endometrium: (1) extensive dirty necrosis; (2) unusually prominent vascular/lymphatic invasion; (3) the presence of a predominant signet ring cell pattern; (4) high-grade nuclear features in a tumor with a predominant glandular pattern; (5) larger amount of tumor in the myometrium than in the endometrium; and (6) tumor infiltrating the endometrial stroma, with entrapment of benign endometrial glands (Fig. 4-41). Immunoperoxidase studies may assist in making the correct diagnosis. Metastatic breast carcinomas are usually positive for gross cystic disease fluid protein (GCDFP-15) and mammaglobin, whereas colorectal adenocarcinomas are usually positive for keratin 20 and negative for keratin 7. Cdx2, an immunomarker usually associated with intestinal differentiation, can be expressed in cases of endometrioid adenocarcinoma, especially in those cases displaying squamous differentiation. Although the expression of Cdx2 in endometrial adenocarcinoma without squamous differentiation is usually focal, rare cases may express this marker diffusely.[103,104] On the other hand, TTF-1, an immunomarker usually expressed

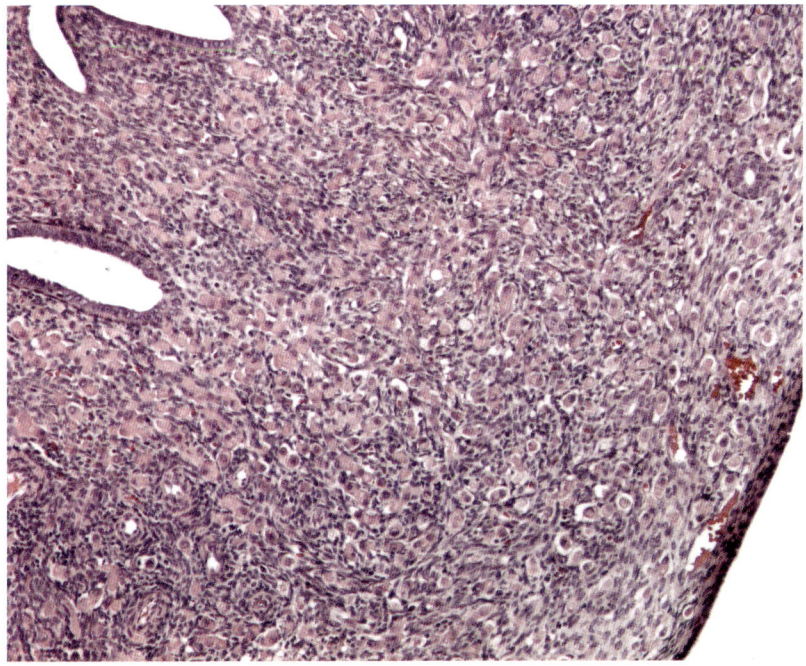

FIGURE 4-41: Metastatic gastric adenocarcinoma to the endometrium.

in lung adenocarcinomas, can be focally or diffusely expressed in adenocarcinomas arising in the endometrium.[105] Because these immunoperoxidase studies are not infallible, good clinicopathologic correlation is important to make the correct diagnosis in challenging cases.

PROGNOSTIC FACTORS AND BEHAVIOR OF ENDOMETRIAL CARCINOMA

Histotypes

Endometrioid Carcinoma[106]

The prognostic value of grading endometrioid adenocarcinoma is well established. The FIGO/International Society of Gynecological Pathologists grading system,[107] with subsequent modifications by Zaino et al.,[108] is as follows:

- Grade 1: Tumors that contain up to 5% of a solid, nonmorular/nonsquamous component (Fig. 4-42).
- Grade 2: Tumors that contain 6% to 50% of a solid, nonmorular/nonsquamous component (Fig. 4-43).
- Grade 3: Tumors that contain >50% of a solid, nonmorular/nonsquamous component (Fig. 4-44).

This system states that a tumor with an architectural pattern of grade 1 but with marked cytologic atypia (grade 3 cytologic atypia) should be designated as a FIGO grade 2 tumor; however, in our experience, this combination of features is exceedingly rare, and when encountered, the diagnosis of glandular variant of serous carcinoma should be entertained.

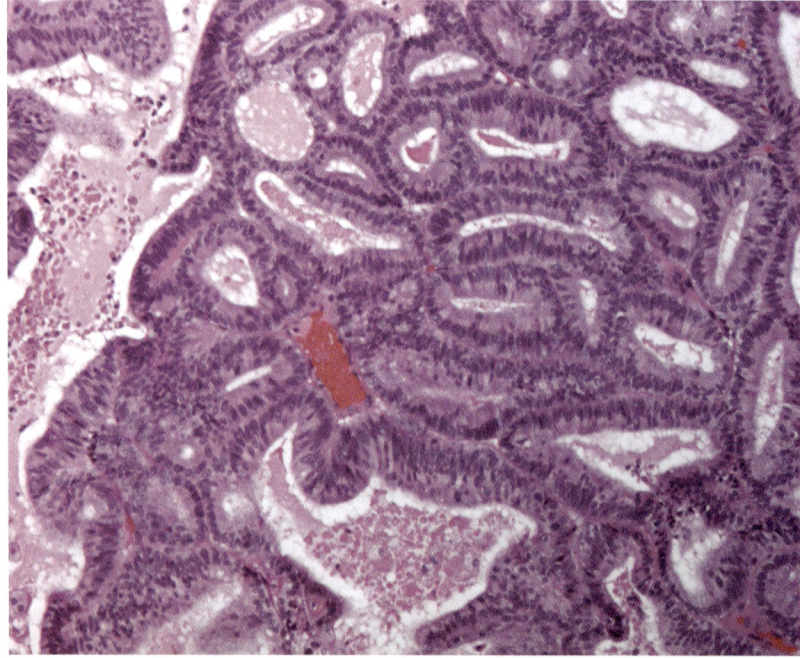

FIGURE 4-42: Endometrioid adenocarcinoma, FIGO grade 1.

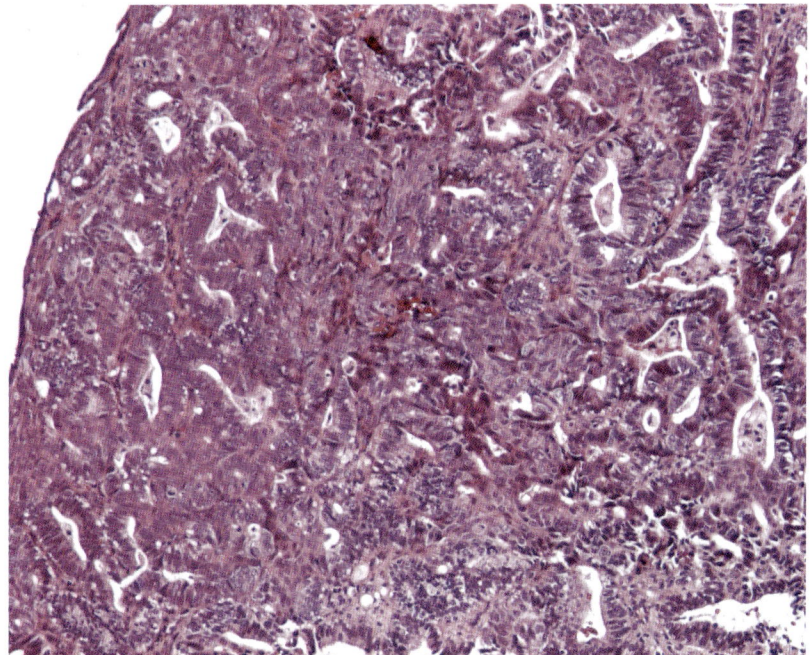

FIGURE 4-43: Endometrioid adenocarcinoma, FIGO grade 2.

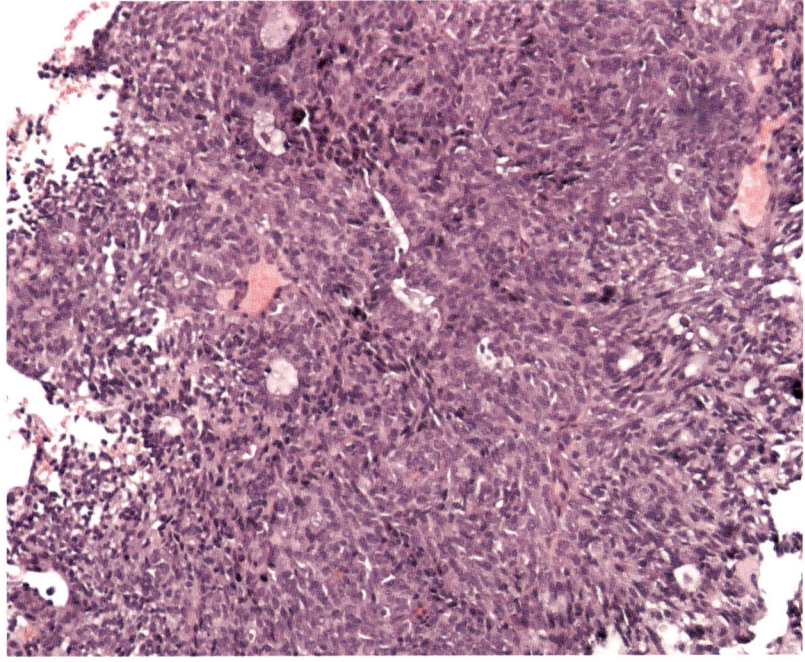

FIGURE 4-44: Endometrioid adenocarcinoma, FIGO grade 3.

The 5-year relative survival for patients with endometrioid adenocarcinoma is as follows: 94% for patients with FIGO grade 1 tumors, 84% for patients with FIGO grade 2 tumors, and 72% for patients with FIGO grade 3 tumors.[106]

Serous Carcinoma

Serous carcinoma is one of the most aggressive types of endometrial carcinoma. The most important prognostic factor is the stage. Patients with tumors confined to the endometrium have approximately an 80% survival rate.[108–112]

Clear Cell Carcinoma

Clear cell carcinoma tends to present as stage I disease; however, once myometrial invasion is present, there is a higher incidence of extrauterine disease as compared to FIGO grade 3 endometrioid adenocarcinoma.[56,113,114] The prognosis depends on the stage of disease, with low-stage cases (FIGO stages I and II) showing a better prognosis than advanced-stage cases. The prognosis of low-stage clear cell carcinoma is better than that of serous carcinoma of similar stage.[115,116]

Mucinous Adenocarcinomas

Mucinous adenocarcinomas are usually FIGO grade 1 or 2, and their clinical behavior does not differ from that of typical endometrioid adenocarcinoma.[6]

Undifferentiated Carcinoma

Undifferentiated carcinoma appears to have a more aggressive behavior than endometrioid adenocarcinoma, FIGO grade 3.[83]

Squamous Carcinoma

Cases of squamous carcinoma confined to the uterus appear to have a good prognosis, whereas stage III cases have a survival rate of only 20%.[68]

Verrucous Carcinoma

Verrucous carcinoma appears to have a favorable prognosis, with no metastases reported thus far.[117]

Transitional Cell Carcinoma

The experience with transitional cell carcinoma of the endometrium is limited; however, in rare cases, patients have had recurrences and died of disease.[71]

Neuroendocrine Carcinoma

Neuroendocrine carcinomas, either small-cell type or large-cell type, are aggressive neoplasms,[84] although more recently, it has been suggested that such tumors arising in polyps or with a polypoid appearance might have a favorable prognosis.[118]

Hepatoid Carcinoma

Hepatoid carcinoma is associated with a poor prognosis; in only two of the eight cases reported have patients survived the disease after treatment with surgery and chemotherapy.[93]

Giant-Cell Carcinoma

Giant-cell carcinoma is an aggressive tumor; patients with tumors that are more than superficially invasive tend to die of disease within 3 years of diagnosis.[89]

Carcinoma with Trophoblastic Differentiation

It has been reported that carcinomas with trophoblastic differentiation showing only syncytiotrophoblastic cells have a better prognosis than those cases with a choriocarcinoma component.[67]

Staging

The new FIGO staging system for endometrial carcinoma is shown in Table 4-3.

Assessment of Myometrial Invasion

Myometrial invasion by endometrial carcinoma correlates with lymph node metastasis and predicts risk for recurrence.[119]

Table 4-3 Updated FIGO Staging for Carcinoma of the Endometrium (2009)

Stage I* Tumor confined to the corpus uteri
IA* No or less than half myometrial invasion
IB* Invasion equal to or more than half of the myometrium
Stage II* Tumor invades cervical stroma but does not extend beyond the uterus†
Stage III* Local and/or regional spread of the tumor
IIIA* Tumor invades the serosa of the corpus uteri and/or adnexae‡
IIIB* Vaginal and parametrial involvement‡
IIIC* Metastases to pelvis and/or para-aortic lymph nodes‡
IIIC1* Positive pelvic lymph nodes
IIIC2* Positive para-aortic lymph nodes with or without positive pelvic lymph nodes
Stage IV* Tumor invades bladder and/or bowel mucosa, and/or distant metastases
IVA* Tumor invasion of bladder and/or bowel mucosa
IVB* Distant metastases, including intra-abdominal metastases and/or inguinal lymph nodes

NOTE. The 5-year relative survival was 94% for the patients with grade 1 tumors, 84% for those with grade 2 tumors, and 72% for those with grade 3 tumors.[120]
* Either grade 1, 2, or 3.
† Endocervical glandular involvement only should be considered as stage I disease and no longer as stage II.
‡ Positive cytology has to be reported separately without changing the stage.
Data from Pecorelli S. Revised FIGO staging for carcinoma of the vulva, cervix, and endometrium. *Int J Gynecol Obstet*. 2009; 105:103–104.

Myometrial invasion can have the following different patterns:

1. Typical pattern: characterized by irregularly shaped glands, single cells, or clusters of cells infiltrating the myometrium, accompanied by changes in the myometrium (i.e., inflammatory response and/or desmoplastic or myxoid changes) (Fig. 4-45).
2. Expansile pattern: characterized by a pushing border with no stromal response in the myometrium.
3. Adenoma malignum-like pattern: characterized by glands infiltrating the myometrium without eliciting an inflammatory response or desmoplastic reaction (Fig. 4-46).
4. Microcystic, elongated, and fragmented (MELF) pattern: characterized by elongated glands or small/cystic glands lined by cuboidal or flattened epithelium. Individual cells and focal tufting are also commonly seen. The stroma can be compact or loose and contains a mixed neutrophilic and lymphocytic infiltrate that can obscure the presence of neoplastic cells (Figs. 4-47 and 4-48).[121] This pattern has been associated with an adverse effect on prognosis, which appears to be due to a higher frequency of vascular invasion.[121] Tumors with MELF pattern are low-grade endometrioid and have a tendency to have areas with mucinous differentiation.[121,122]

The following findings have to be distinguished from myometrial invasion:

1. Tangentially cut endometrial adenocarcinoma confined to an endometrium that has a markedly irregular endomyometrial junction. In this type of case, awareness of the irregularity of the endomyometrial junction and the well-defined shape of the focus of endometrial tissue within the myometrium will facilitate the correct diagnosis.

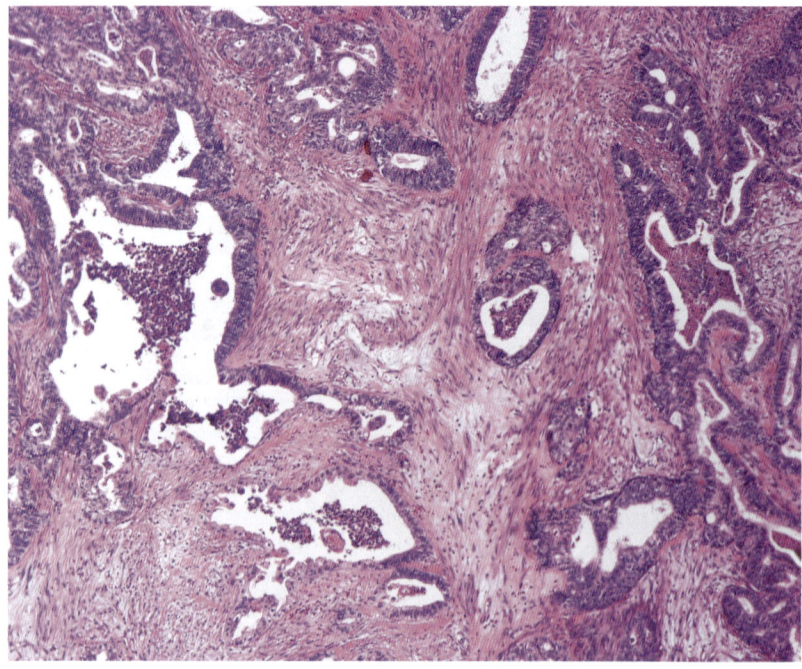

FIGURE 4-45: Endometrial adenocarcinoma; irregularly shaped glands infiltrate the myometrium eliciting a desmoplastic reaction.

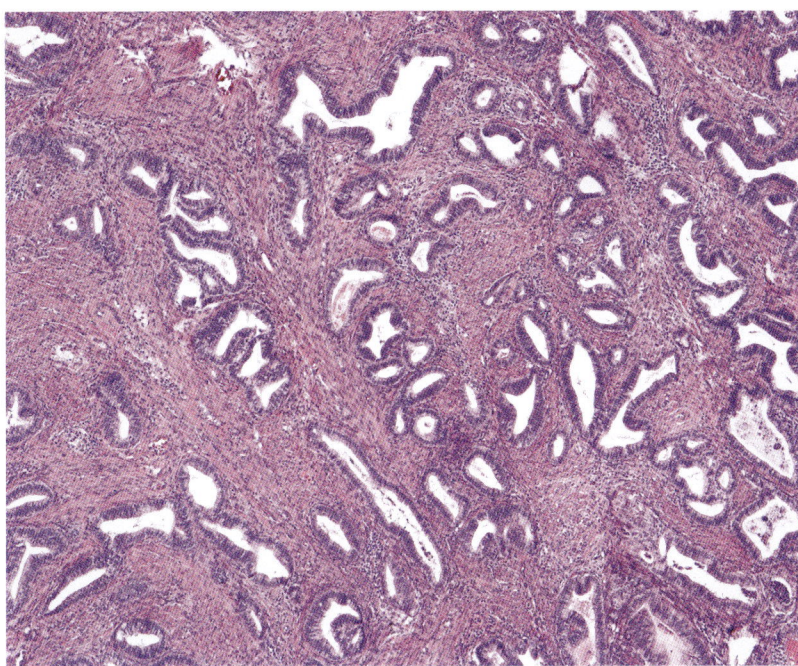

FIGURE 4-46: Endometrial adenocarcinoma; irregularly shaped glands infiltrate the myometrium.

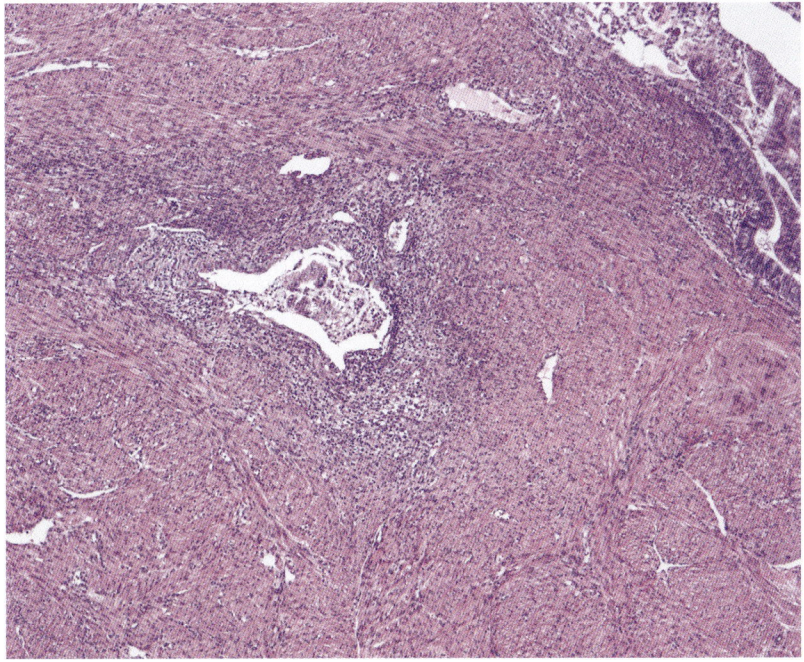

FIGURE 4-47: Endometrial adenocarcinoma; microcystic, elongated, and fragmented glands accompanied by inflammatory cells infiltrating the myometrium.

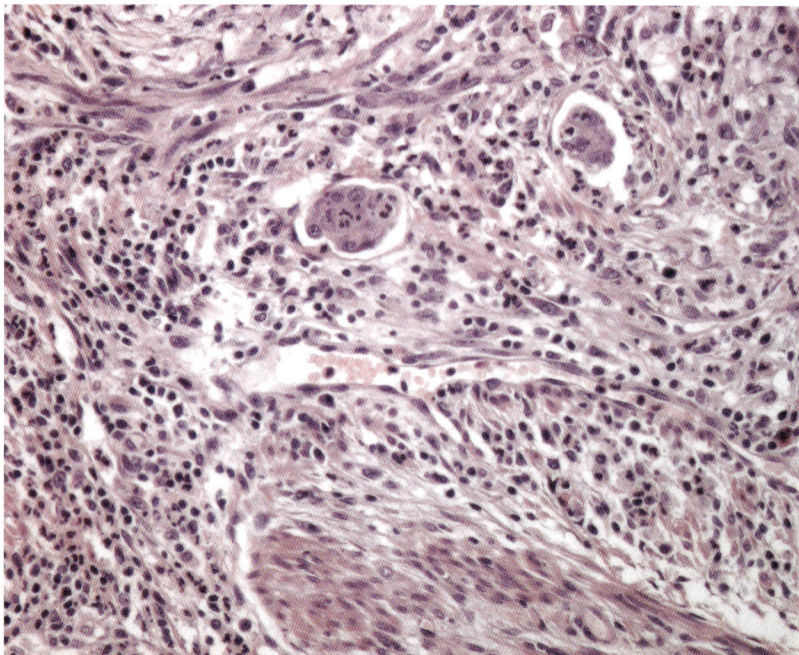

FIGURE 4-48: Endometrial adenocarcinoma; small papillary clusters infiltrate the myometrium.

2. Endometrial adenocarcinoma extending to the intramural portion of the fallopian tube in the uterine wall. This type of case displays a well-defined focus of tumor in the mid or outer portion of the myometrium in a section obtained from the lateral portion of the fundus.
3. Exophytic tumors, especially those cases with smooth muscle metaplasia of the stroma.[123]
4. Extension of the tumor into areas of adenomyosis. In these cases, the areas of concern are well delineated and contain residual endometrial stroma or non-neoplastic glands. In addition, adenomyosis not involved by adenocarcinoma is identified in the vicinity. The use of CD10 immunostaining is not helpful because it is also expressed in the smooth muscle adjacent to foci of myoinvasive adenocarcinoma. Attention has to be paid to the fact that cases involving areas of adenomyosis can be at a higher risk of having bona fide myometrial invasion and are more prone to have invasion into the outer half of the myometrium. Of interest, the latter finding appears to have no adverse impact on prognosis.[124]

Assessment of Vascular/Lymphatic Invasion

Vascular/lymphatic invasion has been shown to be an independent prognostic factor in multiple studies (Fig. 4-49A–B). Even in early-stage, well-differentiated endometrioid adenocarcinoma cases, the presence of vascular/lymphatic invasion appears to be associated with a higher risk of recurrence.[125]

Potential pitfalls in identifying vascular/lymphatic invasion are as follows:

1. The presence of contaminants/floaters within vascular spaces or myometrial clefts.
2. Pseudovascular invasion associated with the intraoperative use of the uterine manipulator in cases of laparoscopically obtained hysterectomies. In these cases,

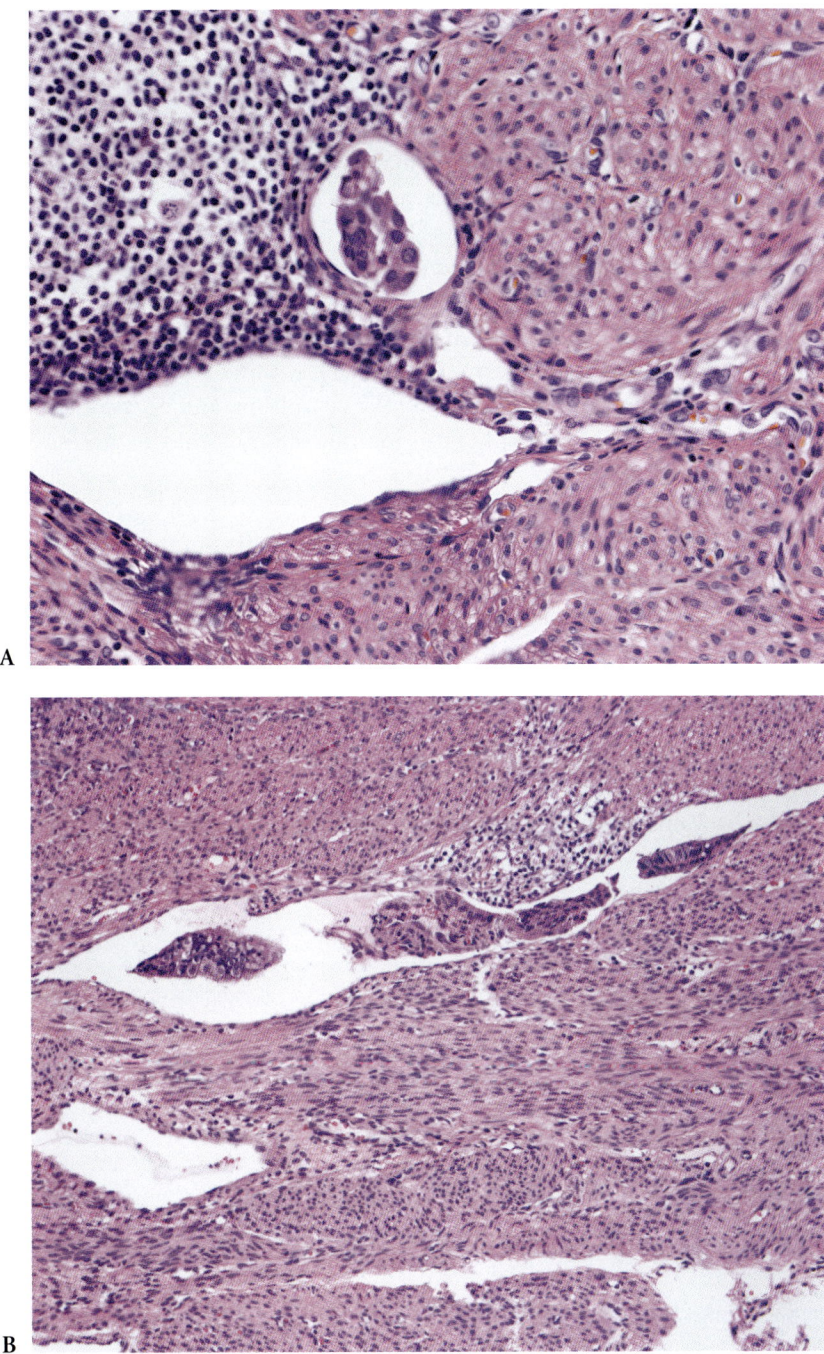

FIGURE 4-49: Vascular/lymphatic invasion in endometrial adenocarcinoma; tumor clusters in vascular spaces are accompanied by a perivascular inflammatory infiltrate (**A and B**).

there are numerous fragments of tumor within small- or large-caliber vessels in the context of a low-grade endometrioid adenocarcinoma. Sometimes the tumor fragments are within vessels in the outer myometrium and myometrial clefts exclusively. These foci of tumor fragments with vascular spaces or myometrial clefts are not associated with an inflammatory infiltrate. There are two theories to explain this phenomenon: (1) an increase of the intrauterine pressure secondary to the use of the uterine manipulator, and (2) a grossing artifact.[126,127]

3. Histiocytic-like vascular/lymphatic invasion. This pattern is characterized by the deceptively bland, histiocytic-like appearance of the neoplastic cells with vascular/lymphatic spaces and the presence of perivascular lymphocytic infiltrate. On hematoxylin and eosin–stained slides, these neoplastic cells can be recognized by their large size, eosinophilic cytoplasm, and occasional intracytoplasmic vacuoles; however, keratin immunostaining may be necessary as a confirmatory study.[128]

Assessment of Cervical Involvement

Cervical involvement by endometrial adenocarcinoma is usually secondary to direct extension to the epithelium or stroma (Fig. 4-50); however, in some cases, it is secondary to implantation or vascular/lymphatic spread. According to the most current FIGO classification, tumors with extension into the cervical epithelium only are considered stage I (Table 4-3).[129] This revision of the staging system has been prompted by the results of studies that demonstrate that invasion into the cervical stroma is associated with a worsened prognosis, whereas involvement of the cervical epithelium is not.[18] An unusual pattern of cervical involvement described as "burrowing" consists of deep involvement of the cervical stroma to the extent that the amount of tumor and depth of the tumor in the cervix can be greater

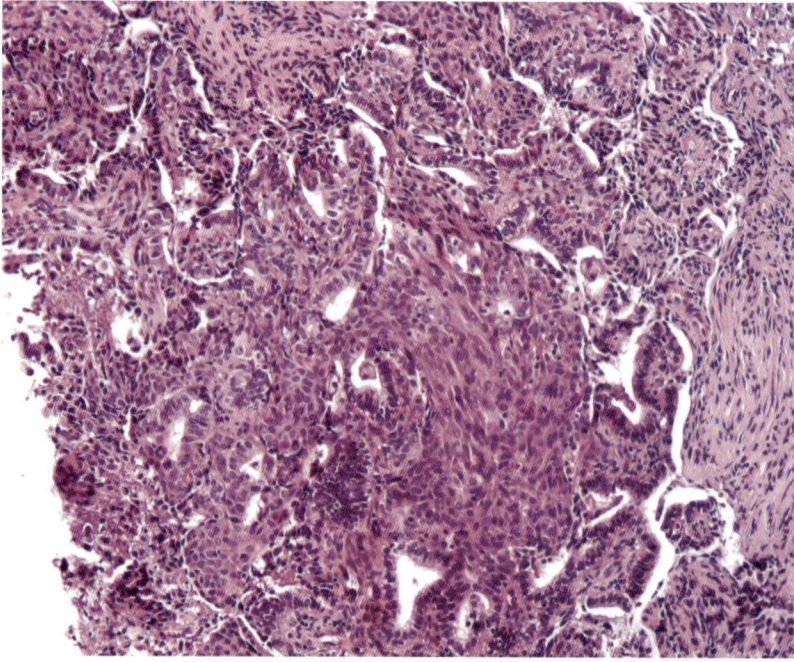

FIGURE 4-50: Endometrial adenocarcinoma in cervical stroma.

than that seen in the myometrium. This pattern can raise the possibility of an independent cervical primary tumor. Other problems associated with this pattern of cervical involvement include the misinterpretation of superficially invasive glands as tuboendometrioid metaplasia, mesonephric hyperplasia, or adenocarcinoma in situ.[130] In difficult cases, the use of immunohistochemical studies, including CEA, vimentin, ER, p16, and in situ hybridization for HPV, will allow for the correct diagnosis.

Peritoneal Cytology

Peritoneal cytology is not part of the most recent FIGO staging system; however, it is still assessed and reported separately (Table 4-3). Currently, there is no definitive consensus on the prognostic significance of positive peritoneal cytology alone; however, it has been reported that even in a low-risk cohort of the former FIGO stage A1 cases, up to 4.1% of the cases with positive peritoneal cytology recurred.[131]

Endometrial Carcinomas Arising in Specific Circumstances

Young Age

Two percent to 14% of endometrial carcinomas occur in patients 40 years of age or younger. Most cases are endometrioid type, well differentiated, have a favorable clinical outcome, and arise in a background of hyperestrogenism secondary to obesity, nulliparity, polycystic ovarian disease, or infertility. More recently, a subset of patients within this age group has been found to have endometrial carcinomas with loss of DNA mismatch repair (MMR) proteins. In this subset, the patients had a low body mass index, and the tumors showed features commonly associated with microsatellite instability, such as undifferentiated or dedifferentiated histology, tumor-infiltrating lymphocytes, and lower uterine segment origin. In addition, these tumors showed lower ER/PR expression compared with tumors that retained staining for MMR protein.[132]

Pregnancy

The association of pregnancy and endometrial carcinoma is rare. Cases have been detected during the first trimester, early in the second trimester, or postpartum. Patients have ranged in age from 21 to 43 years, with a mean age of 33.5 years. The tumors are usually of the endometrioid type, FIGO grade 1, with no or only superficial myometrial invasion and an indolent behavior. However, in the rare cases of advanced-stage disease at presentation, the patients have ultimately died of the disease.[133,134]

Endometrial Polyps

The incidence of carcinoma in endometrial polyps has been reported to range from 0.5% to 4.8%. The risk of endometrial hyperplasia and carcinoma increases with age, with the highest rate seen in women older than 65 years, in whom up to 32% of the endometrial polyps are associated with malignancy.[135] Although a focus carcinoma can be confined to the endometrial polyp, it is important to assess the status of the background endometrium to determine patient management. A group of investigators found that complex endometrial hyperplasia with atypia and endometrioid adenocarcinoma in an endometrial polyp tend to be associated with hyperplasia or carcinoma of the nonpolypoid endometrium in subsequent hysterectomy specimens.[135] In a review of 34 cases of malignant tumors arising in endometrial polyps, it was found that most cases were endometrioid carcinomas followed by serous carcinomas, mixed serous/clear cell/endometrioid carcinoma, and mixed serous/carcinosarcoma.[136]

Atypical Polypoid Adenomyomas

Endometrioid adenocarcinoma can arise in APA. This combination has been designated as APA of low malignant potential (APA-LMP) by some investigators[137]; however, in our practice, we prefer to designate these cases as endometrial endometrioid adenocarcinoma arising in an APA, and the FIGO grade of the adenocarcinoma is provided in the diagnostic line. These cases, when conservatively treated, have a persistence/recurrence rate of 60% (higher than the 33% observed in typical APA).

Adenomyosis

Carcinomas arising in adenomyosis are rare. Most of the cases have been endometrioid adenocarcinomas, with rare reports of clear cell carcinoma.[138–140] Some of these cases, arising in the outer myometrium, have been associated with vascular/lymphatic invasion and/or metastases.[138,139]

Lower Uterine Segment (Uterine Isthmus)

Carcinomas arising in the lower uterine segment are rare, representing 3% to 8% of the cases of endometrial cancer.[141] Tumors arising at this site tend to be of a higher stage and show deeper myometrial invasion than cases arising in the uterine corpus. In addition, they tend to occur in younger patients with a median age of 54.2 years in contrast to the median age of 62.9 years of patients with carcinomas arising in the uterine body.[141] In a recent review, up to 29% of the patients with lower uterine segment carcinoma were confirmed to have Lynch syndrome or were strongly suspected to have Lynch syndrome based on tissue-based molecular assays.[141] Immunohistochemically, these carcinomas tend to express vimentin and ERs. They can express p16 and CEA and are negative for HPV by in situ hybridization.[141]

Synchronous Ovarian and Endometrial Primaries

Synchronous primary carcinomas of the endometrium and ovary occur in approximately 10% of all women with ovarian cancer and in 5% of all women with endometrial cancer.[142] In most cases, the histologic type at both sites is concordant, and the tumor grade at both sites tends to be low (grade 1 or 2). Of interest, a Gynecologic Oncology Group prospective study demonstrated that although almost one-third of the patients had abdominal or pelvic metastasis at the initial surgery, only 15% of the patients suffered a recurrence within 5 years of diagnosis. When the tumor is confined to the uterus and the ovary, the prognosis of these patients is excellent.[142] A more recent study found that patients with synchronous tumors in the endometrium and ovary have a median age of 50 years and tend to be premenopausal, obese, and nulliparous. The prognosis for patients with independent endometrioid carcinomas of the endometrium and ovary is favorable, with a median survival approaching 10 years.[143] Table 4-4 summarizes the features that favor independent primaries in the endometrium and ovary.

Table 4-4	Features That Favor Independent Endometrial and Ovarian Primary Tumors
Young age	
Endometriosis in the ovary	
Endometrial hyperplasia	
Low-grade histology	
Unilateral ovarian tumor	
Absence of ovarian surface involvement	
Absence of vascular/lymphatic invasion in the uterus and ovary	
Absence or superficial myometrial invasion	

Hereditary Nonpolyposis Colorectal Cancer/Lynch Syndrome Related

Hereditary nonpolyposis colorectal cancer (HNPCC)/Lynch syndrome is an autosomal dominant syndrome that causes a predisposition to multiple malignancies, including colorectal, endometrial, and ovarian cancers. In women with this syndrome, the incidence of endometrial cancer equals or exceeds that of colorectal cancer, and in more than 50% of cases, these patients develop a gynecologic cancer as their "sentinel" or first malignancy. Identification of these patients is important because they are at risk of multiple and synchronous tumors. In addition, these patients and their relatives might benefit from appropriate surveillance measures for other HNPCC-associated tumors and genetic counseling.

The following features have been associated with DNA MMR deficiency and endometrial cancer: (1) patient age <50 years, (2) tumor origin in the lower uterine segment, (3) tumor-infiltrating lymphocytes, (4) undifferentiated or dedifferentiated endometrial carcinoma (i.e., a mixed carcinoma composed of endometrioid adenocarcinoma, FIGO grade 1 or 2, and undifferentiated carcinoma), and (5) clear cell carcinoma as a synchronous tumor in the ovary.[144,145]

References

1. Bokham JV. Two pathogenetic types of endometrial carcinoma. *Gynecol Oncol*. 1983;15:10–17.
2. Lax SF. Molecular genetic pathways in various types of endometrial carcinoma: from a phenotypical to a molecular-based classification. *Virchows Arch*. 2004;444:213–223.
3. Amant F, Moerman P, Neven P, et al. Endometrial cancer. *Lancet*. 2005;366:491–505.
4. Velasco A, Pallares J, Santacana M, et al. Loss of heterozygosity in endometrial carcinoma. *Int J Gynecol Pathol*. 2008;27:305–317.
5. Silverberg SG, Kurman RJ, Nogales T, et al. Tumours of the uterine corpus. Epithelial tumours and related lesions. In: Tavassoli FA, Devilee P, eds. *World Health Organization Classification of Tumors, Pathology and Genetics Tumours of the Breast and Female Genital Organs*. Lyon, France: IARC Press; 2003:221–232.
6. Ross JC, Eifel PJ, Cox RS, et al. Primary mucinous adenocarcinoma of the endometrium. A clinicopathologic and histochemical study. *Am J Surg Pathol*. 1983;7:715–729.
7. McCluggage WG, Roberts N, Bharucha H. Enteric differentiation in endometrial adenocarcinomas: a mucin histochemical study. *Int J Gynecol Pathol*. 1995;14:250–254.

8. Haibach H, Oxenhandler RW, Luger AM. Ciliated adenocarcinoma of the endometrium. *Acta Obstet Gynecol Scand*. 1985;64:457–462.
9. Silver SA, Sherman ME. Morphologic and immunophenotypic characterization of foam cells in endometrial lesions. *Int J Gynecol Pathol*. 1998;17:140–145.
10. Mooney EE, Robboy SJ, Hammond CB, et al. Signet-ring carcinoma of the endometrium: a primary tumor masquerading as a metastasis. *Int J Gynecol Pathol*. 1997;16:169–172.
11. Berger G, Fetissof F, Vitre D, et al. Endometrial carcinoma of the intestinal type. A first case report. *Appl Pathol*. 1984;2:63–69.
12. Nogales FF, Gomez-Morales M, Raymundo C, et al. Benign heterologous tissue components associated with endometrial carcinoma. *Int J Gynecol Pathol*. 1982;1:286–291.
13. Parkash V, Carcangiu ML. Endometrioid endometrial adenocarcinoma with psammoma bodies. *Am J Surg Pathol*. 1997;21:399–406.
14. Ambros RA, Ballouk F, Malfetano JH, et al. Significance of papillary (villoglandular) differentiation in endometrioid carcinoma of the uterus. *Am J Surg Pathol*. 1994;18:569–575.
15. Christopherson WM, Alberhasky RC, Connelly PJ. Carcinoma of the endometrium: I. A clinicopathologic study of clear-cell carcinoma and secretory carcinoma. *Cancer*. 1982;49:1511–1523.
16. Tobon H, Watkins GJ. Secretory adenocarcinoma of the endometrium. *Int J Gynecol Pathol*. 1985;4:328–335.
17. Hendrickson MR, Kempson RL. Ciliated carcinoma—a variant of endometrial adenocarcinoma: a report of 10 cases. *Int J Gynecol Pathol*. 1983;2:1–12.
18. Clement PB, Young RH. Endometrioid carcinoma of the uterine corpus: a review of its pathology with emphasis on recent advances and problematic aspects. *Adv Anat Pathol*. 2002;9:145–184.
19. Young RH, Scully RE. Uterine carcinomas simulating microglandular hyperplasia. A report of six cases. *Am J Surg Pathol*. 1992;16:1092–1097.
20. Qiu W, Mittal K. Comparison of morphologic and immunohistochemical features of cervical microglandular hyperplasia with low-grade mucinous adenocarcinoma of the endometrium. *Int J Gynecol Pathol*. 2003;22:261–265.
21. Da Forno PD, McGregor AH, Brown LJR. Microglandular hyperplasia: a pitfall in the diagnosis of microglandular type endometrioid adenocarcinoma. *Histopathology*. 2005;46:346–358.
22. Zaloudek C, Hayashi GM, Ryan IP, et al. Microglandular adenocarcinoma of the endometrium: a form of mucinous adenocarcinoma that may be confused with microglandular hyperplasia of the cervix. *Int J Gynecol Pathol*. 1997;16:52–59.
23. Zamecnik M, Skalova A, Oparny V. Microglandular adenocarcinoma of the uterus mimicking microglandular cervical hyperplasia. *Ann Diagn Pathol*. 2003;7:180–186.
24. Chekmareva M, Ellenson LH, Pirog EC. Immunohistochemical differences between mucinous and microglandular adenocarcinomas of the endometrium and benign endocervical epithelium. *Int J Gynecol Pathol*. 2008;27:547–554.
25. Murray SK, Young RH, Scully RE. Uterine endometrioid carcinoma with small nonvillous papillae: an analysis of 26 cases of a favorable prognosis tumor to be distinguished from serous carcinoma. *Int J Surg Pathol*. 2000;8:279–289.
26. Liang SX, Patel K, Pearl M, et al. Sertoliform endometrioid carcinoma of the endometrium with dual immunophenotypes for epithelial membrane antigen and inhibin alpha: case report and literature review. *Int J Gynecol Pathol*. 2007;26:291–297.
27. Eichhorn JH, Young RH, Clement PB. Sertoliform endometrial adenocarcinoma: a study of four cases. *Int J Gynecol Pathol*. 1996;15:9–26.
28. Usadi RS, Bentley RC. Endometrioid carcinoma of the endometrium with sertoliform differentiation. *Int J Gynecol Pathol*. 1995;14:360–364.
29. Murray SK, Clement PB, Young RH. Endometrioid carcinomas of the uterine corpus with sex cord-like formations, hyalinization, and other unusual morphologic features: a report of 31 cases of a neoplasm that may be confused with carcinosarcoma and other uterine neoplasms. *Am J Surg Pathol*. 2005;29:157–166.

30. Pitman MB, Young RH, Clement PB, et al. Endometrioid carcinoma of the ovary and endometrium, oxyphilic cell type: a report of nine cases. *Int J Gynecol Pathol*. 1994;13:290–301.
31. Fukuoka K, Hirokawa M, Shimizu M, et al. Oxyphilic cell variant of endometrioid adenocarcinoma. *Pathol Int*. 1998;48:754–756.
32. Silver SA, Cheung ANY, Tavassoli FA. Oncocytic metaplasia and carcinoma of the endometrium: an immunohistochemical and ultrastructural study. *Int J Gynecol Pathol*. 1999;18:12–19.
33. Kounelis S, Kapranos N, Kouri E, et al. Immunohistochemical profile of endometrial adenocarcinoma: a study of 61 cases and review of the literature. *Mod Pathol*. 2000;13:379–388.
34. Darvishian F, Hummer AJ, Thaler HT, et al. Serous endometrial cancers that mimic endometrioid adenocarcinomas. A clinicopathologic and immunohistochemical study of a group of problematic cases. *Am J Surg Pathol*. 2004;28:1568–1578.
35. de Brito PA, Silverberg SG, Orenstein JM. Carcinosarcoma (malignant mixed müllerian (mesodermal) tumor) of the female genital tract: immunohistochemical and ultrastructural analysis of 28 cases. *Hum Pathol*. 1993;24:132–142.
36. Sinkre P, Albores-Saavedra J, Miller DS, et al. Endometrial endometrioid carcinomas associated with Ewing sarcoma/peripheral primitive neuroectodermal tumor. *Int J Gynecol Pathol*. 2000;19:127–132.
37. Euscher ED, Deavers MT, Lopez-Terrada D, et al. Uterine tumors with neuroectodermal differentiation. A series of 17 cases and review of the literature. *Am J Surg Pathol*. 2008;32:219–228.
38. Young RH, Treger T, Scully RE. Atypical polypoid adenomyoma of the uterus. *Am J Surg Pathol*. 1986;86:139–145.
39. Zaino RJ. The fruits of our labours: distinguishing endometrial from endocervical adenocarcinoma. *Int J Gynecol Pathol*. 2002;21:1–3.
40. Ansari-Lari MA, Staebler A, Zaino RJ, et al. Distinction of endocervical and endometrial adenocarcinomas: immunohistochemical p16 expression correlated with human papillomavirus (HPV) DNA detection. *Am J Surg Pathol*. 2004;28:160–167.
41. Hording U, Daugaard S, Visfeldt J. Adenocarcinoma of the cervix and adenocarcinoma of the endometrium: distinction with PCR detection of HPV DNA. *APMIS*. 1997;105:313–316.
42. Blancher-Todesca D, Neunteufel W, Williams KE, et al. Influence of postoperative treatment on survival in patients with uterine papillary serous carcinoma. *Gynecol Oncol*. 1998;71:344–347.
43. Liang S, Tornos C, Pearl M, et al. Clinicopathologic features of endometrial serous carcinoma in women younger than 56 years of age. *Mod Pathol*. 2007;20(suppl 2):206A, 940.
44. Liang S, Pearl M, Tornos C, et al. Endometrial serous carcinoma has a strong association with breast cancer, particularly in patients younger than 56 years of age. *Mod Pathol*. 2007; 20(suppl 2):206A, 941.
45. Parkash V, Carcangiu ML. Uterine papillary serous carcinoma after radiation therapy for carcinoma of the cervix. *Cancer*. 1992;69:496–501.
46. Silva EG, Tornos CS, Follen-Mitchell M. Malignant neoplasms of the uterine corpus in patients treated for breast carcinoma: the effects of tamoxifen. *Int J Gynecol Pathol*. 1994;13:248–258.
47. McCluggage WG, Sumathi VP, McManus DT. Uterine serous carcinoma and endometrial intraepithelial carcinoma arising in endometrial polyps: report of 5 cases, including 2 associated with tamoxifen therapy. *Hum Pathol*. 2003;34:939–943.
48. Lavie O, Hornreich G, Arie AB, et al. BRCA1 germline mutations in women with uterine serous papillary carcinoma. *Obstet Gynecol*. 2000;96:28–32.
49. Goshen R, Chu W, Elit L, et al. Is uterine papillary serous adenocarcinoma a manifestation of the hereditary breast–ovarian cancer syndrome? *Gynecol Oncol*. 2000;79:477–481.
50. Hornreich G, Beller U, Lavie O, et al. Is uterine serous papillary carcinoma a BRCA1-related disease? Case report and review of the literature. *Gynecol Oncol*. 1999;75:300–304.
51. Sachmechi I, Kalra J, Molho L, et al. Paraneoplastic hypercalcemia associated with uterine papillary serous carcinoma. *Gynecol Oncol*. 1995;58:378–382.
52. Fukuma K, Miyamura S, Thoya T, et al. Uterine papillary serous carcinoma with high levels of serum carcinoembryonic antigen. Response to chemotherapy. *Cancer*. 1987;59:403–405.

53. Hendrickson M, Ross J, Eifel P, et al. Uterine papillary serous carcinoma: a highly malignant form of endometrial adenocarcinoma. *Am J Surg Pathol.* 1982;6:93–108.
54. Hendrickson MR, Longacre TA, Kemp RL. The uterine corpus. In: *Sternberg's Diagnostic Surgical Pathology.* Vol 2. Philadelphia: Lippincott Williams & Wilkins; 2004:2483.
55. Euscher ED, Malpica A. Papillary endometrioid carcinoma is more aggressive than endometrioid adenocarcinoma FIGO grade 2. *Lab Invest.* 2010;90:242A.
56. Abeler VM, Vergote IB, Kjørstad KE, et al. Clear cell carcinoma of the endometrium: prognosis and metastatic pattern. *Cancer.* 1996;78:1740–1747.
57. Kurman RJ, Scully RE. Clear cell carcinoma of the endometrium: an analysis of 21 cases. *Cancer.* 1976;37:872–882.
58. Kanbour-Shakir A, Tobón H. Primary clear cell carcinoma of the endometrium: a clinicopathologic study of 20 cases. *Int J Gynecol Pathol.* 1991;10:67–78.
59. Lax SF, Pizer ES, Ronnett BM, et al. Clear cell carcinoma of the endometrium is characterized by a distinctive profile of p53, Ki-67, estrogen, and progesterone receptor expression. *Hum Pathol.* 1998;29:551–558.
60. Vang R, Whitaker BP, Farhood AI, et al. Immunohistochemical analysis of clear cell carcinoma of gynecologic tract. *Int J Gynecol Pathol.* 2001;20:252–259.
61. Vang R, Barner R, Wheeler DT, et al. Immunohistochemical staining for Ki-67 and p53 helps to distinguish endometrial Arias-Stella reaction from high-grade carcinoma, including clear cell carcinoma. *Int J Gynecol Pathol.* 2004;23:223–233.
62. Melham MF, Tobon H. Mucinous adenocarcinoma of the endometrium: a clinicopathological review of 18 cases. *Int J Gynecol Pathol.* 1987;6:347–355.
63. Qiu W, Mittal K. Comparison of morphologic and immunohistochemical features of cervical microglandular hyperplasia with low-grade mucinous adenocarcinoma of the endometrium. *Int J Gynecol Pathol.* 2003;22:261–265.
64. Zheng W, Yang GC, Godwin TA, et al. Mucinous adenocarcinoma of the endometrium with intestinal differentiation: a case report. *Hum Pathol.* 1995;26:1385–1388.
65. Nucci MR, Prasad CJ, Crum CP, et al. Mucinous endometrial epithelial proliferations: a morphologic spectrum of changes with diverse clinical significance. *Mod Pathol.* 1999;12:1137–1142.
66. Vang R, Tavassoli FA. Proliferative mucinous lesions of the endometrium: analysis of existing criteria for diagnosing carcinoma in biopsies and curettings. *Int J Surg Pathol.* 2003;11:261–270.
67. Horn LC, Richter CE, Einenkel J, et al. p16, p14, p53, cyclin D1, and steroid hormone receptor expression and human papillomaviruses analysis in primary squamous cell carcinoma of the endometrium. *Ann Diagn Pathol.* 2006;10:193–196.
68. Goodman A, Zukerberg LR, Rice LW, et al. Squamous cell carcinoma of the endometrium: a report of eight cases and a review of the literature. *Gynecol Oncol.* 1996;61:54–60.
69. Seltzer VL, Klein M, Beckman M. The occurrence of squamous metaplasia as a precursor of squamous cell carcinoma of the endometrium. *Obstet Gynecol.* 1977;49(1 suppl):34–37.
70. Yamashina M, Kobara TY. Primary squamous cell carcinoma with its spindle cell variant in the endometrium. A case report and review of literature. *Cancer.* 1986;57:340–345.
71. Marino-Enriquez A, Gonzalez-Rocha T, Burgos E, et al. Transitional cell carcinoma of the endometrium and endometrial carcinoma with transitional cell differentiation: a clinicopathologic study of 5 cases and review of the literature. *Hum Pathol.* 2008;39:1606–1613.
72. Lininger RA, Ashfaq R, Albores-Saavedra J, et al. Transitional cell carcinoma of the endometrium and endometrial carcinoma with transitional cell differentiation. *Cancer.* 1997;79:1933–1943.
73. Ahluwalia M, Light AM, Surampudi K, et al. Transitional cell carcinoma of the endometrium: a case report and review of the literature. *Int J Gynecol Pathol.* 2006;25:378–382.
74. Fukunaga M, Ushigome S. Transitional cell carcinoma of the endometrium. *Histopathology.* 1998;32:284–286.
75. Lininger RA, Wistuba I, Gazdar A, et al. Human papillomavirus type 16 is detected in transitional cell carcinomas and squamotransitional cell carcinomas of the cervix and endometrium. *Cancer.* 1998;83:521–527.

76. Labonte S, Tetu B, Boucher D, et al. Transitional cell carcinoma of the endometrium associated with a benign ovarian Brenner tumor: a case report. *Hum Pathol.* 2001;32:230–232.
77. Giordano G, D'Adda T, Gnetti L, et al. Transitional cell carcinoma of the endometrium associated with benign ovarian Brenner tumor: a case report with immunohistochemistry molecular analysis and a review of the literature. *Int J Gynecol Pathol.* 2007;26:298–304.
78. Huntsman DG, Clement PB, Gilks CB, et al. Small-cell carcinoma of the endometrium: a clinicopathological study of sixteen cases. *Am J Surg Pathol.* 1994;18:364–375.
79. van Hoeven KH, Hudock JA, Woodruff JM, et al. Small cell neuroendocrine carcinoma of the endometrium. *Int J Gynecol Pathol.* 1995;14:21–29.
80. Shaco-Levy R, Manor E, Piura B, et al. An unusual composite endometrial tumor combining papillary serous carcinoma and small cell carcinoma. *Am J Surg Pathol.* 2004;28:1103–1106.
81. Melgoza F, Brewster WR, Wilczynski S, et al. p16 positive small cell neuroendocrine carcinoma of the endometrium. *Int J Gynecol Pathol.* 2006;25:252–256.
82. Katahira A, Akahira J, Nikura H, et al. Small cell carcinoma of the endometrium: report of three cases and literature review. *Int J Gynecol Cancer.* 2004;14:1018–1023.
83. Altrabulsi B, Malpica A, Deavers MT, et al. Undifferentiated carcinoma of the endometrium. *Am J Surg Pathol.* 2005;29:1316–1321.
84. Mulvany NJ, Allen DG. Combined large cell neuroendocrine and endometrioid carcinoma of the endometrium. *Int J Gynecol Pathol.* 2007;27:49–57.
85. Posligua L, Malpica A, Liu J, et al. Combined large cell neuroendocrine carcinoma and papillary serous carcinoma of the endometrium with pagetoid spread. *Arch Pathol Lab Med.* 2008;132:1821–1824.
86. Vargas MP, Merino MJ. Lymphoepithelioma-like carcinoma: an unusual variant of endometrial cancer. *Int J Gynecol Pathol.* 1998;17:272–276.
87. Rahimi S, Lena A, Vittori G. Endometrial lymphoepithelioma-like carcinoma: absence of Epstein-Barr virus genomes. *Int J Gynecol Cancer.* 2007;17:517–535.
88. Young RH, Harris NL, Scully RE. Lymphoma-like lesions of the lower female genital tract: a report of 16 cases. *Int J Gynecol Pathol.* 1985;4:289–299.
89. Jones MA, Young RH, Scully RE. Endometrial adenocarcinoma with a component of giant cell carcinoma. *Int J Gynecol Pathol.* 1991;10:260–270.
90. Mao TL, Kurman RJ, Huang CC, et al. Immunohistochemistry of choriocarcinoma. An aid in differential diagnosis and in elucidating pathogenesis. *Am J Surg Pathol.* 2007;31:1726–1732.
91. Kalhor N, Ramirez PT, Deavers MT, et al. Immunohistochemical studies of trophoblastic tumors. *Am J Surg Pathol.* 2009;33:633–638.
92. Hoshida Y, Nagakawa T, Mano S, et al. Hepatoid adenocarcinoma of the endometrium associated with alpha-fetoprotein production. *Int J Gynecol Pathol.* 1996;15:266–269.
93. Takeuchi K, Kitazawa S, Hamanishi S, et al. A case of alpha-fetoprotein-producing adenocarcinoma of the endometrium with a hepatoid component as a potential source for alpha-fetoprotein in a postmenopausal woman. *Int J Gynecol Cancer.* 2006;16:1439–1478.
94. Yamamoto R, Ishikura H, Azuma M, et al. Alpha-fetoprotein production by a hepatoid adenocarcinoma of the uterus. *J Clin Pathol.* 1996;49:420–422.
95. Toyoda H, Hirai T, Ishii E. Alpha-fetoprotein producing uterine corpus carcinoma: a hepatoid adenocarcinoma of the endometrium. *Pathol Int.* 2000;50:847–852.
96. Adams SF, Yamada SD, Montag A, et al. An alpha-fetoprotein-producing hepatoid adenocarcinoma of the endometrium. *Gynecol Oncol.* 2001;83:418–421.
97. Black K, Sykes P, Östör AG. Trophoblastic differentiation in an endometrial carcinoma. *Aust N Z J Obstet Gynecol.* 1998;38:472–473.
98. Kalir T, Seijo L, Deligdisch, et al. Endometrial adenocarcinoma with choriocarcinomatous differentiation in an elderly virginal woman. *Int J Gynecol Pathol.* 1995;14:266–269.
99. Bradley CS, Benjamin I, Wheeler JE, et al. Endometrial adenocarcinoma with trophoblastic differentiation. *Gynecol Oncol.* 1998;69:74–77.
100. Tunç M, Simsek T, Track B, et al. Endometrium adenocarcinoma with choriocarcinomatous differentiation: a case report. *Eur J Gynaecol Oncol.* 1998;19:489–491.

101. Kumar NB, Hart WR. Metastases to the uterine corpus from extragenital cancers. A clinicopathologic study of 63 cases. *Cancer*. 1982;50:2163–2169.
102. Jordan CD, Andrews SJ, Memoli VA. Well-differentiated papillary neuroendocrine carcinoma metastatic to the endometrium: a case report. *Mod Pathol*. 1996;9:1066–1070.
103. Wani Y, Notohara K, Saegusa M, et al. Aberrant Cdx2 expression in endometrial lesions with squamous differentiation: important role of Cdx2 in squamous morula formation. *Hum Pathol*. 2008;39:1072–1079.
104. Wani Y. Interpretation of diffuse Cdx2 expression in endometrioid adenocarcinoma in the absence of morules. *Histopathology*. 2009;54:495–497.
105. Siami K, McCluggage WG, Ordonez NG, et al. Thyroid transcription factor-1 expression in endometrial and endocervical adenocarcinomas. *Am J Surg Pathol*. 2007;31:1759–1763.
106. Prat J. Prognostic parameters of endometrial carcinoma. *Hum Pathol*. 2004;35:649–662.
107. Announcements. FIGO stages—1988 revision. *Gynecol Oncol*. 1989;35:125–127.
108. Zaino RJ, Kurman RJ, Diana KL, et al. The utility of the revised International Federation of Gynecology and Obstetrics histologic grading of endometrial adenocarcinoma using a defined nuclear grading system. A Gynecology Oncology Group study. *Cancer*. 1995;75:81–86.
109. Slomovitz BM, Burke TW, Eifel PJ, et al. Uterine papillary serous carcinoma (UPSC): a single institution review of 129 cases. *Gynecol Oncol*. 2003;91:463–469.
110. Chan JK, Loizzi V, Youssef M, et al. Significance of comprehensive surgical staging in noninvasive papillary serous carcinoma of the endometrium. *Gynecol Oncol*. 2003;90:181–185.
111. Carcangiu ML, Tan LK, Chambers JT. Stage IA uterine serous carcinoma: a study of 13 cases. *Am J Surg Pathol*. 1997;21:1507–1514.
112. Gehrig PA, Groben PA, Fowler WC Jr, et al. Noninvasive papillary serous carcinoma of the endometrium. *Obstet Gynecol*. 2001;97:153–157.
113. Abeler VM, Kjørstad KE. Clear cell carcinoma of the endometrium: a histopathological and clinical study of 97 cases. *Gynecol Oncol*. 1991;40:207–217.
114. Cirisano FD, Robby SJ, Dodge RK, et al. Epidemiologic and surgicopathologic findings of papillary serous and clear cell endometrial cancers when compared to endometrioid carcinoma. *Gynecol Oncol*. 1999;74:385–394.
115. Malpica A, Tornos C, Burke TW, et al. Low-stage clear-cell carcinoma of the endometrium. *Am J Surg Pathol*. 1995;19:769–774.
116. Carcangiu ML, Chambers JT. Early pathologic stage clear cell carcinoma and uterine papillary serous carcinoma of the endometrium: comparison of clinicopathologic features and survival. *Int J Gynecol Pathol*. 1995;14:30–38.
117. Illanes D, Broman J, Meyer B, et al. Verrucous carcinoma of the endometrium: case history, pathologic findings, brief review of literature and discussion. *Gynecol Oncol*. 2006;102:375–377.
118. Albores-Saavedra J, Martinez-Benitez B, Luevano E. Small cell carcinomas and large cell neuroendocrine carcinomas of the endometrium and cervix: polypoid tumors and those arising in polyps may have a favorable prognosis. *Int J Gynecol Pathol*. 2008;27:333–339.
119. Mariani A, Dowdy SC, Keeney GL, et al. High-risk endometrial cancer subgroups: candidates for target-based adjuvant therapy. *Gynecol Oncol*. 2004;95:120–126.
120. Zaino RJ, Kurman RJ, Herbold D, et al. The significance of squamous differentiation in endometrial carcinoma. *Cancer*. 1991;68:2293–2302.
121. Murray SK, Young RH, Scully RE. Unusual epithelial and stromal changes in myoinvasive endometrioid adenocarcinoma: a study of their frequency, associated diagnostic problems, and prognostic significance. *Int J Gynecol Pathol*. 2003;22:324–333.
122. Stewart CJR, Brennan BA, Leung YC, et al. MELF pattern invasion in endometrial carcinoma: association with low grade, myoinvasive endometrioid tumours, focal mucinous differentiation and vascular invasion. *Pathology*. 2009;41:454–459.
123. Ali A, Black D, Soslow RA. Difficulties in assessing the depth of myometrial invasion in endometrial carcinoma. *Int J Gynecol Pathol*. 2007;26:115–123.

124. Ismiil N, Rasty G, Ghorab Z, et al. Adenomyosis involved by endometrial adenocarcinoma is a significant risk factor for deep myometrial invasion. *Ann Diagn Pathol.* 2007;11:252–257.
125. O'Brien DJ, Flannelly G, Mooney EE, et al. Lymphovascular space involvement in early stage well-differentiated endometrial cancer is associated with increased mortality. *BJOG.* 2009;116:991–994.
126. Logani S, Herdman AV, Little JV, et al. Vascular "pseudo invasion" in laparoscopic hysterectomy specimens: a diagnostic pitfall. *Am J Surg Pathol.* 2008;32:560–565.
127. Kitahara S, Walsh C, Frumovitz M, et al. Vascular pseudoinvasion in laparoscopic hysterectomy specimens for endometrial carcinoma: a grossing artifact? *Am J Surg Pathol.* 2009;33:298–303.
128. McKenney JK, Kong CS, Longacre TA. Endometrial adenocarcinoma associated with subtle lymph-vascular space invasion and lymph node metastasis: a histologic pattern mimicking intravascular and sinusoidal histiocytes. *Int J Gynecol Pathol.* 2004;24:73–78.
129. Pecorelli S. Revised FIGO staging for carcinoma of the vulva, cervix, and endometrium. *Int J Gynecol Obstet.* 2009;105:103–104.
130. Tambouret R, Clement PB, Young RH. Endometrial endometrioid adenocarcinoma with a deceptive pattern of spread to the uterine cervix. A manifestation of stage IIB endometrial carcinoma liable to be misinterpreted as an independent carcinoma or a benign lesion. *Am J Surg Pathol.* 2003;27:1080–1088.
131. Wethington SL, Barrena Medel NI, Wright JD, et al. Prognostic significance and treatment implications of positive peritoneal cytology in endometrial adenocarcinoma: unraveling a mystery. *Gynecol Oncol.* 2009;115:18–25.
132. Garg K, Shih K, Barakat R, et al. Endometrial carcinomas in women aged 40 years and younger: tumors associated with loss of DNA mismatch repair proteins comprise a distinct clinicopathologic subset. *Am J Surg Pathol.* 2009;33:1869–1877.
133. Vaccarello L, Alte SM, Copeland LJ, et al. Endometrial carcinoma associated with pregnancy: a report of three cases and review of the literature. *Gynecol Oncol.* 1999;74:118–122.
134. Yael HK, Lorenza P, Evelina S, et al. Incidental endometrial adenocarcinoma in early pregnancy: a case report and review of the literature. *Int J Gynecol Cancer.* 2009;19:1580–1584.
135. Mittal K, Da Costa D. Endometrial hyperplasia and carcinoma in endometrial polyps: clinicopathologic and follow-up findings. *Int J Gynecol Pathol.* 2007;27:45–48.
136. Farrell R, Scurry J, Otton G, et al. Clinicopathologic review of malignant polyps in stage 1A carcinoma of the endometrium. *Gynecol Oncol.* 2005;98:254–262.
137. Longacre TA, Chung MH, Rouse RV, et al. Atypical polypoid adenomyofibroma (atypical polypoid adenomyoma) of the uterus. A clinicopathologic study of 55 cases. *Am J Surg Pathol.* 1996;20:1–20.
138. Sasaki T, Sugiyama T, Nanjo H, et al. Endometrioid adenocarcinoma arising from adenomyosis: report and immunohistochemical analysis of an unusual case. *Pathol Int.* 2001;51:308–313.
139. Puppa G, Shozu M, Perin T, et al. Small primary adenocarcinoma in adenomyosis with nodal metastasis: a case report. *BMC Cancer.* 2007;7:103.
140. Hirabayashi K, Yasuda M, Kajiwara H, et al. Clear cell adenocarcinoma arising from adenomyosis. *Int J Gynecol Pathol.* 2009;28:262–266.
141. Westin SN, Lacour RA, Urbauer DL, et al. Carcinoma of the lower uterine segment: a newly described association with lynch syndrome. *J Clin Oncol.* 2008;26:5965–5971.
142. Zaino R, Whitney C, Brady MF, et al. Simultaneously detected endometrial and ovarian carcinomas: a prospective clinicopathologic study of 74 cases: a Gynecologic Oncology Group study. *Gynecol Oncol.* 2001;83:355–362.
143. Soliman PT, Slomovitz BM, Broaddus RR, et al. Synchronous primary cancers of the endometrium and ovary: a single institution review of 84 cases. *Gynecol Oncol.* 2004;94:456–462.
144. Broaddus RR, Lynch HT, Chen LM, et al. Pathologic features of endometrial carcinoma associated with HNPCC: a comparison with sporadic endometrial carcinoma. *Cancer.* 2006;106:87–94.
145. Garg K, Leitao M, Kauff N, et al. Selection of endometrial carcinomas for DNA mismatch repair protein immunohistochemistry using patient age and tumor morphology enhances detection of mismatch repair abnormalities. *Am J Surg Pathol.* 2009;33:925–933.

SECTION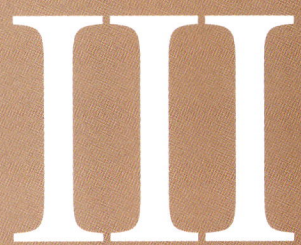

Imaging

▶ CHAPTER 5: Diagnostic Modalities for Endometrial Carcinoma
▶ CHAPTER 6: Current Management and Issues in Treatment of Endometrial Carcinoma

Diagnostic Modalities for Endometrial Carcinoma

5

▶ Reagan Street, MD, and
Tri A. Dinh, MD

Endometrial cancer is more commonly diagnosed than ovarian, cervical, vulvar, and vaginal cancer combined. Management of endometrial cancer, whether conservative or radical, must take into consideration not only the postmenopausal patient, but also the young patient who has not completed her family. Nulligravidity contributes to endometrial cancer risk, so women younger than 40 are often desirous of fertility-sparing treatment.[1] Research into techniques to accurately diagnose and preoperatively evaluate endometrial cancer reflects these concerns. Precise assessment of the extent of disease is augmented by multiple diagnostic modalities.

GENERAL MEDICAL EVALUATION

Endometrial cancer patients are typically obese and postmenopausal and are at high risk for cardiovascular disease and diabetes. Prior to surgical treatment, it is imperative to do a basic preoperative evaluation including electrocardiogram, chest x-ray, and basic laboratory evaluation to assess electrolytes, hemoglobin, and renal function.[2] A chest x-ray can detect cardiopulmonary problems, pleural effusions, and pulmonary metastasis.[2] Along with these essential tests, various imaging modalities may be used to evaluate for myometrial invasion, cervical extension, and lymph node or widespread metastasis (Fig. 5-1).

In cases where early-stage, grade 1 disease is presumed, imaging modalities may not be necessary.[2] Patients with high-risk clear cell or papillary serous histology are more likely to present with extrauterine disease, and preoperative imaging is helpful in presurgical planning.[2] Finally, preoperative imaging is helpful to triage patients who may benefit from consultation with a gynecologic oncologist or extended surgical staging if this is not a procedure that was originally planned.

PRETREATMENT EVALUATION AND DIAGNOSIS

When a patient presents with symptoms consistent with the possibility of endometrial cancer, it is vital for the physician to perform a complete history and physical examination. Family history may elicit conditions such as hereditary nonpolyposis colorectal cancer (HNPCC) or mutations in the *MLH1* and *MSH2* mismatch repair genes.[1] These hereditary conditions

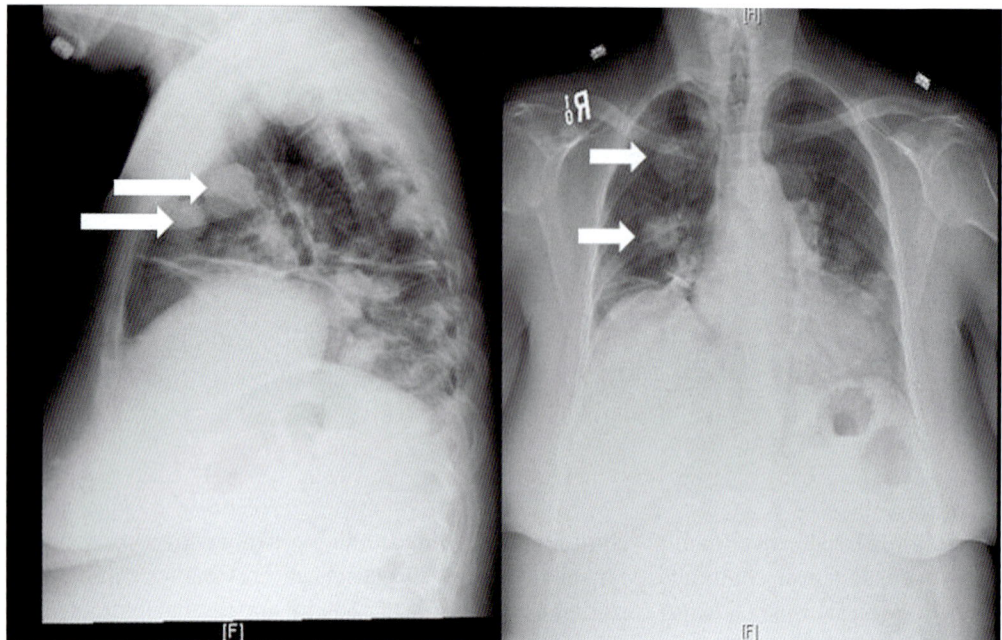

FIGURE 5-1: Pulmonary nodules in a late-stage endometrial cancer on chest x-ray, lateral and anterior-posterior views, respectively.

increase the incidence of early-onset development of endometrial cancer from 0.2% in the general population to 25% in a woman less than 50 years old with these mutations.[1]

A full physical examination will include lymph node survey of the neck, axilla, and groin, as well as complete pelvic and rectal examination to evaluate for pelvic spread of disease.[1] Often, patients are older and have multiple coexisting medical morbidities. These conditions may render a patient a poor surgical candidate and alert the physician to certain findings that may contraindicate a primary surgical treatment.[1] Diabetes and hypertension are common comorbidities, and it is important to have blood glucose levels and blood pressure under control prior to surgery. Anesthetic and surgical risks increase in women who are obese and women with cardiopulmonary disease.[1]

Papanicolaou Smear

The importance of the Papanicolaou (Pap) smear in screening for cervical cancer is well established. Unfortunately, its usefulness in endometrial cancer screening is limited.[3] Several studies have been performed to evaluate the use of Pap smears for endometrial cancer screening, but the average sensitivity is only about 43%.[4] Several small studies report that abnormal Pap smears are found in 100% of papillary serous or clear cell endometrial cancer and in greater than 60% of endometrioid-type cancer.[4] Another study showed a sensitivity of only 26% in detecting endometrial cancer overall; however, the authors note that the Pap smear may have improved sensitivity with higher grade disease.[5] The huge variations in these findings make the clinical utility of the Pap smear in detection of endometrial cancer quite low.

Occasionally, cervical cytology samples show benign endometrial cells. Beal et al.[6] showed that this occurred in approximately 0.9% of women 40 years of age or older; the majority of these women are completely asymptomatic.[6] If benign endometrial cells are an incidental finding in an otherwise asymptomatic premenopausal woman, it is exceedingly rare to find endometrial pathology.[7] No further evaluation is indicated. However, if a woman is symptomatic with irregular or heavy vaginal bleeding, the finding of endometrial cells on Pap smear indicates the need for further investigation.[7] In postmenopausal women, the finding of endometrial cells on Pap smear almost always necessitates endometrial sampling.[8]

The current American Society for Colposcopy and Cervical Pathology recommendations for atypical endometrial cells or abnormal glandular cells provide for further evaluation with colposcopy in conjunction with endocervical curettage, endometrial biopsy, and human papillomavirus testing. More often than not, cervical epithelial neoplasia is found in cases where atypical glandular cells are found on cervical cytology, but the endometrial cavity still warrants evaluation.[8] Endometrial biopsy is indicated if a patient is less than 35 years of age and presents with vaginal bleeding that cannot be explained or has symptoms of chronic anovulation. If the patient is greater than 35 years of age, endometrial biopsy is almost always indicated with the finding of abnormal glandular cells but especially if atypical endometrial cells are noted on cytology. Less than 2% of women younger than 40 years of age have endometrial cells found on Pap smear requiring evaluation. Younger women rarely have pathology associated with the finding of endometrial cells on Pap smear; however, in menopausal women, it is critical to search for a pathologic cause.[8]

Sometimes, women who have had a hysterectomy for benign reasons have Pap smears of the vaginal cuff performed. If this occurs and benign glandular cells are found, no further investigation is needed.[8] However, if a woman has a hysterectomy for cervical or endometrial cancer, Pap smear surveillance of the vaginal cuff is critical to evaluate for evidence of recurrence. Implications of Pap smear in evaluation of recurrent disease will be discussed later.

At time of initial presentation, a positive Pap smear is predictive of poor prognosis and future endometrial cancer recurrence. Histologic subtypes of papillary serous and clear cell endometrial cancer are more likely to be diagnosed after finding abnormal cells on cervical cytology than endometrioid-type endometrial cancer. The presence of abnormal endometrial cells on cervical sampling is also a predictor of poor prognosis, as indicated by the increased likelihood of severe myometrial invasion and nodal metastases.[9] Increased grade of endometrial cancer regardless of histologic subtype is associated with having an abnormal Pap smear.[9] Brown et al.[9] determined that initial abnormal cytology leads to endometrial cancer recurrence in 12% of patients, as opposed to only 4% of patients with normal initial Pap smear findings. The same study showed that 19% of patients who were diagnosed with papillary serous or clear cell subtypes had abnormal cervical cytology compared with only 7% of endometrioid endometrial cancer patients.[9]

Endocervical Curettage

Endocervical curettage (ECC) is another method of evaluating women who present with abnormal cervical cytology or vaginal bleeding. ECC can be positive without any evidence of disease on imaging.[2] This finding may represent microscopic cervical involvement or possible contamination from the uterus.[2] ECC is included in a procedure called a fractional dilation and curettage (D&C), which attempts to isolate endometrial curettage from ECC. Distinguishing cervical involvement from endometrial contamination on fractional D&C is inaccurate. ECC is a poor method for evaluation of cervical extension of endometrial cancer because it has a false-positive rate of up to 50%.[2] False-negative results are also possible, so physicians must use other techniques to determine cervical involvement if there is high suspicion.[2] Cervical involvement does not preclude surgical treatment, and often the presence of cervical involvement is only defined at the time of hysterectomy with frozen section pathology.

Endometrial Sampling

Endometrial sampling is the key step in the diagnosis of endometrial cancer. Premenopausal women who are anovulatory are at higher risk for endometrial neoplasia and require endometrial sampling to work-up abnormal uterine bleeding. All postmenopausal women with vaginal bleeding require endometrial sampling. Ten percent of postmenopausal women who present with this classic symptom will have cancer on biopsy.[2] Combined risk factors of age greater than 70 years, type 2 diabetes, and nulliparity increase risk of neoplasia in women with symptomatic bleeding.[2] Eighty-seven percent of these patients are diagnosed with atypical hyperplasia or endometrial cancer on biopsy.[2] Three percent of women with symptomatic bleeding and none of these risk factors are diagnosed with endometrial cancer on endometrial biopsy.[2] Accurate history and physical prior to endometrial sampling allows a physician to appropriately counsel patients.

Endometrial biopsy is often performed in an outpatient setting with minimal discomfort to the patient and no need for anesthesia. Adequate sampling is a must, and if not obtained, further investigation with more invasive techniques is warranted. Endometrial biopsy in the United States is most often performed with a disposable plastic endometrial suction curette (e.g., Pipelle; CooperSurgical, Trumbull, CT). The patient is placed in lithotomy position, and after placement of a speculum, a curette is inserted through the cervix into the uterine cavity, and a biopsy specimen is obtained.

Risks of endometrial biopsy include pain and bleeding. Infrequently, uterine perforation may occur, but this is almost always benign and does not require any action other than observation. Rarely, a specimen is unobtainable due to cervical stenosis. Endometrial biopsy in the outpatient office setting is a blind procedure and can produce a false-negative result due to lack of tissue representing the entire endometrium. Positive tests are diagnostic, but negative tests often require further endometrial cavity evaluation.[10]

Endometrial biopsy collection fails in approximately 8% of cases when a Pipelle device is used, according to a literature review by Clark et al.[10] They evaluated 11 studies with more than 1,000 patients and found inadequate samples in up to 13% of specimens collected via the Pipelle and 15% of specimens for all methods.[10] Other tools used to collect endometrial samples are the Vabra Aspirator (Berkeley Medevices, Richmond, CA) and the Z sampler device (Zinanti, Chatsworth, CA). The Vabra Aspirator has been found to be less accurate overall in diagnosing hyperplasia and endometrial cancer but is still widely used.[3]

In postmenopausal women, physicians may be unable to perform office endometrial sampling, and even when a sample is obtained, the specimen may still prove inadequate for analysis.[10] Clark et al.[10] found an overall failure rate of 12% but a higher inadequate sampling rate of 22% for all methods in postmenopausal women. The authors concluded that outpatient diagnosis via endometrial biopsy is a valid and valuable tool in the diagnosis of endometrial cancer, especially when negative results are further evaluated in cases where clinical suspicion is high.

The strength of Pipelle endometrial sampling is further demonstrated by Fakhar et al.,[11] who evaluated the sensitivity, specificity, positive predictive value (PPV), and negative predictive value (NPV) of endometrial biopsies in 100 patients. D&C following the biopsy served as the "gold standard" for comparison.[11] If Pipelle sampling indicated endometrial carcinoma, endometrial hyperplasia, or secretory endometrium, then sensitivity, specificity, PPV, and NPV were each 100%.[11] For endometrial hyperplasia with atypia, sensitivity and NPV remained 100%, whereas specificity slightly decreased to 98% and PPV decreased to 80%.[11] These results further authenticate the use of outpatient endometrial sampling with a Pipelle device as a cost-effective, low-risk option with excellent sensitivity and specificity.

Office endometrial biopsy does have limitations in cases where an endometrial polyp is present. Tanriverdi et al.[12] suggest that if a polyp is suspected, D&C is necessary. They also confirmed previous findings that endometrial biopsy in postmenopausal women may produce an inadequate sample in up to 22% of cases and again suggest D&C in such cases.[12] They did not find the high 100% sensitivity and specificity for endometrial carcinoma found by Clark et al.,[10] but they did evaluate the combination of transvaginal ultrasound and Pipelle biopsies, finding close to 100% sensitivity and specificity when these methods are combined.[11,12] Tanriverdi et al.[12] also proposed that outpatient biopsy be used only in low-risk patients without high suspicion of hyperplasia with atypia or endometrial cancer and that patient with high risk for cancer be more carefully and completely evaluated with formal endometrial curettage. Most physicians prefer an attempt at outpatient sampling in all patients, with appropriate follow-up if suspicion remains elevated despite a negative result.

Routine screening for endometrial cancer does not exist, but certain groups warrant some method of evaluation. Patients with known HNPCC should undergo annual endometrial biopsies starting at age 35 according to the American Cancer Society.[2] HNPCC increases the lifetime risk of endometrial cancer from 3% to 20%.[2] Some physicians advocate that women on tamoxifen treatment for breast cancer should undergo endometrial sampling for screening, whereas most physicians advise prompt evaluation only in symptomatic women.[2] Most oncologists and other authorities do not advocate routine evaluation with ultrasound or endometrial biopsy in women on tamoxifen.[2] The American Cancer Society does not recommend endometrial cancer screening for women on tamoxifen.[2]

Dilation and Curettage

D&C is the gold standard for diagnosis of endometrial cancer.[3] A D&C requires general or regional anesthesia in an operating room and is often performed with hysteroscopy to completely evaluate the endometrial cavity. Women with endometrial polyps, cervical stenosis, or insufficient sampling on endometrial biopsy who remain at high suspicion for endometrial cancer require endometrial curettage in the operating room. For patients contemplating medical therapy of endometrial cancer to preserve future fertility, complete evaluation of the endometrium with curettage is crucial.[1] Hysteroscopy involves using a camera inserted into the cervix after adequate dilation. The entire endometrial cavity may be visualized, and directed biopsies may be taken.

The accuracy of office endometrial sampling versus endometrial curettage has been compared, and results are mixed. Larson et al.[13] showed that D&C correctly identified the tumor grade of 77% of endometrial cancers compared with 58% of office samples taken with the Z sampler, one device for outpatient endometrial sampling. Often, the cancers were undergraded (i.e., given a lower tumor grade than the grade found at hysterectomy).[13] Preoperatively, because there is no definitive way to evaluate depth of invasion, tumor grade is of utmost importance to guide the decision of whether or not to perform complete lymphadenectomy for surgical staging.[13] For example, patients with grade 3 endometrial carcinoma, regardless of myometrial invasion, would undergo surgical staging with both pelvic and para-

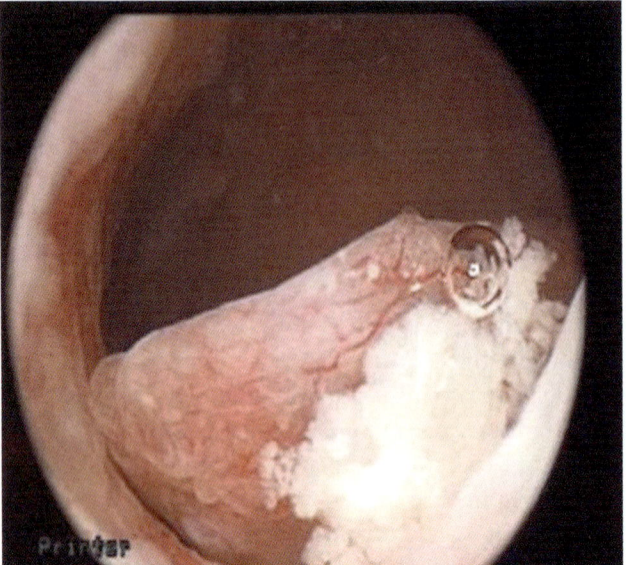

FIGURE 5-2: Hysteroscopy showing polyp suspicious for cancer (later proven serous endometrial cancer by pathology).

aortic lymphadenectomy due to a higher risk of nodal metastasis. In contrast, a patient with grade 1 endometrioid endometrial cancer may be managed with a more conservative surgical procedure.[13]

Hysteroscopy is often performed with D&C. Ben-Yehuda et al.[14] showed that hysteroscopy does not increase the diagnostic accuracy of the endometrial curettage. They reviewed medical records of 403 patients who underwent both uterine curettage and hysteroscopy and noted that there was only 52% concurrence in the diagnosis of hyperplasia via hysteroscopic impression versus final pathology findings. Only 10 patients in their study had endometrial cancer found on D&C, but hysteroscopic impression of carcinoma was only noted in the operative notes of 2 of these patients. Two patients in their study had endometrial cancer diagnosed within 6 months but were not diagnosed with either modality, refuting the idea that hysteroscopy might catch some cancers that curettage may miss[14] (Figs. 5-2 to 5-4).

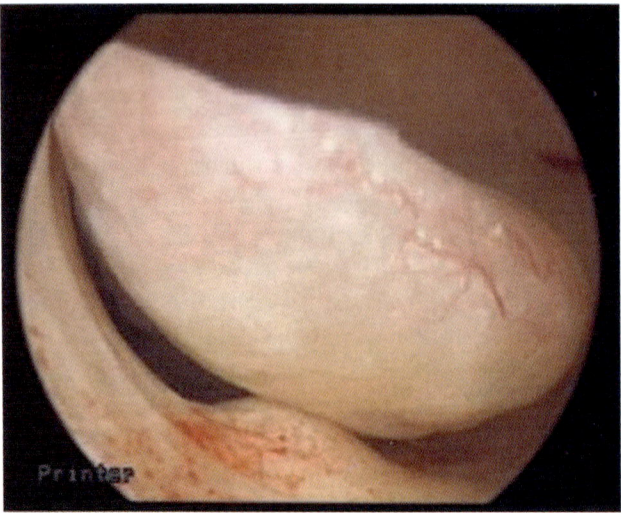

FIGURE 5-3: Hysteroscopy showing endometrial polyp.

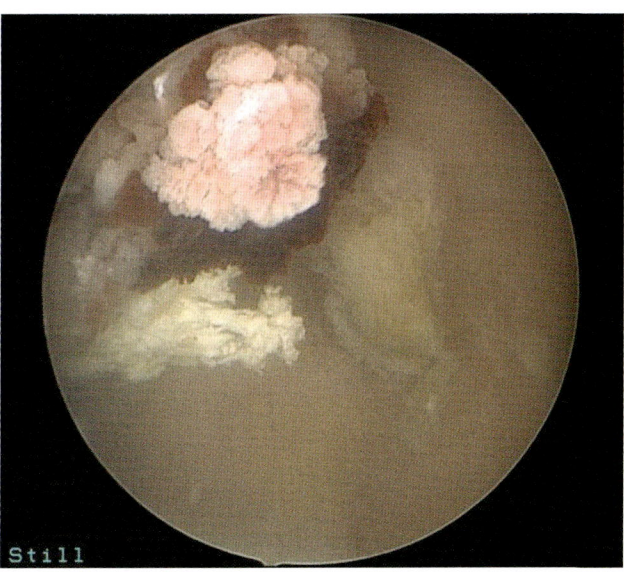

FIGURE 5-4: Hysteroscopy image suspicious for cancer.

In benign gynecologic conditions, when hysteroscopy is used to detect polyps and submucosal leiomyomata, research shows that diagnosis of abnormal uterine bleeding does improve with hysteroscopy combined with endometrial curettage.[14] Uterine curettage was only able to detect 32% of polyps and 6% of leiomyomata in this review, confirming that hysteroscopy aids in diagnosis in some situations.[14] The review by Ben-Yehuda et al.[14] of 403 patients identified three uterine perforations, none of which necessitated exploratory laparotomy. Occasionally, diagnostic laparoscopy may be necessary after uterine perforation to evaluate the intra-abdominal organs for damage.[15] Complications due to general or regional anesthesia can also be encountered during hysteroscopy. In addition, there is the added possibility of complication from the distending media used to visualize the endometrial cavity.[14]

Distending media can be isotonic or hypotonic fluid or carbon dioxide gas. Most gynecologists prefer to use normal saline to distend the uterine cavity to improve visualization. If uterine perforation is encountered, normal saline will not harm the patient unless a large amount is deposited. Pulmonary or cerebral edema from extensive intravascular absorption is a rare complication of excess fluid balance after hysteroscopy, and the patient should be observed postoperatively if this is encountered. Hypotonic fluids such as glycine and sorbitol can lead to electrolyte abnormalities with a relatively minimal amount of positive fluid balance.[15] Accurate assessment of fluid deficits is important in preventing these complications. Carbon dioxide may also be used as a distending media. If the intrauterine pressure is allowed to get too high, venous gas embolism may occur because the gas is forced into the cervical or endometrial vasculature.[15]

PRETREATMENT SERUM MARKER EVALUATION

Physicians treating many different types of cancer use serum markers to evaluate the likelihood of metastasis preoperatively. These markers are also used postoperatively to evaluate for treatment success or recurrence of disease. For example, carcinoembryonic antigen (CEA) is elevated in colon cancer as well as mucinous ovarian cancer.[1] CA19-9 is also elevated in mucinous ovarian cancer, and α-fetoprotein (AFP) is elevated in germ cell ovarian tumors.[2] CA-125 is typically used for diagnosing and following therapy in ovarian cancer, but may also be helpful in the management of endometrial cancer.[16]

Several biomarkers have been studied in relation to endometrial cancer. Biomarkers can be cytokines, growth factors, angiogenesis-promoting factors, cancer antigens, apoptotic proteins, proteases, adhesion molecules, hormones, and adipokines.[17] For example, the cytokine interleukin-6 (IL-6), CA19-9, and matrix metalloproteinase (MMP)-7 are all elevated in endometrial cancer patients.[17] Some biomarkers are seemingly close in function but are found in varied degrees in endometrial cancer. An example is MMP-2, which is decreased in endometrial cancer in contrast to MMP-7, which is elevated as mentioned earlier.[17] An elevated level of CA-125 is a poor prognostic factor associated with decreased survival time.[17] Elevations of CA15-3 and CA19-9 also predict a shorter survival time in patients with endometrial cancer.

Preoperative CA-125 has been proposed as a helpful measure in determining whether a patient will need full lymphadenectomy in the surgical treatment of endometrial cancer or if simple hysterectomy and bilateral salpingo-oophorectomy will suffice.[16] An elevated CA-125 is found in up to 67% of patients with advanced-stage endometrial carcinoma and is thus more likely to be elevated in patients with extrauterine and lymph node disease.[16] For evaluation of recurrent endometrial cancer, distant metastatic disease is associated with elevated CA-125. Unfortunately, any method that may cause peritoneal irritation (e.g., pelvic radiotherapy for a local recurrence or diverticulitis) may artificially elevate CA-125, lowering the sensitivity of this widely used test.[16]

A 2001 Taiwanese study evaluated the preoperative CA-125 values of 124 patients who underwent surgical staging. Their evidence indicates a sensitivity of 78% and specificity of 81% using a CA-125 value of 40 U/mL in screening for lymph node metastasis.[16] In the same study, they noted the median CA-125 value was sixfold higher for stage IV endometrial cancer in comparison with stage I cancer.[16] CA-125 was also noted to be elevated with positive peritoneal washings, adnexal involvement, and distant metastasis and with higher risk histologic types.[16] The study also noted higher levels of preoperative CA-125 with superficial myometrial invasion as opposed to cancer confined to the endometrium. They concluded that full lymphadenectomy should be performed if preoperative CA-125 is greater than 40 U/mL.[16]

Recently, there has been an attempt to develop a multimarker panel to facilitate diagnosis of endometrial cancer.[17] In this study, the authors found that prolactin was the most important biomarker for endometrial cancer.[17] Sensitivity was 98.3% and specificity was 98% when prolactin elevation alone was used for diagnosis.[17] The investigators also measured CA-125, CA15-3, and CEA, noting that these markers were more likely to be elevated in women with stage III or IV endometrial cancer possibly because later stage tumors stimulate cancer antigen shedding.[17] They also found differences in biomarkers for grade 3 tumors, reporting that CA-125, AFP, and adrenocorticotropic hormone (ACTH) were higher with increasing grade of tumor.[17] The study also reported that a combination of prolactin, growth hormone, eotaxin, E-selectin, and thyroid-stimulating hormone (TSH) was helpful in distinguishing endometrial cancer from ovarian cancer and breast cancer.[17]

Prolactin is produced by the endometrial stromal cells during the secretory phase of the menstrual cycle.[17] Tumor growth could trigger stromal cell prolactin secretion.[17] Prolactin has also been implicated in promotion of angiogenesis.[17] Prolactin is at least twice as sensitive in diagnosing endometrial cancer as other biomarker studied by Yurkovetsky et al.[17]

Prolactin was accurate in 93.8% of patients with stage I, 85.8% of patients with stage II, and 96.2% of patients with stage III endometrial cancer.[17] Prolactin levels were compared in patients with endometrial, ovarian, and breast cancers. Prolactin alone could not distinguish these cancers, but in conjunction with eotaxin, growth hormone, E-selectin, and TSH, it was significantly accurate and selective.[17] Future studies of these biomarkers may lead to accurate screening tests for endometrial cancer as well as identification of possible therapeutic value.

Other hormones that have been found to be altered in endometrial cancer in comparison with healthy individuals include TSH, ACTH, and follicle-stimulating hormone (FSH). FSH levels often decrease in endometrial cancer.[17] Increased TSH has been associated with endometrial cancer and may have a derogatory effect on immune function.[17] ACTH is also increased in endometrial cancer and may play a role in tumor cell communication.[17]

Human kallikrein (HK) 6 is a hormone that has been found in papillary serous endometrial cancer. It has been studied as a possible biomarker for cancer surveillance in this histologic subtype.[18] Serum and plasma HK6 is higher in patients with papillary serous endometrial cancer when compared with patients without cancer and patients with endometrioid-type endometrial cancer.[18] HK6 is also being investigated as a prognostic factor in ovarian carcinoma.[18] It has been suggested that elevation of HK6 in both uterine and ovarian malignancies may indicate more aggressive tumors with poor prognosis and resistance to chemotherapy.[18] There are multiple members of the HK family being studied in ovarian cancer that have been identified to have prognostic significance, and it is likely that other types of the HK family will soon be studied as potential biomarkers in papillary serous endometrial cancer.[18]

Inhibins are heterodimeric glycoproteins found in the cell membrane composed of an α and a β subunit.[19] The α subunit is associated with one of two β subunits: βA and βB. The α subunit has recently been found to be a prognostic factor in endometrial cancer.[19] All three subunits have been implicated in endometrial pathogenesis.[19] Increased progression-free survival has been noted with the presence of the inhibin α subunit.[19] Inhibin has been identified as a possible tumor suppressor gene.[19] Advanced-stage and increasing grade tumors demonstrate decreased inhibin α immunoreactivity.[19] Inhibin α loss seems to correlate with an increase in activin A, another hormone that has been implicated in endometrial cancer.[19,20] The presence of inhibin α is an independent prognostic factor indicating increased survival.[19]

Activin A is a homologous protein to inhibin, and both are members of the transforming growth factor-β family, cytokines involved in endometrial cancer.[19,20] Activins are formed by two β subunits.[19] Inhibin α knockout mice show elevated activin levels, and almost all of them develop gonadal tumors.[20] This result could be due to the tumor-suppressing properties of inhibin α or the tumor-enhancing properties of activin.[21] Activin is involved in tumor proliferation and differentiation, but it can also induce apoptosis, suggesting that its action in cancer is multifaceted.[20] Bcl-2 protein is an antiapoptotic protein that is decreased in cells that are high in activin, confirming that activin promotes apoptosis.[20] Activin levels are found to be elevated in women with endometrial cancer prior to surgical removal of tumor.[22] The levels are likely to be directly involved in the tumorigenesis because they decrease after cytoreductive surgery.[21]

There are several MMPs that are associated with various types of cancer. MMP-2 and MMP-9 have been found in up to 88% of endometrial cancers.[2] MMP-2 is associated with unfavorable outcome and decreased survival.[2] CA-125 is thought to be related to MMP because CA-125 levels are higher in patients whose tumors show MMP-2 staining.[2]

PRETREATMENT IMAGING MODALITIES

In the United States, not all patients with endometrial cancer are treated by subspecialist physicians. This pattern of practice often leads to inadequate staging of patients with endometrial cancer because they have surgeries performed by physicians who are not trained to perform lymphadenectomy.[22] Preoperative imaging may lessen, but not completely eliminate, this problem because it may identify the patient who may benefit from a consultation with or transfer of care to a subspecialist physician. Imaging studies may also help a physician determine whether conservative management is an option for patients who want medical management of endometrial cancer in order to preserve future fertility.

Ultrasound

Ultrasound is a cost-effective, virtually risk-free method of evaluating the uterine cavity with minimal patient discomfort.[2] Ultrasound is often used to delineate patients who present with unexplained uterine bleeding but may not need endometrial biopsy. In some cases, ultrasound may help in distinguishing between benign and malignant causes of abnormal uterine bleeding. Occasionally, it may assist in evaluating cervical involvement of cancer or myometrial invasion.

Transvaginal ultrasound is superior to abdominal ultrasound in evaluating the uterus. In the unusual case of a very large uterus, transabdominal ultrasound may be supplementary to transvaginal ultrasound to increase the field of view.[2] Transvaginal ultrasound probes are higher frequency and can be placed closer to the uterus especially when examining obese patients.[23] Transvaginal ultrasound is readily available in most centers and is very cost effective, but it is operator dependent.[23]

Ultrasound can be used to detect uterine myomas, polyps, and endometrial thickness. Increased endometrial thickness, especially in the postmenopausal woman, increases the risk that the patient may have endometrial cancer. If a woman is taking cyclic hormone replacement therapy, it is important to time the ultrasound examination of endometrial thickness to follow a withdrawal bleed. In a premenopausal woman, it is preferable to evaluate during the early proliferative phase of the menstrual cycle. In both of these cases, the endometrium should be at its thinnest.[2] In premenopausal women, after menses, at the beginning of the proliferative phase, the endometrial stripe should measure 2 to 3 mm, increasing up to 8 mm immediately prior to ovulation.[2] Immediately after menses, the endometrial stripe should be echogenic.[2] Prior to ovulation, the endometrium appears trilaminar due to the echogenic appearance of reflective artifact and the presence of a hypoechoic functionalis layer and an echogenic basalis layer.[2] The secretory phase following ovulation involves thickening of the functionalis layer that becomes more echogenic as menstruation gets closer.[2] The endometrial stripe prior to menstruation can be as thick as 15 mm.[2]

Ultrasounds can be transabdominal or transvaginal, and these are often used in combination. Transabdominal ultrasound may also evaluate the entire abdomen and may incidentally find hydronephrosis, ascites, and distant metastasis.[2] Precise ultrasound evaluation of endometrial thickness requires measurement of maximal thickness in a sagittal plane[2] (Figs. 5-5 and 5-6).

Saline infusion sonography (SIS) is a method of enhancing the accuracy of ultrasound in cases where the entire uterine cavity cannot be evaluated easily.[24,25] SIS is also known

Chapter 5 • Diagnostic Modalities for Endometrial Carcinoma

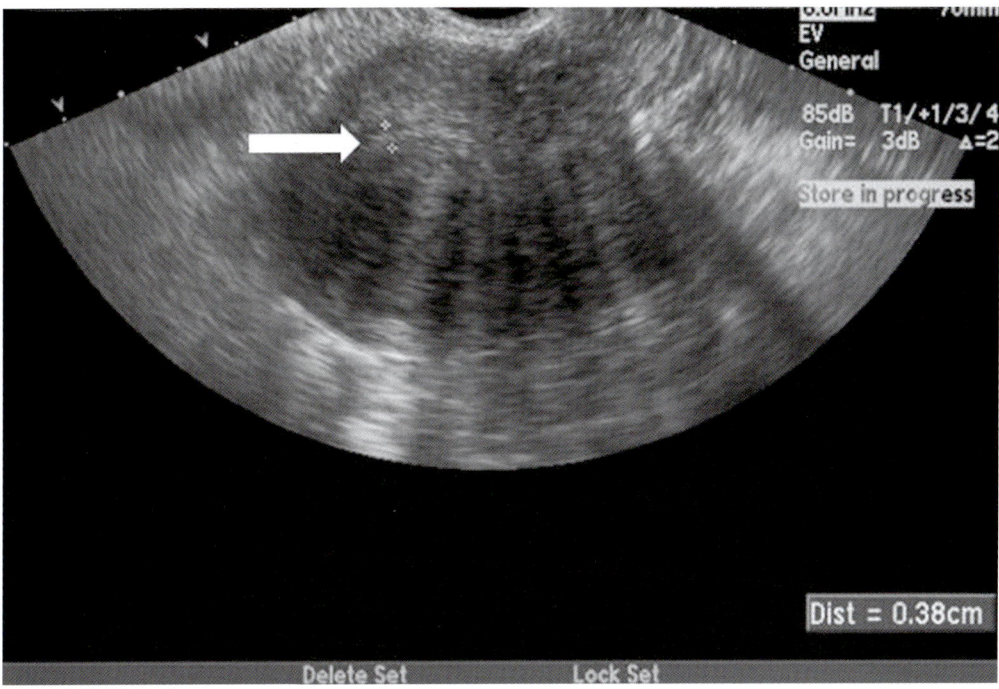

FIGURE 5-5: Ultrasound view of normal endometrial stripe measuring less than 4 mm.

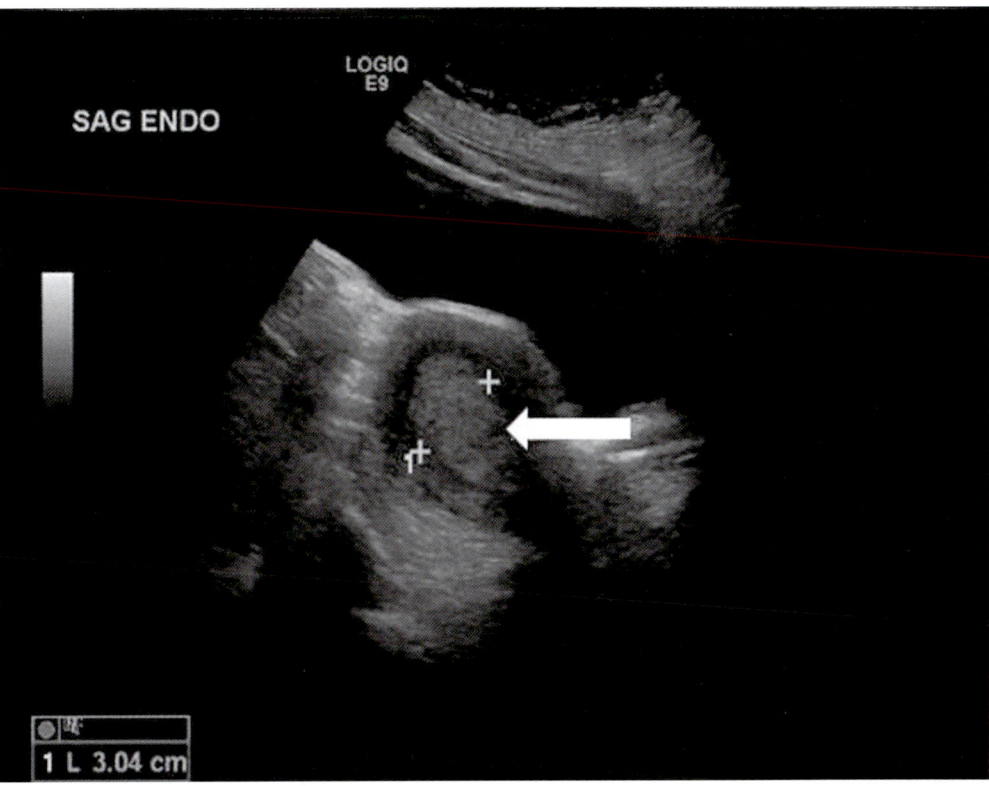

FIGURE 5-6: Transvaginal ultrasound of thickened endometrial stripe measuring 3.04 cm, sagittal view.

as sonohysterosalpingogram. SIS is an office procedure that causes minimal discomfort to the patient. The patient undergoes sterile saline infusion of 5 to 40 mL into the uterus via a small transcervical catheter. Fluid in the endometrial cavity highlights the cavity and allows more distinct outlining of the endometrium.[25] Similar to conventional ultrasonography, SIS measures the thickest part of the endometrium in the midline sagittal image.[2] The cavity is evaluated in terms of shape and lining. If the endometrial lining is irregular or has large focal lesions indicating polyps or fibroids, the result of the SIS is abnormal and requires further evaluation and biopsy. Various studies have reported a wide range of patient tolerance to SIS. Garuti et al.[25] reported only a 60% success rate of performing the entire examination, but other investigators have reported a 92% success rate. SIS cannot be performed in a patient with hematometra, pyometra, or suspected pelvic inflammatory disease.[2] Cervical extension and myometrial invasion are more precisely detected by SIS than ultrasound.[2]

Ultrasound is more valid in the postmenopausal uterus to determine risk of endometrial cancer and need for further investigation. After menopause, the normal endometrium becomes atrophic; similarly, the uterus decreases in size secondary to the hypoestrogenic state of menopause.[26] Studies performed on the same patients 2 years prior to menopause and 2 years after menopause as determined by hormone levels showed that the anteroposterior diameter, uterine width, and endometrial thickness decreased in the postmenopausal women. The endometrial thickness decreased by 28%.[26] Normal postmenopausal endometrial thickness is 2 to 3 mm on average.[27] Ninety-six percent of endometrial cancers will be identified if biopsies are performed after ultrasound detects an endometrial stripe greater than 4 mm.[24]

A meta-analysis performed by Gupta et al.[27] suggests that if a woman presents with postmenopausal bleeding and her endometrial thickness is 5 mm or less, endometrial sampling does not need to be performed. The investigators analyzed 28 studies with over 7,000 patients. Some of these studies used a 4-mm cutoff for endometrial thickness measurement, but most used a 5-mm cutoff. Overall results indicate that risk of endometrial cancer with an ultrasound measurement of endometrial thickness less than 4 mm is 2.4%, increasing to only 5% if the thickness is less than 5 mm.[27] During their analysis, four studies were deemed as good quality studies; in analyzing only those four studies, an ultrasound evaluation of endometrial thickness of 5 mm or less led to a 2.5% posttest probability of endometrial cancer.[27] They note that ultrasound is a test of exclusion and cannot rule in endometrial hyperplasia or cancer.[27]

Another mitigating factor in ultrasound accuracy is postmenopausal use of hormone replacement therapy (HRT). HRT increases the estrogen effect in the uterus, thus thickening the endometrial stripe. Smith-Bindman et al.[28] researched the effectiveness of ultrasound in patients taking and not taking HRT using 5 mm as the threshold for abnormal results. They found that ultrasound was 95% sensitive for identifying endometrial pathology in women not taking HRT and 91% sensitive in women using HRT. The specificity for endometrial pathology was higher in women who were not taking HRT.[28]

In an attempt to make the ultrasound more diagnostic for endometrial malignancy, researchers have investigated the use of Doppler ultrasonography and resistance index (RI) values.[29] The frequencies of ultrasonic waves are used to evaluate the distance from the ultrasound probe to body tissues. The RI value is calculated from these measurements.[29] The RI recognition of myometrial invasion can help identify patients with early-stage disease who can be treated conservatively.[29]

Pektas et al.[29] proposed that the RI can help determine tumor grade, thus helping surgeons in preoperative planning. They evaluated the myometrial invasion in known tumors by comparing the deepest tumor visualized to the surrounding normal endometrium.[29] The RI values in the uterine arteries were measured by Doppler ultrasonography. They noted that in the presence of significant myometrial invasion defined as greater than 50%, the RI values of both uterine arteries were decreased. The RI values of the right and left uterine arteries also reflected tumor grade, decreasing with increasing tumor grade.[29]

Myometrial invasion is an independent predictor of outcome of endometrial cancer.[30] Higher tumor grade and lymph node metastasis are both increased with deeper myometrial invasion.[30] Transvaginal ultrasound alone was found to have a sensitivity of 66% and specificity of 72% for myometrial invasion in known cancers. The extent of myometrial invasion was underestimated in 14% of cases, which may falsely obviate the need for surgical staging.[29] Ultrasound alone is not as accurate in determining myometrial invasion and tumor grade, but when used in conjunction with Doppler measurements, the efficiency improves.[29]

Transvaginal ultrasound has been compared with magnetic resonance imaging (MRI) in prediction of myometrial invasion, and although some studies report comparable efficacy, others find ultrasound to have only 69% accuracy in diagnosis of deep myometrial invasion.[30] Develioglu et al.[30] reported low accuracy in diagnosis as well as low sensitivity and specificity, ultimately resulting in underestimation of deep myometrial invasion by ultrasound.[30] They confirmed that the uterine artery RI can be used to predict deep myometrial invasion.[30] Theoretically, the uterine artery RI can be used along with age and tumor grade to determine the likelihood of deep myometrial invasion and assist in surgical planning.[30]

Recently, advances in technology have led to the invention of three-dimensional (3D) ultrasonography. 3D ultrasonography has been introduced as a superior method of evaluating myometrial invasion in endometrial cancer, compared with two-dimensional ultrasound, with decreased operator dependence.[31] 3D ultrasound allows for improved visualization of the coronal plane of the uterus, thus increasing the detection rate of myometrial invasion.[31] 3D ultrasound also identified cervical involvement correctly in 88% of cases according to a study by Alcazar et al.[31] MRI, as discussed later, remains the superior method of identification of myometrial invasion and assisting in preoperative planning, but 3D ultrasound is helpful in cases where MRI is not available or cannot be performed because of patient reasons.[31] Alcazar et al.[31] note that 3D ultrasound is still in the early stages of research and its application to clinical practice at this time is limited.

Ultrasound evaluation of endometrial thickness in patients using tamoxifen is problematic because tamoxifen causes formation of cystic endometrial changes that make measurement of the endometrial thickness difficult.[32] Previous studies have proposed a 10-mm threshold for normal endometrial thickness because of the changes tamoxifen induces. Although this thicker measurement may prevent unnecessary endometrial biopsies, it comes with a price of false-negative results.[32] Most authorities recommend the continued use of 5 mm as a cutoff point for abnormal endometrial thickness in the postmenopausal woman whether or not she is on tamoxifen.[32]

In conclusion, ultrasound is a valuable tool in evaluating uterine bleeding and helping determine which patients should undergo endometrial sampling. Unfortunately, high-risk histology may be missed on ultrasound if a conventional criterion for endometrial thickness is used.[27] No imaging study is a substitute for good clinical judgment. Follow-up is mandatory, especially if symptoms persist or return.

Computed Tomography, Magnetic Resonance Imaging, and Positron Emission Tomography Scanning

Computed tomography (CT) scanning, MRI, and positron emission tomography (PET) are all available for evaluation of patients with endometrial cancer. These tests may be used to not only determine treatment planning, but also evaluate response to treatment and follow patients for evidence of recurrence.

The American College of Radiology has analyzed the appropriateness of various methods in diagnosing and evaluating the stage of endometrial cancer.[33] They rated the imaging modalities from 1 to 9 in terms of which are most suitable for preoperative evaluation of endometrial cancer. MRI pelvis with contrast is consistently the highest rated study, with a rating of 8 for diagnostic work-up and overall staging, 9 for assessing depth of myometrial invasion, 8 for lymph node evaluation, and 8 for assessing endocervical involvement. CT with contrast was rated 8 for lymph node evaluation, but only received a score of 4 for assessing depth of myometrial invasion, endocervical extension, and overall diagnostic work-up. PET scanning was given a 5 for lymph node evaluation and is not used for other purposes. Lee et al.[33] note that transvaginal ultrasound is ultimately a poor choice as the only preoperative imaging modality when other options are available.

Computed Tomography

CT scanning involves use of intravenous (IV) contrast to enhance images and differentiate blood vessels that fill with contrast from lymph nodes that do not. IV contrast enhances the myometrium and makes tumor boundaries relatively hypodense and thus more visible.[2] CT scans use IV contrast to highlight the bladder and ureters, which can help with delineating tumor involvement. Normally the uterine myometrium enhances with IV contrast more than the endometrium and cervix.[2]

Often a physician is forced to use the imaging modality available rather than the one that is perhaps a better choice. CT scanning is often easier and more cost effective to obtain for endometrial cancer evaluation. CT is accurate for diagnosing depth of myometrial invasion in approximately 60% of cases.[33] If myometrial invasion is identified via CT scan, it is likely involving greater than one-third of the myometrium.[2] CT is only 25% sensitive for cervical extension.[2] Lymph node metastasis is easily evaluated with CT, and this imaging modality is a mainstay for preoperative evaluation.[33] CT can also be used for guided biopsy to confirm extrauterine disease.[2] Fluoroscopy can be used to assist CT-guided biopsy for the most difficult to access sites of suspected metastasis.[2]

Image quality in obese patients is a limit of CT scanning. Some patients are allergic to contrast dye used to enhance imaging, and others may be allergic to the iodine used in the contrast agent.[2] Contrast enhancement of CT is helpful in increasing its accuracy. Endometrial cancer appears the same as myometrial tissue unless contrast is used. With contrast, carcinoma becomes hypodense.[2] CT images can also show a gas pattern in the uterus, which can represent pyometra, necrosis, or a fistula.[2] To diagnose cervical extension on CT, the cervix must be greater than 3.5 cm, and heterogeneous hypodensity must be visualized in the cervical stroma.[2] Absence of pelvic fat may allow for the diagnosis of parametrial or pelvic sidewall extension, which is perhaps the greatest utility of CT scanning for endometrial cancer.[2] Diagnosis of widespread metastases in stage III and IV endometrial cancers, evaluated by CT, is accurate in up to 86% of cases, although accuracy is significantly lower in stage I and II disease.[2] CT accuracy to determine that a patient has early-stage disease has been reported to be as low as 58%[2] (Figs. 5-7 to 5-13).

Chapter 5 • Diagnostic Modalities for Endometrial Carcinoma

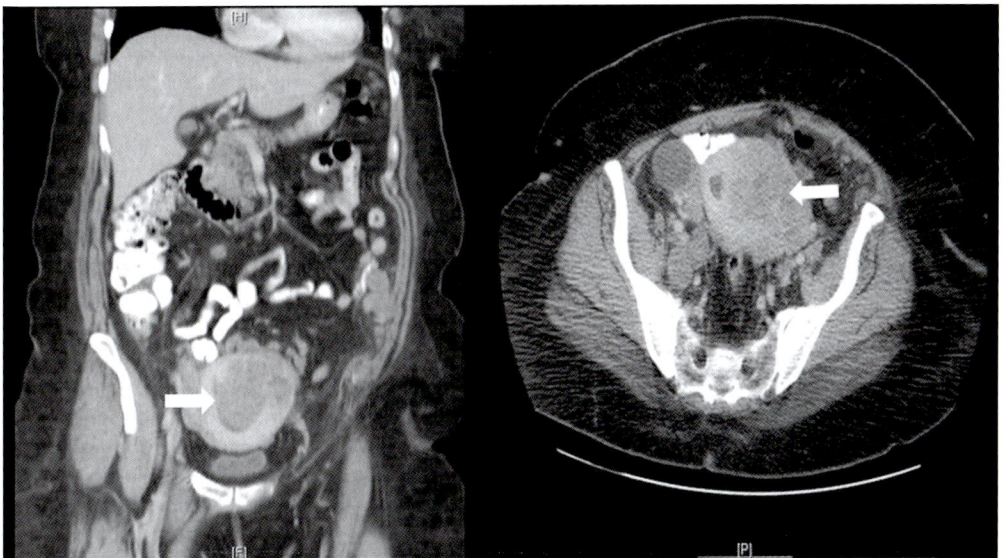

FIGURE 5-7: CT scan showing a large endometrial mass that involves most of the uterus and extends to the level of the cervix, compatible with a large endometrial neoplasm. Note the large heterogenous-appearing endometrial mass in mid-pelvis view.

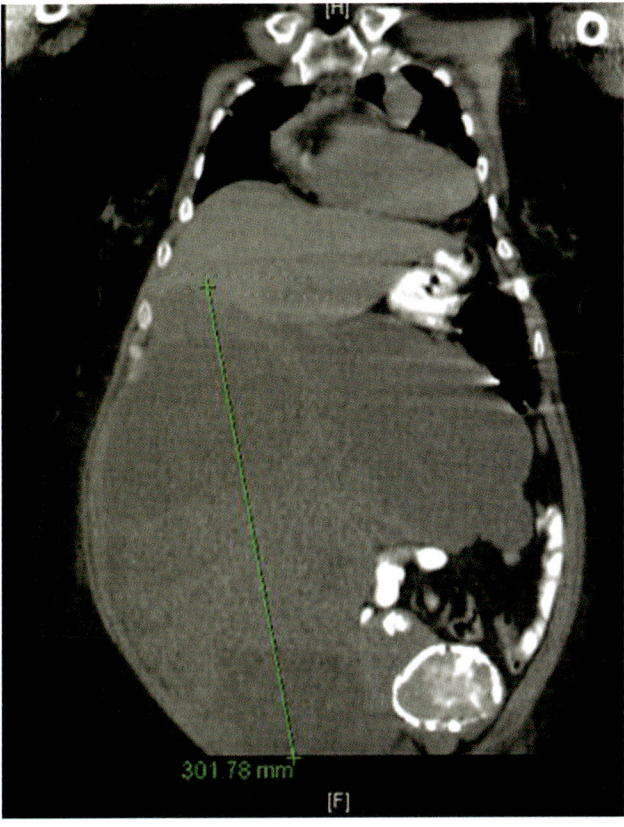

FIGURE 5-8: CT scan of large pelvic mass consistent with late-stage endometrial cancer at time of diagnosis.

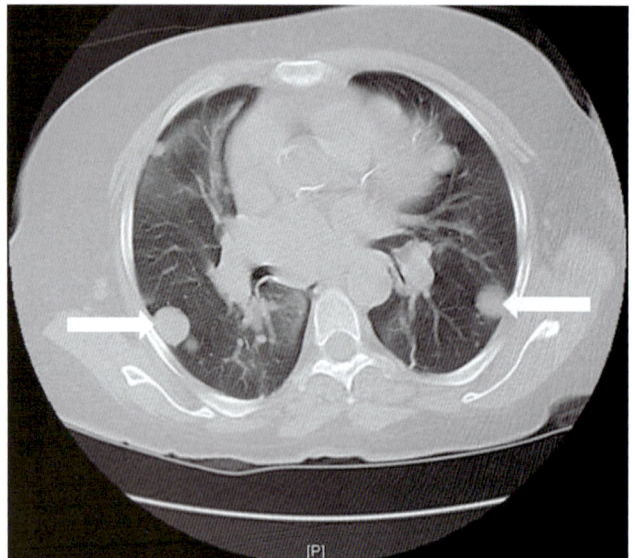

FIGURE 5-9: CT scan showing large pulmonary nodules in a late-stage endometrial cancer.

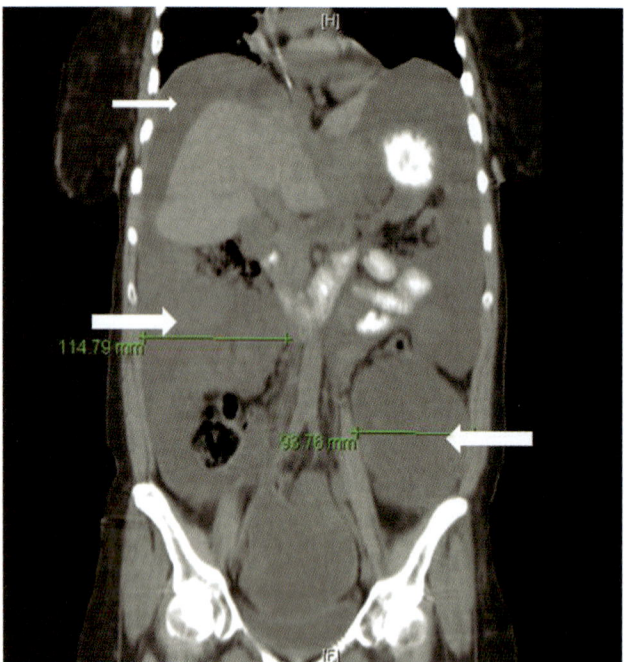

FIGURE 5-10: CT scan showing endometrial cancer recurrence (*large arrows*). Multiple pelvic masses and ascites are noted (*small arrow*).

Chapter 5 • Diagnostic Modalities for Endometrial Carcinoma 121

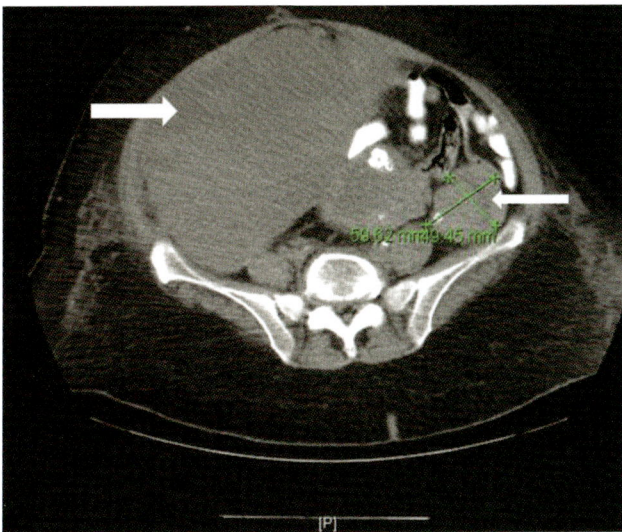

FIGURE 5-11: CT scan showing large pelvic mass, which is diagnosed as late-stage endometrial cancer (*large arrow*). Note the large iliac lymph node on the patient's left side (*small arrow*).

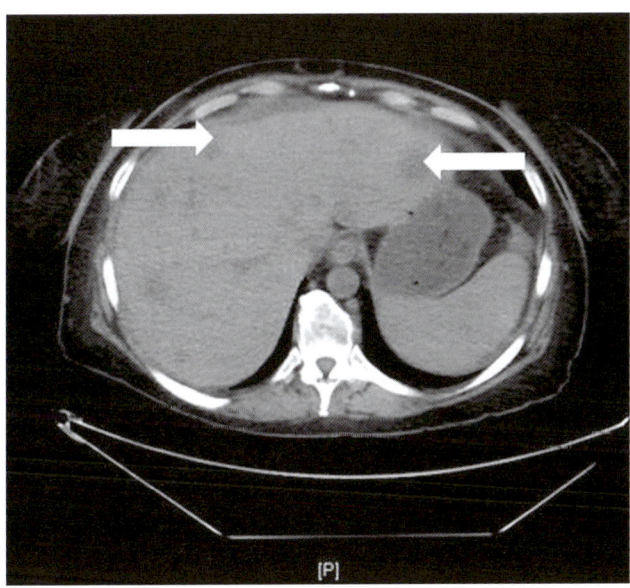

FIGURE 5-12: CT scan showing numerous hypodense masses, which are seen scattered throughout the liver and are consistent with liver metastases. Trace perihepatic ascites is also noted.

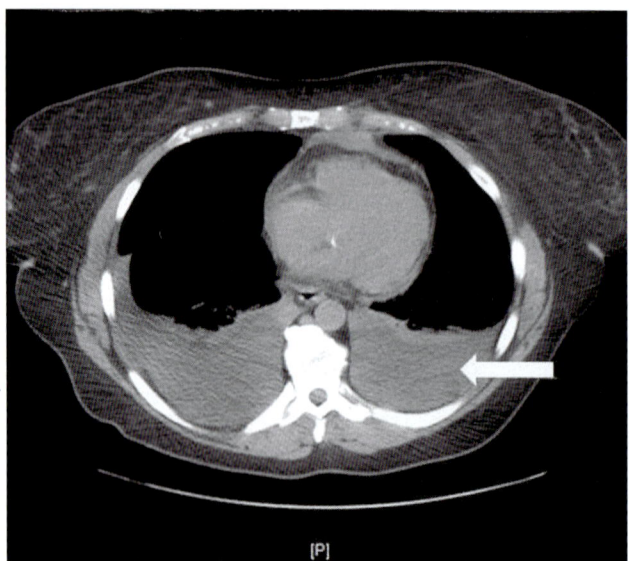

FIGURE 5-13: Pleural effusions seen on CT scan, consistent with late-stage endometrial cancer.

MRI

MRI uses gadolinium contrast intravenously to opacify vessels and to identify the primary tumor, lymph nodes, fistulas, and metastasis.[2] T1-weighted images are fat-saturated and can identify the zones of the uterus by distinguishing the endometrium and the myometrium via greater enhancement than the junctional zone or the space between the two layers.[2] T1-weighted images of cervical mucosa, parametrial tissues, vaginal wall, and submucosa enhance to a greater degree than surrounding tissues after IV contrast administration.[2] T2-weighted images are high-resolution images obtained using the fast spin echo technique.[2] This takes less than 5 minutes, but there are even faster techniques.[2] The faster techniques do not produce the same spatial resolution and are not as helpful in evaluating the pelvis for tumor presence.[2]

MRI is the preferred imaging modality for endometrial cancer preoperative planning.[33,34] MRI consistently performs better in studies comparing it to ultrasound and CT.[2] Both myometrial invasion and cervical extension of tumor are more accurately determined via MRI than ultrasound. MRI is accurate in up to 93% of cases for staging, 95% for cervical extension, and 89% for myometrial invasion.[33] Contrast-enhanced MRI is superior to noncontrast MRI.[35] Overall accuracy for MRI improves from 55% to 83% for noncontrast studies to 85% to 94% for studies with contrast. Gadolinium contrast is used intravenously to improve localization of tumor and depth of myometrial invasion.[35] MRI is typically thought of as an expensive imaging modality, but it is cost effective when used appropriately, as opposed to multiple imaging studies that are often ordered.[2]

MRI is performed in the fasting state with an empty bladder to ensure accuracy of T2-weighted images.[36] Patients are fasting to limit small bowel peristalsis causing artifacts in the images. There are three phases to the MRI evaluation: early enhancement phase at 0 to 1 minute after injection, equilibrium phase at 2 to 3 minutes, and delayed phase at 4 to 5 minutes.[36] Each phase allows identification of important features of endometrial cancer.

T1-weighted images show normal pelvic anatomy in a low- to medium-intensity signal, whereas fat shows a high-intensity signal.[2] T2-weighted images are better suited for soft tissue contrasting and can distinguish layers of vagina, cervix, and uterus by different signal intensity.[2] The T2-weighted MRI shows high-intensity endometrium and medium-intensity myometrium.[2] The use of gadolinium contrast for T1-weighted images further enhances the endometrium and outer myometrium, allowing improved visualization of the junctional zone.[2] The junctional zone helps radiologists evaluate the appearance of myometrial invasion. T1-weighted images are used to evaluate the entire abdomen and pelvis, and the higher resolution T2-weighted images are better suited for imaging the primary tumor.[36] T1 images are suitable for evaluating cervical involvement, and both T1- and T2-weighted images are helpful in determining myometrial invasion[36] (Fig. 5-14).

Myometrial invasion is the one of the most important prognostic factors in endometrial cancer.[33] Patients with stage IB disease (>50% myometrial invasion) have a higher incidence of para-aortic lymph node metastasis. Therefore, for stage IA disease (invasion <50%) and low-grade histology, a surgeon may forego lymph node dissection, whereas for stage IB disease, many surgeons will perform full lymph node dissection.[36] Preoperative determination of myometrial invasion can be extremely helpful in determining extent of surgery, especially in a poor surgical candidate or in a patient who desires fertility-sparing treatment.

MRI is substantially more accurate at identifying deep myometrial invasion than superficial myometrial invasion.[37] The junctional zone is a low-intensity band separating the endometrium from the myometrium, allowing assessment of myometrial invasion.[23] The use of the junctional zone to identify myometrial invasion is limited by the fact that it is most often identified in premenopausal women who do not represent the majority of endometrial cancer cases.[38] In postmenopausal women with thin atrophic endometrium, overestimation of myometrial invasion is more likely than underestimation.[38] This is problematic because older patients who are possibly poor surgical candidates may be subjected to more extensive surgery than necessary if deeper myometrial invasion is suspected on imaging.[38] These mild inaccuracies have been mostly overcome with the use of contrast-enhanced MRI.

Superficial myometrial invasion is seen immediately after injection during the enhancement phase of the MRI, which allows visualization of the subendometrial zone.[36] Deep myometrial invasion is best evaluated during the equilibrium phase of MRI imaging approximately 2 to 3 minutes after injection.[36] Sensitivity and specificity of MRI in assessing

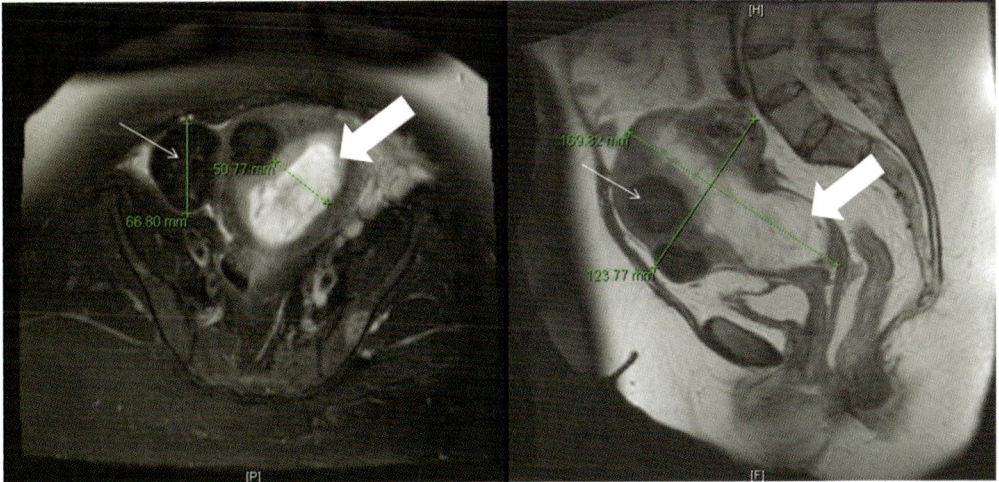

FIGURE 5-14: T2-weighted MRI of pelvis showing fibroids (*small arrow*) and endometrial cancer (*large arrow*).

deep myometrial invasion have been studied, with a sensitivity range of 69% to 94% and a specificity range of 64% to 100% in various studies.[36]

Errors occur when polyps, adenomyosis, leiomyomas, or congenital anomalies obstruct the images.[36,38] Specifically, these findings often lead to underestimation of myometrial invasion.[37] Tumor involvement of the uterine cornua also makes MRI less accurate.[36] Previous uterine curettage also skews results of imaging studies either by causing inflammation in the area or by removing the majority of the tumor.[37] Blood in the uterine cavity can also lead to incorrect MRI findings.[36,38] Large, polypoid tumors also make evaluation by MRI more difficult because they decrease the overall myometrial thickness, making differentiation of deep myometrial invasion problematic.[37,38]

Accurate determination of cervical involvement is critical in determining a surgical plan. A more extensive hysterectomy, such as the radical hysterectomy typically performed for cervical cancer, may be planned for a patient with cervical involvement of cancer. Radiation may be a more appropriate primary treatment plan if extensive parametrial involvement is present.[34] MRI is more accurate than CT in determining presence and extent of cervical involvement.[34] Superficial cervical invasion is not a prognostic factor, but cervical stromal invasion upstages endometrial cancer. Radiologists reading MRI studies look for enhancement of cervical mucosa to rule out cervical stromal invasion during the delayed phase.[36] High-intensity T2-weighted images show abnormal fibrocervical stroma indicating cervical extension.[36] MRI is 92% accurate, 80% sensitive, and 96% specific in visualizing cervical invasion.[36]

Lymph node metastasis is another crucial finding of imaging modalities. Both MRI and CT accurately detect lymph node metastasis in up to 90% of cases when using size criteria (abnormal >1 cm) to detect adenopathy.[2,36] Size criteria mean that tumor invasion should be suspected in nodes greater than 1 cm in size. Recently, the introduction of an MRI contrast agent called ultrasmall superparamagnetic iron oxide (USPIO) particles has increased the lymph node–specific findings of MRI.[36] USPIO is packaged in a contrast agent called ferumoxtran-10.[39] Substantial increases in sensitivity of MRI lymph node evaluation have occurred with this new technology.[36] Specificity remained at almost 100%. MRI previously was not helpful for nodes less than 1 cm in size, and often additional evaluation via PET scanning was required for best accuracy. The USPIO nanoparticles are eaten by macrophages of normal cells and do not show T1 and T2 signal enhancement within lymph nodes because of an artifact from the iron.[39] If malignant tissue is present in the lymph node, the macrophages are displaced so the darkening of the lymph node does not occur and the lymph node with metastatic disease remains bright.[39] Dark lymph nodes are read as benign.[39] Traditional MRI evaluation used size of lymph node greater than 1 cm to suggest malignant transformation, but USPIO allows evaluation of lymph nodes regardless of size.[40] Malignant lymph nodes less than 1 cm can be identified with this method.[40] This technique increased sensitivity from 29% to 93%.[39] The authors of this study suggest that if MRI using USPIO is negative, surgeons could avoid lymph node dissection, especially in morbidly obese or otherwise high-risk patients.[39]

PET

PET scanning is used in a variety of gynecologic cancers, especially in posttreatment surveillance. PET for initial staging of endometrial cancer is not adequately studied, but PET combined with MRI or CT is superior for detection of recurrent disease.[2] PET works by measuring the metabolic activity of cancer cells by injecting radiolabeled molecules, often 18-fluoro-2-deoxy-D-glucose (FDG), to image biologic processes.[41] Glycolysis is increased in cancer cells, so the radiolabeled glucose analog FDG undergoes increased uptake by tumor cells, which can then be visualized.[41] PET can use other compounds to measure different biologic mechanisms if FDG is not available or glucose use is problematic.[42] Different PET compounds can measure fatty acid metabolism or choline metabolism in tumor cells, or they can be used to measure tumor hypoxia.[42]

FDG uptake in normal tissues must be differentiated from areas suspicious for malignancy. In premenopausal patients, ovarian FDG uptake is more intense midcycle, and endometrial FDG uptake is increased during the beginning of the menstrual cycle.[2] Postmenopausal patients do not have physiologic uptake of the FDG in the uterus or ovaries, and any highlighted areas should be suspected as malignant[2] (Fig. 5-15).

PET scanning itself cannot localize the tumor accurately, so it is often combined with CT to increase diagnostic precision.[41,43,44] A CT scan may be performed before and after PET scanning, initially to help with attenuation and subsequently for actual diagnosis.[42] In most cases, CT for attenuation correction is performed prior to PET scanning, but diagnostic CT after PET scanning is unnecessary.[42] Specificity is higher with PET/CT than with PET alone.[44] PET/CT can identify cancerous lesions less than 7 mm in size, even if the FDG uptake is minimal.[42] PET/CT has a high specificity and NPV in lymph node metastasis, but cannot replace surgical staging.[41] False-positive results are high with PET/CT, especially after biopsy causing reactive lymphadenopathy, but this does not take away from its primary purpose in correctly diagnosing distant metastasis.[41,44]

PET imaging requires 4 hours of fasting prior to the scan to keep insulin levels low to prevent a nondiagnostic examination.[2] Because FDG is a glucose derivative, high insulin levels would cause skeletal muscle to uptake the FDG, preventing it from reaching the metabolically active tumor cells.[2] FDG administration in diabetic patients must be undertaken carefully, and often, protocols call for holding the examination if glucose levels are greater than 200 mg/dL.[2] Patients are injected with the FDG intravenously, and then PET scanning occurs approximately 1 hour later.[2] Patients are often given diuretics or catheterized to reduce bladder activity that could disturb the results.[42]

False-positive FDG uptake can occur in premenopausal women depending on the phase of the menstrual cycle. Preferably imaging occurs a week prior to menstruation because

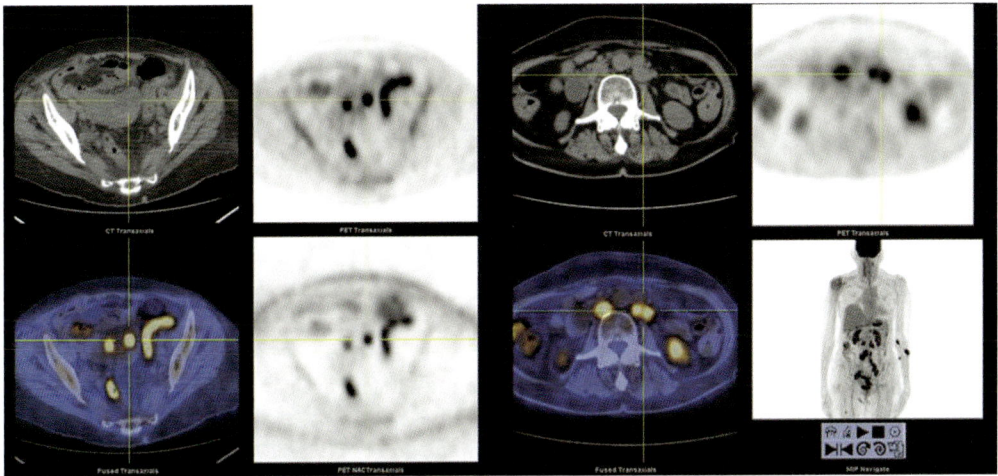

FIGURE 5-15: PET scan (**left**) showing abnormal FDG uptake in two uterine masses. Physiologic bowel uptake is noted. PET scan (**right**) showing enlarge lymph nodes with abnormal FDG uptake.

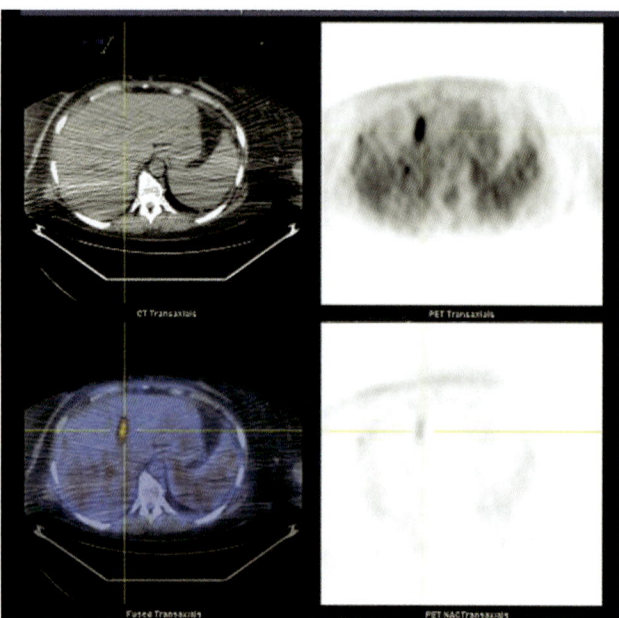

FIGURE 5-16: PET scan showing FDG uptake in a liver nodule, indicating metastasis.

the highest FDG uptake occurs during menses.[2] Postmenopausal women can undergo PET scanning at any time. Women who are taking HRT or tamoxifen are treated as postmenopausal women because there are no studies on the subject.[2]

PET scanning is rarely used for initial preoperative planning for endometrial cancer but is often used for posttreatment surveillance. Microscopic tumor properties detected by increased metabolic activity can be recognized by PET earlier than macroscopic tumor foci identified with CT or MRI.[43] It is helpful in detecting recurrence when a patient does not have symptoms, and a negative PET scan correlates well with patient survival.[33] Park et al.[43] showed that PET and PET/CT combined had 96% accuracy in diagnosing recurrence in 24 symptomatic patients. In 66 asymptomatic patients who underwent PET/CT scanning as part of routine surveillance, the accuracy was 100%, with no false-positive or false-negative results.[43] Another study found that FDG-PET was 96% sensitive and 78% specific in posttreatment cancer surveillance.[42] PET scanning contributes to treatment planning by helping physicians determine the need for chemotherapy versus radiation therapy for recurrence. It is also helpful in mapping the radiation field needed to adequately treat a recurrence.[43] PET scanning can also help a physician determine whether salvage surgery such as pelvic exenteration is feasible[43] (Fig. 5-16).

References

1. Benshushan A. Endometrial adenocarcinoma in young patients: evaluation and fertility-preserving treatment. *Eur J Obstet Gynecol Reprod Biol.* 2004;117:132–137.
2. Barakat R, Markman M, Randall M. *Principles and Practice of Gynecologic Oncology.* 5th ed. Philadelphia: Lippincott Williams & Wilkins; 2009:96–104, 153–156, 197–216, 683–722.
3. Bakkum-Gamez J, Gonzalez-Bosquet J, Laack N, et al. Current issues in the management of endometrial cancer. *Mayo Clin Proc.* 2008;83:97–112.

4. Zhou J, Tomashefski J, Khiyami A. ThinPrep Pap tests in patients with endometrial cancer: a histo-cytological correlation. *Diagn Cytopathol*. 2007;35:448–453.
5. Thrall M, Kjeldahl K, Gulbahce J, et al. Liquid based Papanicolaou test (Surepath) interpretations before histologic diagnosis of endometrial hyperplasias and carcinomas. *Cancer*. 2007;111:217–223.
6. Beal H, Stone J, Beckmann M, et al. Endometrial cells identified in cervical cytology in women > 40 years of age: criteria for appropriate endometrial evaluation. *Am J Obstet Gynecol*. 2007;196:568.e1–568.e6.
7. Frable W. Screening for endometrial cancer? *Cancer*. 2008;114:219–222.
8. Wright T, Massad L, Dunton C, et al. 2006 consensus guidelines for the management of women with abnormal cervical cancer screening tests. *Am J Obstet Gynecol*. 2007;197:346–355.
9. Brown AK, Gillis S, Deuel C, et al. Abnormal cervical cytology: a risk factor for endometrial cancer recurrence. *Int J Gynecol Cancer*. 2005;15:517–522.
10. Clark T, Mann C, Shah N, et al. Accuracy of outpatient endometrial biopsy in the diagnosis of endometrial cancer: a systematic quantitative review. *BJOG*. 2002;109:313–321.
11. Fakhar S, Saeed G, Khan A, et al. Validity of Pipelle endometrial sampling in patients with abnormal uterine bleeding. *Ann Saudi Med*. 2008;28:188–191.
12. Tanriverdi J, Barut A, Gun B, et al. Is Pipelle biopsy really adequate for diagnosing endometrial disease? *Med Sci Monit*. 2004;10:271–274.
13. Larson DM, Johnson KK, Broste SK, et al. Comparison of D&C and office endometrial biopsy in predicting final histopathologic grade in endometrial cancer. *Obstet Gynecol*. 1995;86:38–42.
14. Ben-Yehuda OM, Kim YB, Leuchter RS. Does hysteroscopy improve upon the sensitivity of dilation and curettage in the diagnosis of endometrial hyperplasia or carcinoma? *Gynecol Oncol*. 1998;68:4–7.
15. Schorge J, Schaffer J, Halvorson L, et al. *Williams Gynecology*. New York: McGraw-Hill; 2008: 950–953.
16. Hsieh C, ChangChien C, Lin H, et al. Can a preoperative CA-125 level be a criterion for full pelvic lymphadenectomy in surgical staging of endometrial cancer? *Gynecol Oncol*. 2002;86:28–33.
17. Yurkovetsky Z, Ta'asan S, Skates S, et al. Development of multimarker panel for early detection of endometrial cancer. High diagnostic power of prolactin. *Gynecol Oncol*. 2007;107:58–65.
18. Santin A, Diamandis E, Bellone S, et al. Human kallikrein 6: a new potential serum biomarker for uterine serous papillary cancer. *Clin Cancer Res*. 2005;11:3320–3325.
19. Mylonas I, Worbs S, Shabani N, et al. Inhibin-alpha subunit is an independent prognostic parameter in human endometrial carcinomas: analysis of inhibin/activin-alpha, -betaA, -betaB subunits in 302 cases. *Eur J Cancer*. 2006;45:1304–1314.
20. Di Simone N, Schneyer A, Caliandro D, et al. Regulation of endometrial adenocarcinoma cell proliferation by activin-a and its modulation by 17B-estradiol. *Mol Cell Endocrinol*. 2002;192:187–195.
21. Petraglia F, Florio P, Luisi S, et al. Expression and secretion of inhibin and activin in normal and neoplastic uterine tissues. High levels of serum activin A in women with endometrial and cervical carcinoma. *Endocrinol Metab*. 1998;83:1194–1200.
22. Barakat R, Hricak H. What do we expect from imaging? *Radiol Clin North Am*. 2002;40:521–526.
23. Cagnazzo G, Addario V, Martinelli G, et al. Depth of myometrial invasion in endometrial cancer: preoperative assessment by transvaginal ultrasonography and magnetic resonance imaging. *Ultrasound Obstet Gynecol*. 1992;1:40–43.
24. Bosch T, Schourbroeck D, Domali E, et al. A thin and regular endometrium on ultrasound is very unlikely in patients with endometrial malignancy. *Ultrasound Obstet Gynecol*. 2007;29:674–679.
25. Garuti G, Cellani F, Grossi F, et al. Saline infusion sonography and office hysteroscopy to assess endometrial morbidity associated with tamoxifen intake. *Gynecol Oncol*. 2002;86:323–329.
26. Sokalaska A, Valentin L. Changes in ultrasound morphology of the uterus and ovaries during the menopausal transition and early postmenopause: a 4-year longitudinal study. *Ultrasound Obstet Gynecol*. 2008;31:210–217.
27. Gupta J, Chien P, Voit D, et al. Ultrasonographic endometrial thickness for diagnosing endometrial pathology in women with postmenopausal bleeding: a meta-analysis. *Acta Obstet Gynecol Scand*. 2002;81:799–816.

28. Smith-Bindman R, Kerlikowske K, Feldstein V, et al. Endovaginal ultrasound to exclude endometrial cancer and other endometrial abnormalities. *JAMA*. 1998;280:1510–1517.
29. Pektas M, Gungor T, Mollamahmutoglu L. The evaluation of endometrial tumors by transvaginal and Doppler ultrasonography. *Arch Gynecol Obstet*. 2008;277:495–499.
30. Develioglu O, Bilgin T, Yalcin O, et al. Adjunctive use of the uterine artery resistance index in the preoperative prediction of myometrial invasion in endometrial carcinoma. *Gynecol Oncol*. 1999;72:26–31.
31. Alcazar J, Galvan R, Albela S, et al. Assessing myometrial infiltration by endometrial cancer: uterine virtual navigation with three dimensional US. *Radiology*. 2009;250:776–783.
32. Weaver J, McHugo J, Clark T. Accuracy of transvaginal ultrasound in diagnosing endometrial pathology in women with post-menopausal bleeding on tamoxifen. *Br J Radiol*. 2005;78:394–397.
33. Lee S, Andreotti R, Angtuaco T, et al. American College of Radiology Appropriateness Criteria: endometrial cancer of the uterus. Reviewed 2007. Available at http://www.acr.org/SecondaryMainMenuCategories/quality_safety/app_criteria.aspx.
34. Kinkel K, Kaji Y, Yu K, et al. Radiologic staging in patients with endometrial cancer: a meta-analysis. *Radiology*. 1999;212:711–718.
35. Hricak H, Hamm B, Semelka R, et al. Carcinoma of the uterus: use of gadopentetate dimeglumine in MR imaging. *Radiology*. 1991;181:95–106.
36. Sala E, Wakely S, Senior E, et al. MRI of malignant neoplasms of the uterine corpus and cervix. *Am J Radiol*. 2007;188:1577–1587.
37. Chung H, Kang S, Cho J, et al. Accuracy of MR imaging for the prediction of myometrial invasion of endometrial carcinoma. *Gynecol Oncol*. 2007;104:654–659.
38. Sironi S, Taccagni G, Garancini P, et al. Myometrial invasion by endometrial carcinoma: assessment by MR imaging. *Am J Radiol*. 1992;158:565–569.
39. Rockall A, Sohaib A, Harisinghani M, et al. Diagnostic performance of nanoparticle-enhanced magnetic resonance imaging in the diagnosis of lymph node metastases in patients with endometrial and cervical cancer. *J Clin Oncol*. 2005;23:2813–2821.
40. Manfredi R, Mirk P, Maresca G, et al. Local-regional staging of endometrial carcinoma: role of MR imaging in surgical planning. *Radiology*. 2004;231:372–378.
41. Park J-Y, Kim E, Kim D-Y, et al. Comparison of the validity of magnetic resonance imaging and positron emission tomography/computed tomography in the preoperative evaluation of patients with uterine corpus cancer. *Gynecol Oncol*. 2008;108:486–492.
42. Lai C, Yen T, Chang T. Positron emission tomography imaging for gynecologic malignancy. *Curr Opin Obstet Gynecol*. 2007;19:37–41.
43. Park J-Y, Kim E, Kim D-Y, et al. Clinical impact of positron emission tomography or positron emission tomography/computed tomography in the posttherapy surveillance of endometrial carcinoma: evaluation of 88 patients. *Int J Gynecol Cancer*. 2008;18:1332–1338.
44. Sironi S, Picchio M, Landoni C, et al. Post therapy surveillance of patients with uterine cancer: value of integrated FDG PET/CT in the detection of recurrence. *Eur J Nucl Med Mol Imaging*. 2007;34:472–479.

Current Management and Issues in Treatment of Endometrial Carcinoma

▶ Tri A. Dinh, MD, and
Reagan Street, MD

Endometrial cancer is the leading cause of gynecologic cancer in the United States, with approximately 40,000 cases diagnosed per year. Endometrial cancer follows only lung, breast, and colon cancers as a cause of cancer in women. It is the most common of the gynecologic cancers.[1] Seventy-five percent of patients with endometrial cancer are postmenopausal, but 3% to 5% are younger than 40 years old.[2] Management of endometrial cancer, whether surgical or medical, must take into consideration the histology of the cancer, the stage of the disease at presentation, and the patient's comorbidities; in young women with early-stage endometrioid carcinoma, the patient's desire for future fertility is also considered.

Ninety percent of endometrial cancers arise in the endometrial glands as opposed to the endometrial stroma or myometrium.[3] There are two types of endometrial cancers that are subdivided by histology. Type I accounts for 80% of endometrial cancer, is caused by hyperestrogenism, usually in the setting of obesity, and arises in a background of atypical hyperplasia. A European study reported that obesity is the cause of up to 39% of all endometrial cancers.[4] Large amounts of adipose tissue aromatize estrogen, leading to increased estrogen effects on the uterus. Endometrial proliferation caused by estrogen may cause neoplastic change in the absence of progesterone, either endogenous or exogenous.[4] Type II endometrial cancer develops in a population without a history of long-term unopposed estrogen, usually in nonobese women. Type II cancer occurs in the setting of an atrophic endometrium.[4] Type I is usually low-grade endometrioid histology, whereas type II includes more aggressive clear cell and papillary serous cancers. Type I is almost always confined to the uterus, and outcomes of survival are considerably better than type II cancer, which has often metastasized prior to diagnosis even without evidence of extensive myometrial invasion.[3]

Endometrial cancer patients are typically obese and postmenopausal and are at high risk for cardiovascular disease and diabetes. Because the majority of patients diagnosed with endometrial cancer are older and have multiple associated comorbidities, surgical planning must consider issues of cardiac and pulmonary tolerance for major surgery, wound healing, and subsequent ability to tolerate adjuvant therapy, if needed.

HISTOLOGY AND CLINICAL CORRELATION

Endometrial Hyperplasia

Endometrial hyperplasia carries a reasonably high risk of progression to endometrial cancer if not adequately treated. Simple hyperplasia without cytologic atypia carries a less than 1% chance of progression to cancer, whereas complex hyperplasia without atypia has a 2% to 3% chance of progression to cancer. Thus, these two entities are usually treated medically using progesterone therapy. With cytologic atypia, simple hyperplasia and complex hyperplasia carry an 8% and 27% to 28% chance of progression to cancer, respectively. With cytologic atypia, hysterectomy is usually the treatment of choice unless future fertility is still desired.[5]

With a diagnosis of complex endometrial hyperplasia with atypia found on either in-office endometrial sampling or dilation and curettage, there is a significant risk of concurrent endometrial cancer at the time of hysterectomy. The Gynecologic Oncology Group (GOG), in a study with 302 patients diagnosed in the community with atypical endometrial hyperplasia (GOG Protocol 167A), found that there is poor reproducibility of the diagnosis when a panel of GOG pathologists reviewed the original biopsy slides. These patients, treated with hysterectomy within 12 weeks of study entry without other intervening treatments, had a 43% incidence of concurrent endometrial cancer.[6] In a recent study using the extensive patient database of the Kaiser Permanente Group, Suh-Burgmann et al.[7] found that there is a 48% incidence of endometrial cancer when the patient had a preoperative diagnosis of atypical endometrial hyperplasia.

The high incidence of endometrial cancer when the patient undergoes hysterectomy for atypical endometrial hyperplasia underscores two dilemmas in diagnosis. First, it is often difficult to distinguish histologically between atypical endometrial hyperplasia and well-differentiated endometrioid cancer. Second, typical office endometrial biopsy instruments sample only a small proportion of the entire uterine cavity, giving rise to the possibility of error due to sampling inadequacy.[8] Clinically, it is important to ascertain the diagnosis preoperatively because the majority of patients with atypical endometrial hyperplasia are treated surgically by general gynecologic surgeons who may not be trained to perform lymphadenectomy to complete surgical staging of an endometrial cancer.

Endometrioid Carcinoma

Preoperative grade of disease and depth of myometrial invasion are key factors in determination of extent of surgical staging (Tables 6-1 and 6-2). Patients with low-grade disease (grades 1 and 2) and minimal myometrial invasion have low risk ($\leq 5\%$) of lymph nodal metastasis.[9] Although pelvic and para-aortic lymphadenectomy to stage endometrial cancer is routinely performed by gynecologic oncologists, the procedure does have inherent risks of blood loss, infection associated with prolonging surgical time, injury to nearby nerves and vasculature, lymphocyst formation, and lymphedema. Surgery is more challenging due to the anatomic constraints of morbid obesity, a common characteristic of patients with endometrial cancer. Thus, the risk of complications due to the procedure must be weighed with the benefits of diagnosis of lymphadenopathy to diagnose and remove metastatic disease.

Although surgical staging has been advocated since 1988 with the inclusion of surgical criteria in the International Federation of Gynecology and Obstetrics (FIGO) staging guidelines, only 40% of patients in the United States are surgically staged. This dichotomy between

Table 6-1	Histologic Grade and Depth of Invasion			
	Grade			
Depth	G1 (%)	G2 (%)	G3 (%)	Total (%)
Endometrium only	44 (24)	31 (11)	11 (7)	86 (14)
Superficial	96 (53)	131 (45)	54 (35)	281 (45)
Middle	22 (12)	69 (24)	24 (16)	115 (19)
Deep	18 (10)	57 (20)	64 (42)	139 (22)
Total	180 (100)	288 (100)	153 (100)	621 (100)

Reprinted from Creasman WT, Morro CP, Bundy BN, et al. Surgical pathologic spread patterns of endometrial cancer. A Gynecologic Oncology Group study. *Cancer*. 1987;60(8 suppl):2035–2041.

what is advocated and what is actually done is due to the previously stated fact that the majority of patients with endometrial cancer are treated by general gynecologic surgeons who are not trained in necessary techniques to complete surgical staging.[10] In a multicenter study of 9,000 patients, only 30% of patients undergoing surgical treatment of endometrial cancer received lymph node assessment. In the same study, 28% of patients received postoperative radiation treatment despite lack of adequate staging information indicating the need for adjuvant radiation. Adequate surgical staging can identify as many as 20% of patients with extrauterine disease previously thought to have stage I disease based on clinical evaluation.[11]

Table 6-2	Frequency of Nodal Metastasis in Lymph Nodes Based on Uterine Risk Factors			
	Grade			
Depth of Invasion	G1	G2	G3
	(N = 180)	(N = 288)	(N = 153)
Pelvic Lymph Nodes			
Endometrium only (N = 86)	0 (0%)	1 (3%)	0 (0%)
Inner (N = 281)	3 (3%)	7 (5%)	5 (9%)
Middle (N = 115)	0 (0%)	6 (9%)	1 (4%)
Deep (N = 139)	2 (11%)	11 (19%)	22 (34%)
Aortic Lymph Nodes			
Endometrium only (N = 86)	0 (0%)	1 (3%)	0 (0%)
Inner (N = 281)	1 (1%)	5 (4%)	2 (4%)
Middle (N = 115)	1 (5%)	0 (0%)	0 (0%)
Deep (N =139)	1 (6%)	8 (14%)	15 (23%)

Reprinted from Creasman WT, Morro CP, Bundy BN, et al. Surgical pathologic spread patterns of endometrial cancer. A Gynecologic Oncology Group study. *Cancer*. 1987;60(8 suppl):2035–2041.

Many gynecologic surgeons practice selective lymphadenectomy, believing that full lymph node dissection should be reserved for those at highest risk for metastatic disease. Data from the surgicopathologic study by the GOG (Protocol 33) suggest that uterine parameters including grade, depth of invasion, and cervical involvement may be used to determine the risk of lymph node involvement to decide whether or not to perform lymphadenectomy[9] (see Table 6-2). Surgeons must decide for themselves their cutoff value for deciding to perform lymphadenectomy, taking into consideration the risk of positive lymph nodes, their own incidence and experience with complications, and the published risk of serious complications from the literature of less than 6%.[12]

High-Risk Histologies

Routine surgical staging for endometrial cancer, including total abdominal hysterectomy, bilateral salpingo-oophorectomy, and pelvic and para-aortic lymphadenectomy, may not be adequate for patients with high-risk histologies such as clear cell or serous carcinomas. Serous or clear cell histology carries a higher risk of positive lymph nodes.[13] Chan et al.[14] found that omentectomy may be needed to find the 25% of patients who present with stage IVB serous endometrial carcinoma. They advocate that patients with serous endometrial carcinoma undergo "extended" surgical staging similar to that done for patients with ovarian carcinoma, with the inclusion of omentectomy and peritoneal biopsies in addition to routine lymphadenectomy.

Carcinosarcoma

Carcinosarcoma (malignant mixed müllerian tumor) is histologically defined as having both malignant epithelial (carcinoma) as well as mesodermal (sarcoma) components. Many studies confirm that these cancers arise from a single clonal cell population and should be considered anaplastic carcinomas. Clinically, the behavior of the tumor is driven by the carcinomatous component of the cancer; most metastatic sites include only the carcinoma component. The carcinomatous components are more likely to appear more aggressive, invading into the myometrium or lymphovascular spaces.[15] Clinical treatment for this cancer is typically geared toward treating the carcinomatous element.

FIGO STAGING FOR ENDOMETRIAL CANCER

In 2009, FIGO revised its staging criteria for endometrial cancer (Table 6-3). The new revision reflects improved understanding of the natural history of endometrial cancer and the survival and recurrence data obtained from decades of treating the disease. The changes may be summed up in several general statements. First, patients with minimally invasive cancer uniformly do well. Second, the prognosis of patients with cervical glandular involvement is dependent on other uterine factors (depth of invasion, grade, and the presence of lymphovascular invasion). Similarly, the presence of positive peritoneal cytology does not portend a bad prognosis without other histologic high-risk factors. Prior to 2009, uterine sarcoma (e.g., leiomyosarcoma), endometrial sarcoma, adenosarcomas, and carcinosarcomas have been staged using the same criteria as for endometrial carcinomas. In 2009, FIGO devised a separate staging guideline for sarcomas. Carcinosarcomas will continue to be staged using carcinoma guidelines.

Table 6-3	Revised 2009 FIGO Staging for Endometrial Carcinoma (changes from 1988 FIGO guidelines)
Stage I*: Tumor confined to the corpus uteri	
IA*: No or less than half myometrial invasion	
IB*: Invasion equal to or more than half of the myometrium	
(New guideline eliminates endometrium-confined cancer as a specific category.)	
Stage II*: Tumor invades cervical stroma but does not extend beyond the uterus†	
(New guideline eliminates cervical glandular involvement as a specific category [stage IIA] in the 1988 guideline.)	
Stage III*: Local and/or regional spread of the tumor	
IIIA*: Tumor invades the serosa of the corpus uteri and/or adnexae‡	
IIIB*: Vaginal and/or parametrial involvement‡	
IIIC*: Metastases to pelvic and/or para-aortic lymph nodes‡	
IIIC1*: Positive pelvic nodes	
IIIC2*: Positive para-aortic lymph nodes with or without positive pelvic lymph nodes	
(New guideline eliminates positive cytology as part of stage IIIA. It also subcategorizes pelvic and para-aortic lymph nodes as subsets of stage IIIC.)	
Stage IV*: Tumor invades bladder and/or bowel mucosa, and/or distant metastases	
IVA*: Tumor invasion of bladder and/or bowel mucosa	
IVB*: Distant metastases, including intra-abdominal metastases and/or inguinal lymph nodes	

FIGO, International Federation of Gynecology and Obstetrics.
*Either G1, G2, or G3.
†Endocervical glandular involvement only should be considered as stage I and no longer as stage II.
‡Positive cytology has to be reported separately without changing the stage.

INITIAL TREATMENT FOR ENDOMETRIAL CANCER

Surgery

The mainstay for treatment of endometrial cancer is surgery. Typically, the surgery includes removal of the uterus and bilateral adnexal, pelvic, and para-aortic lymph nodes. Peritoneal cytology is also done, and the presence or absence of abnormal cells is noted, but this is no longer included as part of the staging criteria. For high-risk histologies, omentectomy and peritoneal biopsies are also done as part of "extended" surgical staging.

Minimally Invasive Surgery

Over the last decade, there has been a shift toward minimally invasive surgery for many gynecologic conditions. The same trend is true for the surgical treatment of endometrial cancer. Laparoscopic hysterectomy and bilateral salpingo-oophorectomy have been done routinely since the 1980s for benign indications. These procedures, as well as laparoscopic lymphadenectomy, have been adopted by gynecologic oncologists for the treatment of their patients with endometrial cancer. Recently, outcomes of patients with endometrial cancer treated with conventional laparotomy versus laparoscopy have been compared. In the LAP-2 study by the

GOG, 1,696 patients with stage I and IIA disease (cervical glandular involvement without stromal involvement by 1988 FIGO staging criteria) were randomized between laparotomy and laparoscopy for surgical staging. Laparoscopy was successful in 74.2% of patients, requiring conversion to laparotomy in 25.8% of patients; both groups had similar intraoperative complication rates. The most common reason for conversion from laparoscopy to laparotomy was poor visibility (14.6%). Other reasons include advanced disease requiring laparotomy to complete the surgery (4.1%), excessive bleeding (2.9%), and other reasons (4.2%). Increasing age, higher body mass index, and advanced disease are statistically significant predictors of conversion to laparotomy. The use of laparoscopy shortened the hospital length of stay but increased the time in the operating room. In 8% of patients in the laparoscopy group, pelvic and para-aortic lymph nodes were not removed, in contrast to only 4% of patients in the laparotomy group.[16] In early 2010, the results were updated to include survival and recurrence data. At 3 years, there was no difference between the two groups in terms of survival, with nearly 90% of patients alive in both the laparoscopy and laparotomy arms.[17] In terms of quality of life, patients who underwent laparoscopic treatment for endometrial cancer reported a better quality of life at 6 weeks after surgery; however, the differences between the two groups were not statistically significant by 6 months except for an improved body image score in the laparoscopy group.[18]

The use of the robotic surgical platform is now common in the treatment of endometrial cancer. For many gynecologic surgeons, the use of the robotic platform with its three-dimensional view allows use of conventional surgical techniques within the confines of a minimally invasive procedure. This increase in laparoscopic dexterity comes at a price of loss of tactile feel; however, the lack of haptic sense is offset by the increased vision of the camera technology of the robotic platform. Although there are no randomized trials to compare robotic surgery for endometrial cancer to conventional laparoscopy or laparotomy, a preponderance of large case series suggest that robotically assisted laparoscopic surgery is very similar to conventional laparoscopic surgery for the treatment of endometrial cancer in terms of blood loss, complication rate, postoperative recovery time, and probably outcome.[19]

The Role of Lymphadenectomy

Pelvic and para-aortic lymphadenectomy are typically done as part of comprehensive surgical staging for endometrial cancer. This is standard practice in the United States, but not in many European countries. Proponents of lymphadenectomy cite that reasons supporting the procedure are to define a subset of patient who may not benefit from adjuvant therapy, to define the field of radiation, and possibly, to improve outcome by removal of metastatic disease. There is good evidence to suggest that lymphadenectomy may lead to more treatment with radiation and yet does not improve overall survival.[20]

For preoperative grade 1 endometrial cancer, two management strategies, one favoring routine lymphadenectomy and one not, were compared in terms of recurrence-free and overall survival. At Duke University, patients were surgically staged unless the patient had grade 1 disease, limited to one-half myometrial invasion. At Toronto Sunnybrook Regional Cancer Center (TSRCC), patients were not routinely staged. Thus, nearly 50% of patients had lymphadenectomy at Duke, whereas only 12% of patients had lymphadenectomy at TSRCC. More patients (21%) at TSRCC received adjuvant radiation therapy versus 7% of patients at Duke. At 3 years, overall and recurrence-free survival rates of patients at both institutions were similar (96% versus 96% for overall survival and 96% versus 95% for recurrence-free survival).[21]

The ASTEC trial conducted in 85 centers in four countries (United Kingdom, Poland, South Africa, and New Zealand) randomized 1,408 women to receive either hysterectomy with pelvic lymphadenectomy (lymphadenectomy group) or hysterectomy with nodal sampling only if clinically suspicious (standard surgery group). In 1,369 women who were confirmed to have endometrial cancer (39 women did not have endometrial cancer after pathology review), 5% of women in the standard surgery group had lymphadenectomy (median number of nodes, 2), and 90% of women in the lymphadenectomy group ultimately had lymphadenectomy (median number of nodes, 12). At a median follow-up of 37 months, there was no difference in overall survival between the two groups when adjuvant pelvic radiation was given based on uterine risk factors (stage IA; stage IB with grade 3, serous or clear cell histology; stage IC; or stage IIA, based on 1988 FIGO staging). The hazard ratios for 5-year overall survival and recurrence-free survival were not different between the two groups ($P = .83$ and $P = .14$, respectively). Based on the results of this large randomized surgical trial, the authors suggest that pelvic lymphadenectomy is not necessary or recommended for patients with clinical stage I endometrial cancer, unless the procedure is part of a clinical trial.[22]

There is some nonrandomized evidence to suggest that there is a therapeutic benefit to lymphadenectomy. Kilgore et al.[23] reviewed their data at the University of Alabama at Birmingham involving 649 patients with endometrial cancer. Two hundred twelve patients underwent "multiple-site" pelvic lymph node sampling, defined as removal of lymph nodes from at least four sites including the common iliac, external and internal iliacs, and obturator nodal chains (mean node count, 11), whereas 205 patients underwent limited node sampling, defined as removal of lymph nodes from fewer than four sites (mean node count, 4), and 208 patients had no node sampling. Patients with multiple-site lymph node sampling had better survival than those who had no lymph node sampling. In the group that received pelvic radiation, those who had multiple-site lymph node sampling still had better survival than those who had no lymph node sampling. For low-risk and high-risk patients (high risk defined as disease outside the uterine corpus), patients who underwent multiple-site lymph node sampling had better survival than low-risk patients who were given pelvic radiation without lymph node sampling.[23] Cragun et al.[24] from Duke, in a retrospective study of 509 patients, found that removal of more than 11 pelvic lymph nodes confers a survival advantage over removal of less than 11 pelvic lymph nodes in patients with poorly differentiated endometrial cancer. Even when the patients with positive lymph nodes were removed from the data set, patients with more than 11 lymph nodes removed as part of their surgical treatment had better overall survival.[24]

Although these studies suggest a therapeutic effect to lymphadenectomy for patients with endometrial cancer, their conclusion should be interpreted in view of their retrospective nature. Retrospective surgical studies are prone to bias due to the differences in the cohort that does or does not receive the surgical intervention. It is entirely possible that the improved survival seen in the patients who had lymphadenectomy is related to their overall fitness, which allowed them to have the surgery in the first place. In addition, these types of studies are prone to the "stage migration" effect because there will be a cohort of patients not surgically staged who actually may have occult undetected metastatic disease.

Selective lymph node dissection is practiced by some gynecologic surgeons who will remove palpably abnormal lymph nodes. This method is not supported by the literature. Arango et al.[25] reported on their experience with 126 women undergoing lymphadenectomy for endometrial cancer. Experienced surgeons in practice for a mean of 9.3 years removed 2,138 nodes. Sensitivity and specificity for this group of surgeons were 72% and 81%, respectively.[25] Similar results were found by Eltabbakh,[26] who suggests that palpation is not a substitute for histologic examination.

"Debulking" Surgery for Advanced-Stage Disease at Initial Presentation

Although the majority of patients with endometrial cancer will have disease confined to the uterus, it is not uncommon for patients with poorly differentiated cancer or high-risk histologies to initially present with bulky metastatic disease. Using the same paradigm as in ovarian cancer, gynecologic oncologists have applied a similar surgical principle of optimal cytoreduction. There is consistent evidence in many case series that removal of visible disease improves overall survival. These studies define optimal cytoreduction differently (residual disease <2 cm or <1 cm or no visible disease). Patients who are optimally cytoreduced have a better overall survival than patients who are not able to achieve optimal cytoreduction. In one study by Lambrou et al.,[27] patients with stage IIIC and IV disease who were optimally cytoreduced to less than 2 cm had a median survival of 17.8 months versus a median survival of 6.7 months in patients who did not approach optimal status. Whether this finding reflects surgical skill or inherent differences in tumor, biology is a source of ongoing debate.

Radiation Therapy

Some patients with endometrial cancer are not surgical candidates due to medical comorbidities. In these patients, the risk of death or serious complications from surgery may outweigh the risk of death from the cancer itself. However, in many instances, there is the need for palliation of symptoms such as vaginal bleeding. Radiation therapy is an option that may be used with curative intent as well as a method to palliate symptoms.

The American Brachytherapy Society has published recommendations for treatment of patients with endometrial cancer who are not surgical candidates. Most patients are candidates for external-beam radiation therapy followed by brachytherapy. In a subset of patients who clinically have early disease (grade 1 or 2, limited to the endometrium), treatment may consist of brachytherapy only. Preoperative treatment planning may be done with either computed tomography or magnetic resonance imaging (MRI). For evaluation of depth of myometrial invasion, MRI may offer better resolution.[28]

Several institutional case series have reported good results for primary radiation therapy for patients who were inoperable. Fishman et al.[29] from Yale reported on 54 patients who were treated between 1975 and 1992. In these patients with endometrial cancer clinically confined to the uterus, the 5-year, cancer-specific survival rates were 80% and 85% for patients with stage I and II disease, respectively. This is only slightly lower than the rate of a similar cohort treated with primary surgery. However, the 5-year overall survival was much lower in the cohort who was treated with primary radiation for clinical stage I disease (30%) compared with patients treated with surgery (88%). This suggests that for inoperable patients, medical issues and comorbidities may play a bigger role in survival than endometrial cancer.[29]

A large series of 325 patients from Vienna treated with primary radiation therapy for inoperable endometrial cancer confirmed the above findings. The 5-year overall survival rate ranged from 40% to 63% for early-stage cancer confined to the uterus. At 10 years, the survival rate was between 21% and 35% for the same group of patients.[30]

Hormonal Therapy

Five percent of endometrial cancer cases occur in women under the age of 40 years. As women delay childbearing until later in their reproductive life, there are more patients with endometrial cancer who are still desirous of uterine preservation for future fertility. An option for therapy is hormonal treatment with high-dose progestins or the progestin-containing intrauterine device. In a review article, Ramirez et al.[31] reported on 81 patients treated at different institutions. Overall, 76% of patients showed a response to treatment with progestin therapy, with a median time to response of 12 weeks. Twenty-four percent of patients who initially responded to therapy had a recurrence at a median time of 19 months, with 67% of patients who had a recurrence being treated finally with hysterectomy. There were no deaths due to endometrial cancer in this cohort. Twenty patients were able to become pregnant after successful treatment of their cancer.[31]

Careful counseling and informed consent of the patient prior to treatment of endometrial cancer with hormonal therapy are of paramount importance. The patient is initially evaluated with a dilation and curettage procedure to confirm histologic grade (if initial diagnosis is done with in-office endometrial biopsy). An MRI is usually performed to rule out metastatic disease or myometrial involvement. Usually, patients with grade 1 histology and no myometrial involvement of cancer are candidates for hormonal therapy. After 3 to 6 months of treatment, a repeat curettage procedure is done to confirm grade and evaluate for therapeutic efficacy. Continued presence of cancer after a course of hormonal therapy is considered a therapeutic failure, and hysterectomy is a reasonable next step.

ADJUVANT THERAPY FOR ENDOMETRIAL CANCER

"High Intermediate Risk" Endometrioid Histology

The surgical pathologic study on endometrial cancer by the GOG (Protocol 33) defined a group of patients with uterine-confined cancer of endometrioid histology of any grade with myometrial invasion as an intermediate-risk group with a 20% to 25% risk of recurrence within the first 2 years after diagnosis.[9] Based on this finding, the GOG embarked on a trial to compare pelvic radiation therapy with no further therapy in this intermediate-risk group. This trial, GOG Protocol 99, conducted between 1987 and 1995, continues to be a source of debate among gynecologic oncologists who still use the data to guide adjuvant therapy for endometrial cancer, at least in the United States. Thus, 392 patients were finally enrolled onto the trial with FIGO 1988 stages IB, IC, and II (microscopic involvement only) endometrioid uterine cancer. Patients who received pelvic radiation therapy had a 58% hazard reduction in the risk of recurrent cancer. The absolute incidence of recurrence in the adjuvant pelvic radiation group was 3%, in contrast to 12% in the "no further therapy (NFT)" group, with the major difference between the two groups being the number of vaginal recurrence. There were 13 vaginal recurrences in the NFT group versus 2 in the pelvic radiation group. As the trial went on, it appears that the original definition of "intermediate risk" for inclusion onto the trial identified a group with only a 12% risk of recurrence at 2 years for those receiving no further therapy. Subgroup analysis within this trial identified a group who accounted for two-thirds of the recurrences and two-thirds of the deaths in the trial, despite comprising only one-third of the total number of trial patients (n = 132). The NFT treatment arm in this subgroup, which was called "high intermediate risk (HIR)," had a 24% risk of recurrence at 2 years, which is more in line with the original statistical calculations for the trial. This HIR group is characterized as follows: (1) age greater than 70 years with one of the three risk factors identified in GOG 33 (grade 2 or 3, outer third myometrial invasion, or lymphovascular invasion), (2) age 50 to 69 years with two risk factors, or younger than age 50 with all three risk factors. Considering patients in this HIR group alone, the reduction in recurrence at 2 years was statistically significant (relative hazard, 0.42; 95% confidence interval, 0.21 to 0.83). There was also reduction in mortality in the HIR group; however, this did not reach statistical significance. Until the recent publication of the ASTEC trial, this was the only prospective randomized trial on the question of radiation therapy. In addition, one of the major findings in this trial was that vaginal recurrences make up the majority of cases of recurrent endometrial cancer for patients with uterine-confined disease. Thus, treatment with vaginal brachytherapy alone may offer a higher therapeutic index than conventional pelvic radiation.[32]

The argument for treatment with vaginal brachytherapy only is further supported by the recently published PORTEC-2 trial. In this randomized, noninferiority trial, 427 patients with HIR endometrioid endometrial cancer (defined differently than GOG 99 criteria as age >60 and FIGO 1988 stage IC, grade 1 or 2, or stage IB, grade 3; or any age with FIGO 1988 stage IIA, except patients with grade 3 and >50% myometrial invasion) were treated with either vaginal brachytherapy or pelvic external-beam radiation therapy. At a median follow-up of 45 months, patients in both groups had similar low rates of vaginal recurrent disease (1.6% and 1.8% for external-beam radiation therapy and vaginal brachytherapy, respectively) and locoregional recurrent disease (2.1% and 5.1%, respectively). There was a statistically significant difference between the two groups in terms of pelvic recurrence, favoring the external-beam radiation group (0.5% versus 3.8% for the vaginal brachytherapy group). However, the majority of patients with pelvic recurrences also had concurrent distant metastases. Disease-free survival and overall survival were not different between the two groups. Regarding side effects of treatment, patients in the external-beam radiation therapy group had more minor (grade 1 to 2) gastrointestinal toxicity than those in the brachytherapy group. This difference decreased with time after completion of therapy and was not statistically significant at 2 years. The PORTEC-2 trial lends further support to the findings of the GOG 99 and the PORTEC-1 trials, which both found that recurrences in the vagina account for about 75% of all recurrent disease in this subgroup of patients with endometrial cancer. Thus, vaginal brachytherapy may offer adequate protection without incurring significant toxicity or cost.[33]

A Japanese GOG study suggested that chemotherapy may be at least as efficacious as pelvic radiation therapy for early-stage, high-risk disease. Three hundred eighty-five patients were randomized between pelvic radiation and combination chemotherapy with cyclophosphamide, doxorubicin, and cisplatin. Overall, there were no differences in progression-free and overall survival between the two groups. However, in a subgroup analysis of patients over the age of 70 with grade 3 histology or patients with stage II or IIIA disease, the use of chemotherapy improved progression-free and overall survival.[34]

Early-Stage, High-Risk Histology

For patients with uterine-confined disease of high-risk histology (e.g., papillary serous, clear cell), chemotherapy is the usual adjuvant treatment of choice. Although there is no consensus treatment, most patients will receive adjuvant chemotherapy. Adjuvant radiation therapy, in the form of vaginal brachytherapy, is often prescribed. Kelly et al.[35] reported on the Yale experience with uterine-confined serous carcinoma. In the Yale experience, patients who received adjuvant chemotherapy after surgery had a significantly lower chance of recurrence than patients who received no chemotherapy. The overall recurrence rate for stage I serous endometrial cancer is 28% in their series. Only 1 patient in a cohort of 31 patients who received platinum-based chemotherapy had a recurrence of cancer, as compared with 20 of 43 patients who did not receive adjuvant chemotherapy (most patients in this "no chemotherapy" cohort received expectant management, pelvic radiation, vaginal radiation, whole abdominal radiation, or a combination of radiation therapy). The majority of patients who received vaginal brachytherapy also received adjuvant chemotherapy. In only one cohort, the addition of chemotherapy did not influence recurrence. In patients with disease confined to the endometrium and in whom curettage had completely removed the cancer mass, additional chemotherapy did not influence recurrence rate. Based on their data, the authors favor platinum-based chemotherapy and vaginal brachytherapy for patients with uterine-confined serous carcinoma.[35]

Advanced-Stage Disease

For patients who have extrauterine disease at the time of initial diagnosis, chemotherapy is the mainstay of adjuvant therapy. Until the publication of the results of GOG Protocol 122, there was no real consensus treatment for advanced-stage disease of any histology. Whole abdominal radiation (WAR), reported in many case series, was used with variable success with tolerable toxicity and long-term survival.[36,37] In an earlier study completed in the mid-1990s and reported in 2005 by the GOG, WAR as single-modality adjuvant therapy achieved a 3-year survival rate of 31% for endometrioid histology and 35% for papillary serous and clear cell histologies. This study also highlighted the need for complete cytoreduction in advanced endometrial cancer. There were no long-term survivors in the group of patients who had gross residual disease after surgery, whereas there were long-term survivors in both cohorts of patients who either did not have gross disease or who were cytoreduced to no visible disease.[37] GOG 122 compared chemotherapy using the combination of doxorubicin and cisplatin versus WAR. At 60 months, combination chemotherapy improved progression-free survival by 12% (50% for doxorubicin and cisplatin versus 38% for WAR) and overall survival by 13% (55% for doxorubicin and cisplatin versus 42% for WAR).[38] The question of the ideal chemotherapeutic regimen is still a subject of debate. The combination of doxorubicin and cisplatin was compared with the triplet of paclitaxel, doxorubicin, and cisplatin (TAP) in stage III, stage IV, or recurrent endometrial cancer. The TAP regimen was superior in terms of rate of recurrence, progression-free survival, and overall survival at the cost of increased peripheral neuropathy. The enthusiasm with TAP was tempered as a result of five treatment-related deaths on this arm in 134 treated patients.[39] Currently, many patients with advanced or recurrent endometrial cancer are treated with a variation of the TAP regimen or the combination of paclitaxel and carboplatin. Paclitaxel and carboplatin is a well-tolerated regimen and has been widely used for ovarian cancer for over a decade. Although there are no large published trials comparing paclitaxel and carboplatin with other chemotherapy combinations, many case series suggest that the combination is reasonably efficacious.[40] A protocol by the GOG to compare TAP with paclitaxel and carboplatin has completed accrual; however, data have not been published at the time of this writing.

Carcinosarcoma

Data to guide adjuvant therapy for carcinosarcoma are lacking. For uterine-confined disease, patients are treated in a similar manner as patients with high-risk histologies (serous and clear cell carcinomas). Even in early-stage disease, chemotherapy is used, often in conjunction with adjuvant radiation therapy. In Protocol 150, the GOG compared WAR versus combination chemotherapy with doxorubicin and ifosfamide with mesna. Despite allowing enrollment of patients with all stages of disease, it took 12 years to complete the study. The results show a non–statistically significant trend toward improvement in progression-free and overall survival, favoring chemotherapy. More vaginal recurrences occurred in the chemotherapy group, which suggested a benefit to adding vaginal brachytherapy to chemotherapy in future trials.[41] Research in this disease is hampered by its low incidence and poor accrual. A trial by the European Organisation for Research and Treatment of Cancer (EORTC) randomized stage I and II patients between pelvic radiation therapy and expectant management. Despite the inclusion of leiomyosarcoma and endometrial stromal sarcoma in addition to carcinosarcoma, the trial needed 13 years to complete accrual. The conclusion of the trial is that pelvic radiation decreased local recurrence rate with no impact on recurrence-free or overall survival.[42]

ONGOING TRIALS FOR ENDOMETRIAL CANCER

As of the summer of 2011, phase III trials actively accruing patients with endometrial cancer include the following:

1. GOG 249: A phase III trial of pelvic radiation therapy versus vaginal cuff brachytherapy followed by paclitaxel/carboplatin chemotherapy in patients with high-risk, early-stage endometrial carcinoma. This trial further evaluates the role and duration of chemotherapy for adjuvant therapy of early-stage endometrial cancer. It builds on the Japan GOG data, summarized earlier, suggesting that chemotherapy is at least equally efficacious as pelvic radiotherapy in intermediate-risk patients and may actually be better in older patients with more worrisome pathologic features (age >70, grade 3 with deep myometrial invasion, cervical involvement, or positive peritoneal cytology).
2. GOG 258: A randomized phase III trial of cisplatin and tumor volume–directed irradiation followed by carboplatin and paclitaxel versus carboplatin and paclitaxel for optimally debulked, advanced endometrial carcinoma. This trial assesses both the efficacy and the tolerability of multimodality therapy for advanced endometrial carcinoma.
3. EORTC 55984: A randomized trial of doxorubicin and cisplatin versus paclitaxel, doxorubicin, and cisplatin in patients with relapsed or locally advanced inoperable endometrial cancer. This trial compares two established, active regimens in endometrial cancer.
4. EORTC 55991: A randomized trial of adjuvant treatment with radiation plus chemotherapy versus radiation alone in high-risk endometrial carcinoma. This trial answers similar questions as GOG 249 in a slightly different high-risk subgroup (serous, clear cell, undifferentiated, or grade 3 with deep myometrial invasion histologies).

References

1. Jemal A, Siegel R, Ward E, et al. Cancer statistics 2009. *CA Cancer J Clin*. 2009;59:225–249.
2. Benshushan A. Endometrial adenocarcinoma in young patients: evaluation and fertility-preserving treatment. *Eur J Obstet Gynecol Reprod Biol*. 2004;117:132–137.
3. Bakkum-Gamez JN, Gonzalez-Bosquet J, Laack NN, et al. Current issues in the management of endometrial cancer. *Mayo Clinic Proc*. 2008;83:97–112.

4. Modesitt SC, van Nagell JR. The impact of obesity on the incidence and treatment of gynecologic cancers: a review. *Obstet Gynecol Surv*. 2005;60:683–692.
5. Kurman RJ, Kaminski PF, Norris HJ. The behaviour of endometrial hyperplasia. A long-term study of "untreated" hyperplasia in 179 patients. *Cancer*. 1985;56:403–411.
6. Trimble CL. Atypical endometrial hyperplasia: a tough call. *Int J Gynecol Cancer*. 2005;15:401.
7. Suh-Burgmann E, Hung YY, Armstrong MA. Complex atypical endometrial hyperplasia: the risk of unrecognized adenocarcinoma and value of preoperative dilation and curettage. *Obstet Gynecol*. 2009;114:523–529.
8. Batool T, Reginald PW, Hughes JH. Outpatient pipelle endometrial biopsy in the investigation of postmenopausal bleeding. *Br J Obstet Gynaecol*. 1994;101:545–546.
9. Creasman WT, Morro CP, Bundy BN, et al. Surgical pathologic spread patterns of endometrial cancer. A Gynecologic Oncology Group study. *Cancer*. 1987;60(8 suppl):2035–2041.
10. Partridge EE, Shingleton HM, Menck HR. The National Cancer Data Base report on endometrial cancer. *J Surg Oncol*. 1996;61:111–123.
11. Roland PY, Kelly FJ, Kulwicki CY, et al. The benefits of a gynecologic oncologist: a pattern of care study for endometrial cancer treatment. *Gynecol Oncol*. 2004;93:125–130.
12. Homesley HD, Kadar N, Barrett RJ, et al. Selective pelvic and periaortic lymphadenectomy does not increase morbidity in surgical staging of endometrial carcinoma. *Am J Obstet Gynecol*. 1992;167:1225–1230.
13. Goff BA, Kato D, Schmidt RA, et al. Uterine papillary serous carcinoma: patterns of metastatic spread. *Gynecol Oncol*. 1994;54:264–268.
14. Chan JK, Loizzi V, Youssef M, et al. Significance of comprehensive surgical staging in noninvasive papillary serous carcinoma of the endometrium. *Gynecol Oncol*. 2003;90:181–185.
15. Ferguson SE, Tornos C, Hummer A, et al. Prognostic features of surgical stage I uterine carcinosarcoma. *Am J Surg Pathol*. 2007;31:1653–1661.
16. Walker JL, Piedmonte MR, Spirtos NM, et al. Laparoscopy compared with laparotomy for comprehensive surgical staging of uterine cancer. Gynecologic Oncology Group Study LAP 2. *J Clin Oncol*. 2009;27:5331–5336.
17. Walker JL, Piedmonte MR, Spirtos NM, et al. Recurrence and survival after randomization to laparoscopy versus laparotomy for comprehensive surgical staging of uterine cancer (Gynecologic Oncology Group LAP2). *Gynecol Oncol*. 2010;117:393–395.
18. Kornblith AB, Huang HQ, Walker JL, et al. Quality of life of patients with endometrial cancer undergoing laparoscopic International Federation of Gynecology and Obstetrics staging compared with laparotomy: a Gynecologic Oncology Group study. *J Clin Oncol*. 2009;27: 5337–5342.
19. Bell MC, Torgerson J, Seshadri-Kreaden U, et al. Comparison of outcomes and cost for endometrial cancer staging via traditional laparotomy, standard laparoscopy and robotic techniques. *Gynecol Oncol*. 2008;111:407–411.
20. Panici PB, Basile S, Maneschir F, et al. Systematic pelvic lymphadenectomy vs. no lymphadenectomy in early-stage endometrial carcinoma: a randomized clinical trial. *J Natl Cancer Inst*. 2008;100:1707–1716.
21. Bernardini MQ, May T, Khalifa MA, et al. Evaluation of two management strategies for preoperative grade 1 endometrial cancer. *Obstet Gynecol*. 2009;114:7–15.
22. The Writing Committee on Behalf of the ASTEC Study Group. Efficacy of systemic pelvic lymphadenectomy in endometrial cancer (MRC ASTEC trial): a randomized study. *Lancet*. 2009;373:125–136.
23. Kilgore LC, Partridge EE, Alvarez RD, et al. Adenocarcinoma of the endometrium: survival comparisons of patients with and without pelvic node sampling. *Gynecol Oncol*. 1995;56:29–33.
24. Cragun JM, Havrilesky LJ, Calingaert B, et al. Retrospective analysis of selective lymphadenectomy in apparent early-stage endometrial cancer. *J Clin Oncol*. 2005;23:3668–3675.
25. Arango HA, Hoffman MS, Roberts WS, et al. Accuracy of lymph node palpation to determine need for lymphadenectomy in gynecologic malignancies. *Obstet Gynecol*. 2000;95:553–556.

26. Eltabbakh GH. Intraoperative clinical evaluation of lymph nodes in women with gynecologic cancer. *Am J Obstet Gynecol.* 2001;184:1177–1181.
27. Lambrou NC, Gomez-Marin O, Mirhashemi R, et al. Optimal surgical cytoreduction in patients with stage III and stage IV endometrial carcinoma: a study of morbidity and survival. *Gynecol Obstet.* 2004;93:653–658.
28. Nag S, Erickson B, Parikh S, et al. The American Brachytherapy Society recommendations for the high dose rate brachytherapy for carcinoma of the endometrium. *Int J Radiat Oncol Biol Phys.* 2000;48:779–790.
29. Fishman DA, Roberts KB, Chambers JT, et al. Radiation therapy as exclusive treatment for medically inoperable patients with stage I and II endometrioid carcinoma of the endometrium. *Gynecol Oncol.* 1996;61:189–196.
30. Knocke TH, Kucera H, Weidinger B, et al. Primary treatment of endometrial carcinoma with high-dose rate brachytherapy: results of 12 years of experience with 280 patients. *Int J Radiat Oncol Biol Phys.* 1997;37:359–365.
31. Ramirez PT, Frumovitz M, Bodurka DC, et al. Hormonal therapy for the management of grade 1 endometrial adenocarcinoma: a literature review. *Gynecol Oncol.* 2004;95:133–138.
32. Keys HM, Roberts JA, Brunetto VL, et al. A phase III trial of surgery with or without adjunctive external pelvic radiation therapy in intermediate risk endometrial adenocarcinoma: a Gynecologic Oncology Group study. *Gynecol Oncol.* 2004;92:744–751.
33. Nout RA, Smit VT, Putter H, et al. Vaginal brachytherapy versus pelvic external beam radiotherapy for patients with endometrial cancer of high-intermediate risk (PORTEC-2): an open-label, non-inferiority, randomised trial. *Lancet.* 2010;375:816–823.
34. Susumu N, Sagae S, Udagawa Y, et al. Randomized phase III trial of pelvic radiotherapy versus cisplatin-based combined chemotherapy in patients with intermediate and high-risk endometrial cancer: a Japanese Gynecologic Oncology Group study. *Gyncol Oncol.* 2008;108:226–233.
35. Kelly MG, O'Malley DM, Hui P, et al. Improved survival in surgical stage I patients with uterine papillary serous carcinoma (UPSC) treated with adjuvant platinum-based chemotherapy. *Gynecol Oncol.* 2006;98:353–359.
36. Lee SW, Russell AH, Kinney WK. Whole abdomen radiotherapy for patients with peritoneal dissemination of endometrial adenocarcinoma. *Int J Rad Oncol Biol Phys.* 2003;56:788–792.
37. Sutton G, Axelrod JH, Bundy BN, et al. Whole abdominal radiotherapy in the adjuvant treatment of patients with stage III and IV endometrial cancer: a Gynecologic Oncology Group study. *Gynecol Oncol.* 2005;97:755–763.
38. Randall ME, Filiaci VL, Muss H, et al. Randomized phase III trial of whole-abdominal irradiation versus doxorubicin and cisplatin chemotherapy in advanced endometrial carcinoma: a Gynecologic Oncology Group study. *J Clin Oncol.* 2006;24:36–44.
39. Fleming GF, Brunetto VL, Cella D, et al. Phase III trial of doxorubicin plus cisplatin with or without paclitaxel plus filgrastim in advanced endometrial carcinoma: a Gynecologic Oncology Group study. *J Clin Oncol.* 2004;22:2159–2166.
40. Sovak MA, Hensley ML, Dupont J, et al. Paclitaxel and carboplatin in the adjuvant treatment of patients with high-risk stage III and IV endometrial cancer: a retrospective study. *Gynecol Oncol.* 2006;103:451–457.
41. Wolfson AH, Brady MF, Rocereto T, et al. A Gynecologic Oncology Group randomized phase III trial of whole abdominal irradiation (WAI) vs. cisplatin-ifosfamide and mesna (CIM) as post-surgical therapy in stage I-IV carcinosarcoma (CS) of the uterus. *Gynecol Oncol.* 2007;107:77–185.
42. Reed NS, Mangioni C, Malmstrom H, et al. Phase III randomized study to evaluate the role of adjuvant pelvic radiotherapy in the treatment of uterine sarcomas stages I and II: an EORTC Gynaecological Cancer Group Study (protocol 55874). *Eur J Cancer.* 2008;44:808–818.

SECTION IV

Molecular Pathology

- ▶ CHAPTER 7: Molecular Pathogenesis of Endometrial Carcinoma
- ▶ CHAPTER 8: High-Risk Endometrial Carcinoma
- ▶ CHAPTER 9: Endometrial Sarcomas

Molecular Pathogenesis of Endometrial Carcinoma

▶ Martin Kobel, MD

The collective of endometrial carcinomas is increasingly recognized to comprise a number of distinct diseases.[1] The major histologic types of endometrial carcinomas are associated with distinct molecular alterations. Phenotypic criteria, which are used to type endometrial carcinomas, have been defined on an architectural and cellular, nuclear level. These morphologic features are directly related to distinct molecular events that determine the lineage of differentiation and the oncogenic pathway. Serous carcinomas are characterized by anaplastic nuclear features, which correlate with the underlying chromosomal instability, whereas other alterations (e.g., *PTEN/PI3K* and *Wnt/CTNNB1* pathways) are associated with low-grade nuclear features.[2]

Three decades ago, the first characteristic molecular features for specific types of endometrial carcinomas were reported, with landmark papers describing *TP53* mutation in "nonendometrioid" (serous) carcinomas,[3] the identification of microsatellite instability in a significant portion of sporadic endometrial carcinomas,[4] and *PTEN* mutation[5,6] and *CTNNB1* mutation in endometrioid types.[7] Initially based on clinical features[8] and later on histopathologic and molecular features,[9] a binary classification system for endometrial carcinomas has been proposed that divides these tumors into type I (endometrioid, mucinous) and type II (serous, clear cell). This model clearly delineates endometrial carcinomas with respect to their relation to estrogen stimulation. However, the model obscures some of the significant differences within these groups (i.e., between low-grade endometrioid and high-grade endometrioid carcinoma and between serous and clear cell carcinoma). The molecular characterization of endometrial carcinomas has been evolving, and an overview on the mutational landscape across histologic types as known today is given in Table 7-1.[10–16]

There are four major clinicopathologic variants of endometrial carcinomas that account for more than 95% of cases that differ with respect to molecular alterations, phenotype, biomarker expression, and clinical behavior. These types include low-grade (grade 1 and grade 2) endometrioid, high-grade (grade 3) endometrioid, serous, and clear cell carcinoma.

Most of the alterations shown in Table 7-1 were identified as candidate genes by analogy with tumors from other organ systems. These numbers may represent an underestimate due to the limited sensitivity of conventional Sanger sequencing; however, these case series might also be subject to selection bias. Unbiased comprehensive new genomic and epigenomic analysis is needed to broaden our understanding of the complex molecular basis of these

Table 7-1	Frequencies of Selected Mutations and Microsatellite Instability (MSI) Across Different Histologic Types			
Gene	EC-1/2	EC-3	SC	CCC
PTEN	55%[10]	59%[10]	0[10]	2/9[11]
PIK3CA	19/73; 26%[12]	10/29; 34%[12]	4/13; 31%[10]	6/13; 46%[10]
CTNNB1	41/60; 68%[13]		0[14]	
ARID1A	10/25; 40%*		0/12*	
KRAS	18/109; 17%[12]		1/45; 2%	
MSI	118/543; 28%[15]		0/34[16]	1/9[11]
TP53	1/60; 2%[10]	5/29; 17%[10]	25/27; 93%[16]	1/11[11]
PPP2R1A	3/60; 5%[†]		20/49; 41%[†]	

CCC, clear cell carcinoma; EC-1/2, low-grade (grades 1 and 2) endometrioid carcinoma; EC-3, high-grade (grade 3) endometrioid carcinoma; SC, serous carcinoma.
*Data from Guan B, Mao TL, Panuganti PK, et al. Mutation and loss of expression of ARID1A in uterine low-grade endometrioid carcinoma. *Am J Surg Pathol.* 2011;35:625–632.
†McConechy MK, Anglesio MS, Kalloger SE, et al. Subtype-specific mutation of PPP2R1A in endometrial and ovarian carcinomas. *J Pathol.* 2011;223:567–573.

diseases. Comparison of tumor-type specific mRNA expression profiles has further provided insight into the biologic differences of these distinct tumor types,[17-20] and some candidate biomarkers are being used in diagnostic practice (see below).

LOW-GRADE ENDOMETRIAL CARCINOMA

Low-grade (grade 1 or 2) endometrial carcinomas of endometrioid or mucinous type are associated with low stage at diagnosis and usually a rather favorable outcome. Because pure mucinous carcinomas are rare, the following discussion is restricted to low-grade endometrioid carcinomas irrespective of morphologic variant.

Molecular Pathways

PTEN/PI3K Pathway

Mutations in the tumor suppressor gene *PTEN* occur in the majority of endometrioid carcinomas with a frequency of 83% in a selected series of endometrioid carcinomas that were associated with a precursor lesion such as endometrial intraepithelial neoplasia.[21] *PTEN* is a dual specific phosphatase that is able to dephosphorylate both proteins and phospholipids. The main substrate of *PTEN* is phosphatidylinositol-3,4,5-triphosphate (PIP3). *PTEN* antagonizes the action of phosphatidylinositol 3-kinase (PI3K) on PIP3 with inhibitory effects on the *PI3K/AKT* signaling pathway. Loss of *PTEN* function accelerates signaling through the *PI3K/AKT* pathway. Activation of this pathway results in prevention of apoptosis, in addition to many other cellular effects (Fig. 7-1).[22] The *PI3K/AKT* pathway acts predominantly via the downstream TSC1/TSC2 and rapamycin-sensitive mammalian target of rapamycin (mTOR)

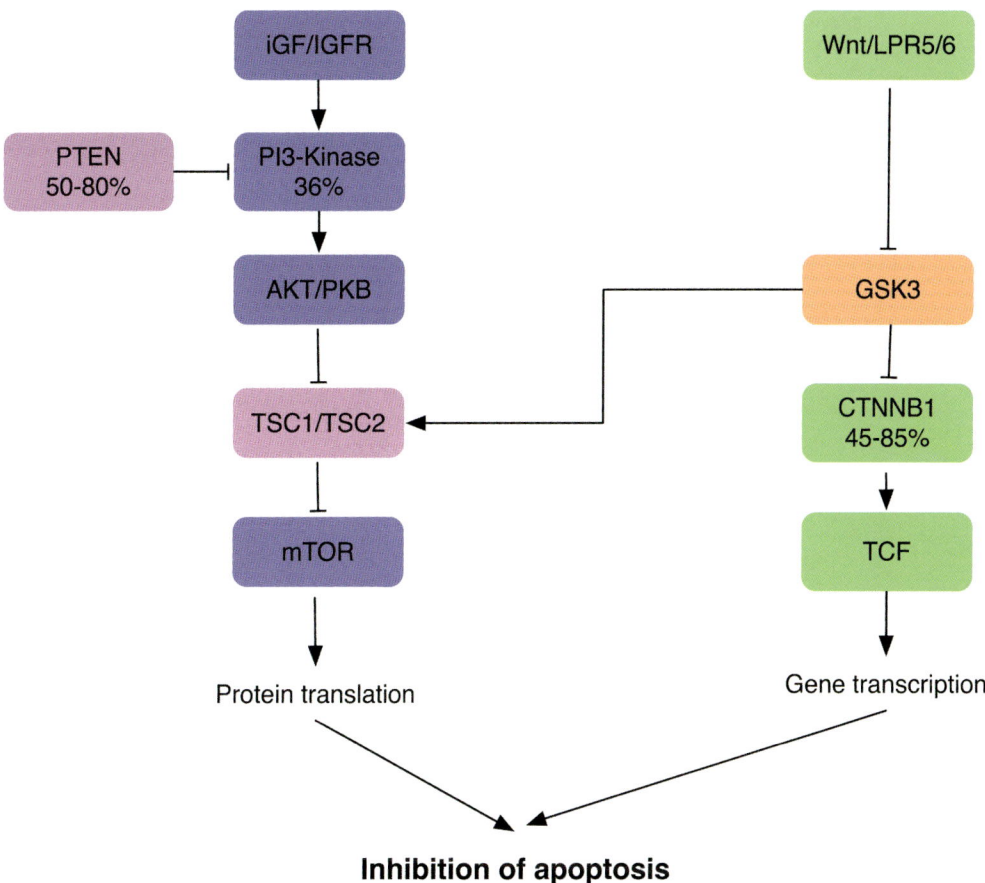

FIGURE 7-1: Simplified *PTEN/PI3K* (**left**) and *Wnt/CTNNB1* (**right**) signaling pathways including example crossover. Prevalence rates of common mutated genes in endometrioid carcinomas are indicated in percentages.

complex. The mTOR complex is a major regulator of ribosome and therefore protein synthesis. External activation of the *PI3K* pathway can occur via insulin and other growth factors by binding through their receptors. Epidemiologic studies have linked endometrioid carcinomas to individuals with obesity. Obesity is caused by numerous lifestyle factors including high-fat diet and hyperinsulinemia.

PTEN mutations result in loss of function due to frameshift mutations such as insertions or deletions (so called indels), which alter the reading frame (frameshift). A shift in reading frame may lead to nonsense or premature stop codons (nonsense mutation). Nonsense mutation theoretically translates into a nonfunctional or truncated protein. Yet such nonfunctional proteins do not occur due to the nonsense-mediated mRNA decay pathway, which degrades mRNAs containing nonsense mutations before they are translated. Some *PTEN* mutations are missense mutations that result from a point mutation that leads to substitution of an amino acid. The phosphatase catalytic domain that is encoded on exon 5 of the *PTEN* gene and missense mutations in this exon are important for loss of *PTEN* gene function that is accompanied by retained *PTEN* expression (Fig. 7-2).

Hemizygous *PTEN* mutations are accompanied by additional genetic alterations of the second allele, such as loss of heterozygosity at chromosome 10q23 leading to biallelic *PTEN*

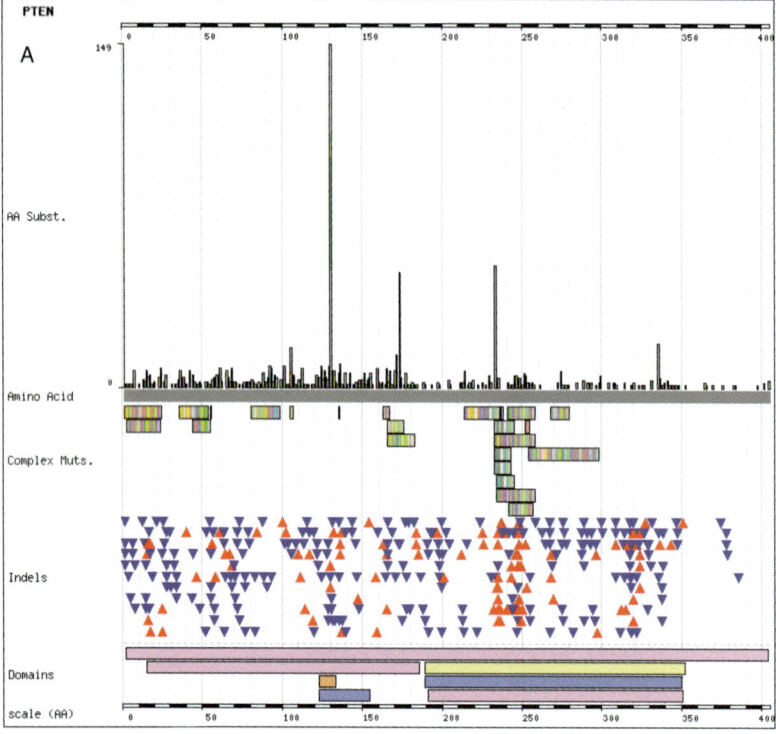

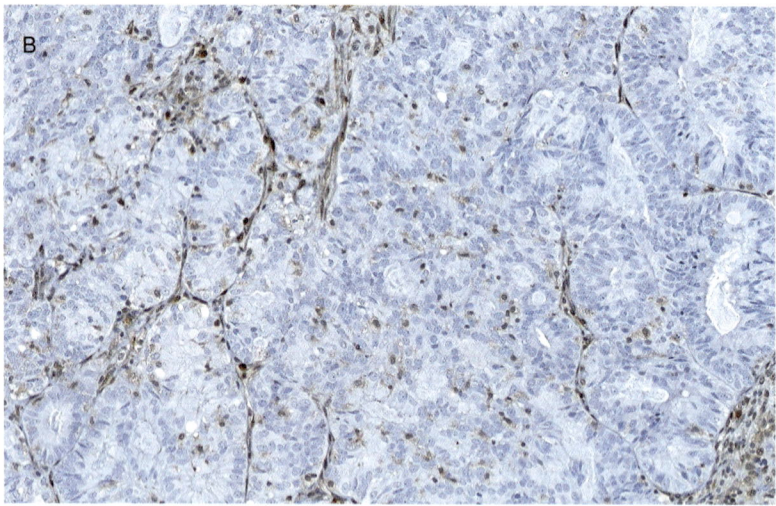

FIGURE 7-2: A: Mutations found in the *PTEN* gene in a variety of tumor entities and the distribution of these mutations along the protein the gene encodes. The scale represents the 403 amino acids of the PTEN protein. Most mutations are "indels" (i.e., insertion or deletions), which result in a frameshift and a loss of *PTEN* expression (see part B). Complex mutations result in loss of *PTEN* expression. There is a small peak of 149 missense mutations ("AA subst") in exon 5 encoding the phosphatase domain of the gene, which results in a nonfunctional but expressed *PTEN* protein. (Mutation data obtained from the Sanger Institute Catalogue of Somatic Mutations in Cancer website, http://www.sanger.ac.uk/cosmic; and Bamford S, Dawson E, Forbes S, et al. The COSMIC [Catalogue of Somatic Mutations in Cancer] database and website. *Br J Cancer*. 2004;91:355–358.) **B:** *PTEN* expression by immunohistochemistry can be used as an imperfect surrogate for the *PTEN* mutational status (i.e., absence of *PTEN* expression suggests loss of function mutation).

inactivation and loss of *PTEN* expression.[21] Loss of *PTEN* expression is seen in approximately half of endometrioid carcinomas. It is possible that some of the *PTEN* inactivation is hemizygous. In mice, heterozygous *PTEN* inactivation produces an abnormal endometrial phenotype in mice, with 100% of mice developing hyperplastic lesions and 20% of animals progressing to endometrial carcinoma.[23] The significance of this *PTEN* haploinsufficiency remains to be elucidated for humans.

Inherited germ line mutation of *PTEN* causes a spectrum of hamartoma syndromes including Cowden syndrome. Besides being associated with benign lesions such as trichilemmomas and thyroid follicular adenomas, Cowden syndrome involves a slightly increased risk for endometrial endometrioid carcinomas, estimated as an increase of 5% to 10% compared to the risk in the general population, with 3% of patients[24] indicating a low penetrance of *PTEN* germ line mutations.[25]

PTEN mutations have been detected in endometrial hyperplasias, and focal loss of *PTEN* expression has been observed in approximately half of endometrial hyperplasia, either atypical or nonatypical. Notably, there was no difference in loss of *PTEN* expression between endometrial hyperplasias that progressed to carcinoma compared with those that did not progress.[26] These data suggest that *PTEN* alterations are common, occur early, and provide a susceptibility background. Loss of *PTEN* function might be necessary but not sufficient for initiation of endometrioid carcinogenesis. In other words, a few *PTEN*-negative glands may indicate a low-risk lesion that is likely being shed during subsequent ovulation; however, an expanded field as defined as 1 mm by Mutter (http://www.endometrium.org) may possess the capacity to progress and acquire additional events.

PI3K is another pathway member that is frequently (36%)[27] altered by activating mutations. *PI3K* mutation cluster in exon 9 and exon 20 of the gene *PIK3CA* encodes the regulatory subunit of class IaA *PI3K*, p110α. In the study by Oda et al.,[27] 26% of tumors showed concomitant *PTEN* and *PI3K* mutations, indicating a synergistic effect. *PI3K* mutations, unlike *PTEN* mutations, were found only rarely in endometrial hyperplasia.[28] Histologic grade varied according to location of the *PIK3CA* mutations. Exon 9 (helical domain) mutations were more often detected in low-grade endometrioid carcinomas compared with high-grade endometrioid carcinomas, which were more often mutated in exon 20 (kinase domain).[17] This suggests that *PI3K* mutations are associated with differentiation of endometrioid carcinomas.

Wnt/CTNNB1 Pathway

Activating mutations in exon 3 of *CTNNB1* have been reported in 45% of endometrioid carcinomas.[29] Hot spots for mutations are phosphorylation sites of serine-threonine residues coded in exon 3 of *CTNNB1* targeted by *GSK3* (Fig. 7-3). GSK3 is activated in response to wingless-type mouse mammary tumor virus integration site (Wnt) through the LPR5/6 or frizzled receptors. *GSK3* tightly regulates *CTNNB1* levels. *GSK3* inhibition by lithium increases cytoplasmic *CTNNB1* levels.[30] Phosphorylation of specific exon 3 residues by *GSK3* requires a multiprotein complex including APC and axin, among others, and induces *CTNNB1* degradation through ubiquitin-proteasome process. Mutated *CTNNB1* escapes this degradation, resulting in increased cytoplasmic level of *CTNNB1*, nuclear translocation, and enhanced participation in transcriptional regulation through the formation of bipartite complex with the TCF transcription factor. Target genes of *Wnt/CTNNB1* signaling include *MYC*, *CCND1*, and *MMP7*.[31] The *Wnt* signaling pathway is involved in pleiotropic cellular functions including differentiation. During embryologic

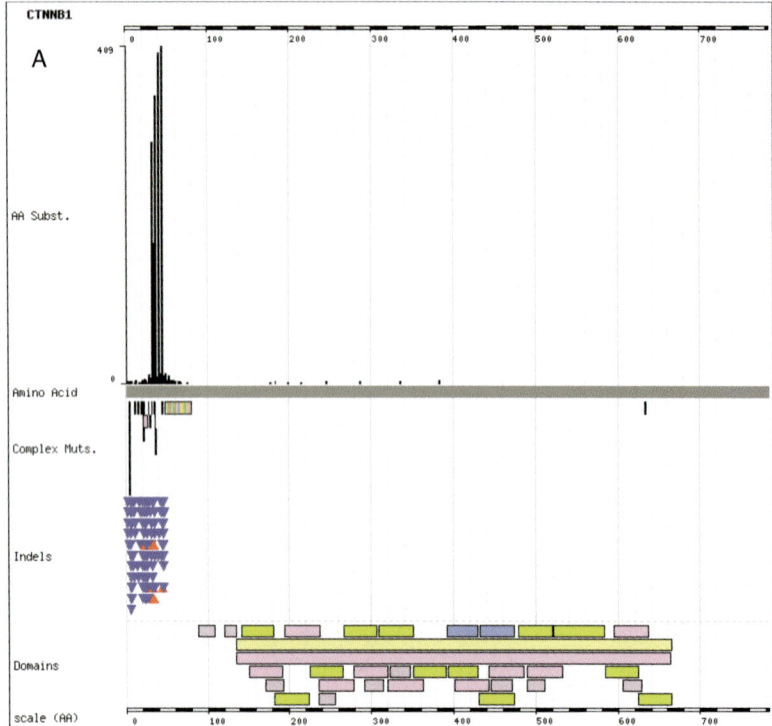

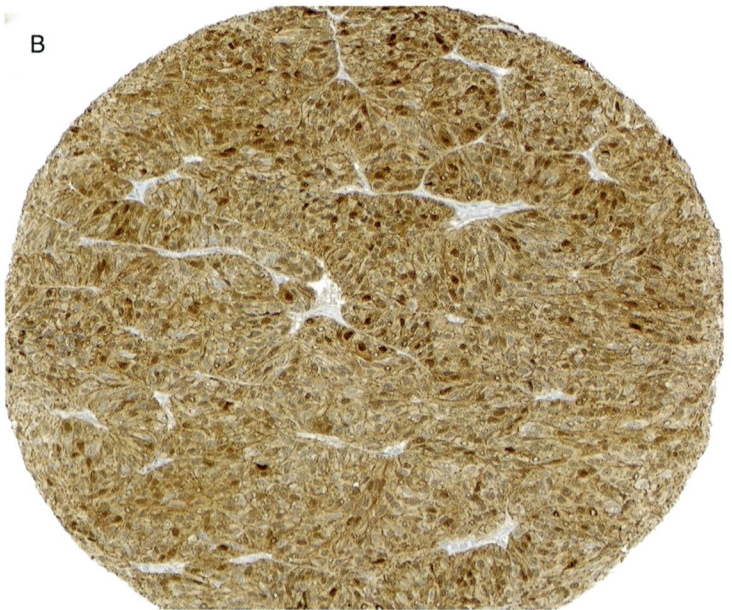

FIGURE 7-3: **A:** Mutations found in the *CTNNB1* gene in a variety of tumor entities and the distribution of these mutations along the protein the gene encodes. *CTNNB1* mutations cluster in exon 3 at phosphorylation sites targeted by GSK3. (Mutation data obtained from the Sanger Institute Catalogue of Somatic Mutations in Cancer website, http://www.sanger.ac.uk/cosmic; and Bamford S, Dawson E, Forbes S, et al. The COSMIC [Catalogue of Somatic Mutations in Cancer] database and website. *Br J Cancer*. 2004;91:355–358.) **B:** *CTNNB1* expression by immunohistochemistry can be used as an imperfect surrogate for the *CTNNB1* mutational status (i.e., nuclear and/or cytoplasmic *CTNNB1* expression suggests activating *CTNNB1* mutation).

differentiation, a tight regulation of cellular division and apoptosis is required. With respect to carcinogenesis, the antiapoptotic effects of the *CTNNB1* mutation may be the major outcome of aberrant *Wnt* signaling.

Furthermore, *GSK3* provides a cross-link to the tumor suppressor complex *TSC1/2*. Inhibition of *GSK3* will lead to inactivation of *TSC1/2*, followed by mTOR activation (see Fig. 7-1). This is one example for the complexity of cross talks between the *Wnt* pathway and other pathways such as the *PI3K* pathway. We are far from understanding how these pathways cooperate during oncogenesis. Application of system biology, the integrative rather than reductive approach to complex interactions in biologic systems using functional data (phosphorylation status, not just simple protein expression), will provide insight into this network to identify the major players involved.

Because direct sequencing is cumbersome, immunohistochemistry has been suggested as a surrogate marker for mutational status of *CTNNB1*. *CTNNB1* is also a submembrane component of the cadherin-mediated cell–cell adhesion system, strengthening the linkage of *CDH1* and *CTNNA1* to the actin cytoskeleton, maintaining epithelial cell composite. Normal *CTNNB1* is primarily located submembranally, resulting in a membranous staining pattern by immunohistochemistry. *CTNNB1* mutations correlate with increasing cytoplasmic and nuclear staining pattern, although the alteration is often seen only focally. Nuclear *CTNNB1* accumulation is often found in areas of squamous differentiation, which are associated with *CTNNB1* mutation. *CTNNB1* mutations have been detected in up to 85% of low-grade endometrioid carcinomas with squamous morules.[13] Moreover, *CTNNB1* mutations are generally identical to those in surrounding glandular carcinoma tissue. This suggests that *CTNNB1* mutation may promote squamous differentiation and that squamous differentiation might serve as a surrogate marker for underlying *CTNNB1* mutation. Given the often focal nuclear expression of *CTNNB1* in endometrioid carcinomas, there is a need for a more reliable test to infer the molecular status of *CTNNB1*. For example, Dickkopf-1 (*DKK-1*) encodes a secreted *Wnt* antagonist that binds to LRP5/6 and induces its endocytosis, leading to inhibition of the *Wnt* pathway, a mechanism that is lost in endometrioid carcinomas due to constitutive downstream activation.[32] *DKK-1* overexpression in endometrioid carcinomas with *CTNNB1* mutation might be a futile attempt to control this signaling pathway and may be used as surrogate marker for *Wnt* pathway activation.[33]

Mismatch Repair Deficiency

Approximately 20% of endometrioid carcinomas carry defects in their mismatch repair (MMR) machinery; of those defects, approximately 90% are sporadic, somatically acquired defects in one of the MMR genes, and 10% are inherited within the Lynch syndrome, or hereditary nonpolyposis colorectal cancer (HNPCC).[15,34]

MMR is one form of single-stranded DNA repair that corrects errors that escaped proofreading during DNA replication. Other forms of single-stranded DNA repair are base excision and nucleotide excision. The MMR machinery corrects mismatch base pairs within the newly synthesized strand using the template. Examples of mismatched bases include a G/T or A/C pairing. The cause of MMR deficiency is due to genetic or epigenetic perturbations of one of the six known human DNA MMR genes: *MLH1*, *PMS2*, *MSH2*, *MSH6*, *MSH3*, and *PMS1*. For the function of the MMR machinery, the presence and function of all partners are essential; hence, MMR deficiency occurs if one partner is lost, but both alleles must be inactivated. Inactivation can be either genetic (mutation and/or loss of heterozygosity) or epigenetic (promoter hypermethylation). In the sporadic setting, the most common mechanism for MMR deficiency is due to biallelic promoter hypermethylation of *MLH1* with subsequent loss of MLH1 expression and function.[35,36] Somatic mutations of one the MMR genes are rare but may occur secondarily to MLH1 inactivation. A minority of cases (10%) with MMR deficiency are caused by hereditary germ line mutations within those genes and are associated with HNPCC.

Oncogenic Consequences

MMR deficiency itself does not cause cancer but reduces DNA sequence stability and increases significantly the risk of acquiring secondary oncogenic mutations. Defects in MMR affect genomic stability on the sequence level, and this is sometimes referred as "mutator phenotype." Mutator phenotype describes an accumulation of mutations in coding and noncoding DNA sequences. MMR deficiency is prone to special sequences (i.e., mononucleotide repeats). This presumably occurs because DNA polymerase has a higher propensity to "slip" at repetitive sequences during DNA synthesis. In case of noncoding DNA, this affects microsatellites (see below). In case of coding DNA or genes, MMR deficiency targets specifically genes that contain long repetitive sequences. Some candidates have been suggested,[37] including mutations in the DNA damage response gene *ATR* that were found exclusively in 12 of 144 tumors with MMR deficiency.[38] *PTEN* mutations also occur more often in MMR-deficient tumors (78% versus 40%).[39]

MMR deficiency is also prone to a particular type of mutation. The type of mutation is insertion or deletion (indels), which alters the reading frame (frameshift). DNA polymerase slippage occurs when the nascent strand (the strand being synthesized) and the template strand transiently dissociate and then re-anneal incorrectly, resulting in the presence of one or more extrahelical nucleotides in either the nascent or the template strand. A failure to repair the resulting loop before the next round of DNA replication will result in a deletion if the unpaired base (deletion) is on the template strand or an addition if the unpaired base (insertion) is on the nascent strand. The incorporation of incorrect nucleotides by DNA polymerase is corrected by the exonucleolytic proofreading activity of DNA polymerase itself and by the MMR system, which removes replication errors that escape the proofreading activity of DNA polymerases. Such a shift in reading frame has significant impact on the presence of the gene product and/or its function. Stop codons in the alternative reading frame usually result in truncation of the protein. Unlike the majority of base substitutions, frameshift mutations almost invariably destroy or drastically alter the function of a protein. Because of their deleterious nature, it is particularly important for cells to recognize and remove frameshift intermediates.[40]

Because MMR deficiency is associated with a particular pattern of mutation, the mutation may be prone to specific target genes; our understanding, however, is still limited by the candidate approach. The identification of actual driver mutations that are supposed to be evident in every cell (except the rare event of backward mutation) within these tumors will be challenging and needs a comprehensive approach using novel techniques such as new-generation sequencing. In tumors with a mutator phenotype, thousands of mutations without significant functional consequence occur (so-called passenger mutations). It has been shown that these secondary mutations in coding mononucleotide tracts are heterogeneously distributed within the tumors and are found in some tumor areas but not in others.[41] Yet some of these mutations might induce progression of molecularly and phenotypically distinct tumor subclones. As a result, these tumors are more likely to develop intratumoral heterogeneity morphologically appreciated as mixed endometrial carcinomas or as dedifferentiated carcinoma as the prototype for tumor progression.[42] MMR-deficient tumors often generate novel tumor-specific carboxy-terminal frameshift peptides, which attract an immune response that might be used as a morphologic diagnostic feature.

Lynch Syndrome

Lynch syndrome (HNPCC) is associated with a germ line mutation in one of the MMR genes and is associated with an increased risk for the development of colorectal, endometrial, and ovarian cancers. The estimated lifetime risk for patients with Lynch syndrome to develop endometrial carcinoma is 40%,[43] which is the equivalent risk for colorectal carcinoma. The cumulative risk to develop both is 80%. The frequency of MMR germ line mutations among women with colorectal and endometrial carcinomas has been reported as 2%.[15,44] In patients with endometrial carcinoma younger than age 50 years, the incidence is increased to 9%.[45] Identification of women with HNPCC is desirable given their family risk for a variety of carcinomas, but an efficient strategy is hampered by the low prevalence. Direct sequencing of the MMR genes is the gold standard. Mutational analysis, however, is still expensive, time consuming, and cumbersome given the number of MMR genes and the heterogeneity of mutations. Alternative techniques include testing for microsatellite instability (MSI), MMR gene expression by immunohistochemistry, and assessment of the MLH1 promoter methylation status.

MSI can be used as a surrogate marker for MMR deficiency. MSI refers to an abnormal length of certain microsatellites in cells with MMR deficiency compared to normal cells from the same individual. Microsatellites are noncoding repeated DNA sequences (e.g., dinucleotide repeat). The most common dinucleotide sequence in eukaryotes is the (CA)n repeat, and there are 50,000 to 100,000 (CA)n repeats in the entire human genome. MSI testing is accomplished by polymerase chain reaction using five conventional primers, two mononucleotide repeats (BAT25 and BAT26), and three dinucleotide repeats (D2S123, D5S346, and D17S250). A tumor is classified as MSI high when two or more of the five markers show MSI.

Because MMR deficiency is, in almost all cases, associated with lack of MMR protein expression, the utility of immunohistochemistry has been investigated using four-marker panels of the most common affected proteins. Recently, a two-marker panel consisting of PMS2 and MSH6 has been suggested as being sufficient to detect MMR deficiency.[46] This is based on the assumption that MMR proteins dimerize and loss of one partner is almost always coupled with concurrent loss of the secondary partner.

Both methods have a similar performance despite the fact that *MSH6* mutations do not necessarily result in high levels of MSI. Endometrial carcinomas associated with HNPCC are relatively more frequently associated with *MSH6* mutations than colorectal cancers. In other words, MSI might miss some HNPCC cases associated with *MSH6* mutation. Immunohistochemistry is also advantageous because it can pinpoint the affected gene or genes, leading to an ability to target specific genes for sequencing. For example, loss of MLH1/PMS2 expression can be followed by MLH1 promoter hypermethylation and, only in the case of nonmethylated status, subjected to direct sequencing, whereas loss of *MSH2/MSH6* will be directly followed by sequencing with restriction to those two genes (Fig. 7-4). MSI and immunohistochemistry have shortcomings because they do not distinguish between inherited and somatic alterations that result in MMR deficiency. Both techniques will identify sporadic, MMR-associated endometrial carcinomas and hereditary cases in an estimated ratio of 9:1. However, the limitation of both techniques is that mostly sporadic, MMR-deficient carcinomas will be detected, with only a few cases that arise in a hereditary setting detected. Because it is neither practical nor feasible to analyze all endometrial carcinomas for the possibility of MMR defects, it has become important to identify additional criteria that effectively narrow

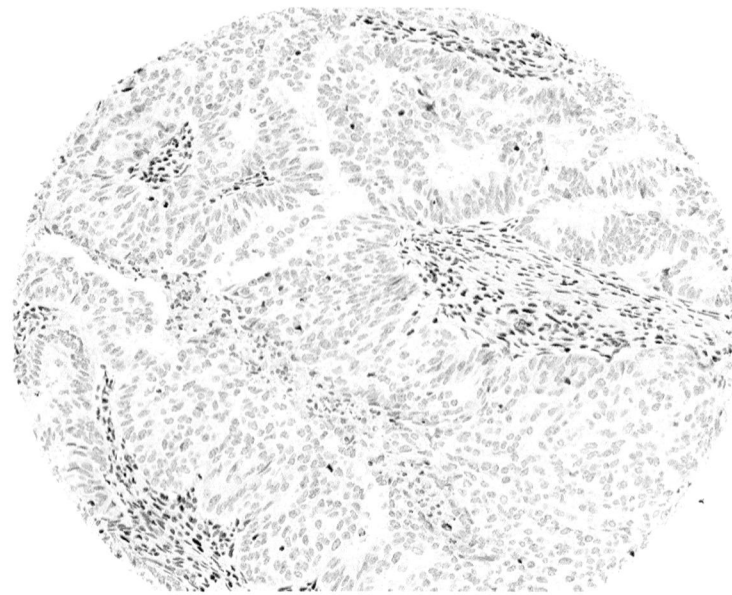

FIGURE 7-4: Endometrioid carcinoma with loss of MSH2 expression. Note retained expression in stromal and inflammatory cells as positive internal control.

the pool of patients. Candidate cases can then undergo further testing with one or more assays, with analysis for germ line mutation in the DNA-MMR genes being the confirmatory test for diagnosing Lynch syndrome.

Investigation for the most effective screening has been performed using criteria equivalent to the Bethesda guidelines used for colorectal cancer. In the series by Hampel et al.,[15] age-based screening would have failed to detect 6 of 10 patients with HNPCC-defining germ line mutations, and family history–based screening would have missed 7 of 10 patients with HNPCC. In particular, patients with *MSH6* mutations frequently present at an older age. In contrast, 7 of 10 HNPCC patients had MSI-high tumors, and 8 of 10 HNPCC patients had abnormal MMR immunohistochemistry. Two of 10 patients with normal immunohistochemistry had missense mutations.[15]

Other criteria recommended for more effective screening would be particular morphologic features associated with MMR deficiency. Tumors with MMR deficiency frequently show tumor-specific morphologic characteristics, including tumor-infiltrating lymphocytes, and intratumoral heterogeneity such as high-grade endometrioid or undifferentiated components (so called dedifferentiated carcinoma[42]), admixed or synchronous clear cell carcinoma (including ovarian clear cell carcinoma), and lower uterine segment origin.[45] Such phenotypic criteria may trigger the application of a screening test. However, the sensitivity of a morphologic selection has to be determined.

Ras Pathway

The *KRAS-BRAF-MAPK* pathway is altered in a small portion of endometrioid carcinomas. The frequency of *KRAS* mutation is 17%.[12,47] *BRAF* mutations are a rare event in endometrioid carcinomas, with a frequency of approximately 4%. Alternative promoter hypermethylation of the *KRAS* inhibitor RASSF1A might contribute to activation of this pathway in approximately one-third of cases.⁴⁷ Downstream signaling via *MAPK* provokes prevention of apoptosis, as a possible alternative or synergistic effect to the aforementioned alterations.

Model of Endometrioid Carcinogenesis

The earliest morphologically recognizable precursor lesions for endometrioid carcinomas are designated as complex atypical hyperplasia (World Health Organization) or endometrioid intraepithelial carcinoma.[48] The molecular alterations already described for carcinoma, with the exception of *PI3K* mutation, have been detected in these lesions, justifying their classification as precancers.[49] Comparison of the frequency of genomic changes from precursor to carcinoma usually indicates an increase, which has been interpreted as progression.[21] However, it does not make sense that a difference in frequencies is interpreted as a qualitative difference between precursor and carcinoma in one subgroup but not the other group. Alternatively, an increase in mutation frequency may just be explained by technical limitations. The portion of neoplastic cells in precursor lesions is limited, and the sensitivity of direct sequencing might miss a significant portion of mutations. Novel techniques will clarify this issue.

Carcinogenesis is defined by one or more genetic hits that lead to uncontrolled cell proliferation (i.e., disrupted balance of cell division and apoptosis). It is important to note that the risk of acquiring such defects is not equally distributed among the population. Several factors can create a field of increased susceptibility. One mechanism is to increase the amount of susceptible tissue that would correlate with an increased chance for a random molecular event (e.g., mutation) to occur. Clinicians observed the frequent relation of endometrioid carcinomas with obesity and hyperestrogenism. Medical conditions in which there is increased insulin-like growth factors or unopposed estrogen increase the amount of endometrium recognizable as a morphologic continuum in diagnostic categories such as disordered proliferative endometrium or simple or complex hyperplasia without atypia, which are alternatively combined as benign endometrial hyperplasia. It is also accepted that hormonal factors positively (estrogen) or negatively (progestin) modulate growth. Increasing the rate of mutation by deterioration of DNA repair, such as MMR deficiency, is an example of another mechanism.

Within the hyperplastic background endometrium, a focal initiation event is acquired that then expands by clonal growth to a premalignant neoplastic precursor lesion. One molecular event that has been extensively studied in these localized monoclonal proliferations of endometrial glands with nuclear atypia is the loss of *PTEN*. Mutter et al.[48] reported scattered *PTEN* loss (null glands) by immunohistochemistry and then demonstrated the *PTEN* mutation by microdissection studies. The loss of *PTEN* is present in the proliferative phase in 40% of endometrial biopsies.[48] These mutant cells escape menstrual regeneration. Precancerous lesions persist if located within the noncycling basalis endometrium or endometrial polyps. Anovulatory cycles associated with unopposed estrogen prolong the interval between shedding episodes, providing conditions that favor outgrowth of precancerous lesions. It also became clear that *PTEN* alterations alone are not sufficient for carcinoma progression. The term "latent precancer" has been applied to conditions with loss of *PTEN* to emphasize that endometrial cancer risk is not necessarily increased without additional genetic change and onset of morphologic change. Alternatively, *PTEN* loss can be viewed as low-risk lesion, and therefore could be coined as "*PTEN* signature" in analogy to the "*p53* signature." It is difficult to draw the line between molecular alterations that increase susceptibility and tumor suppressors/oncogenes. Likely, further mutations such as *CTNNB1* mutations are required

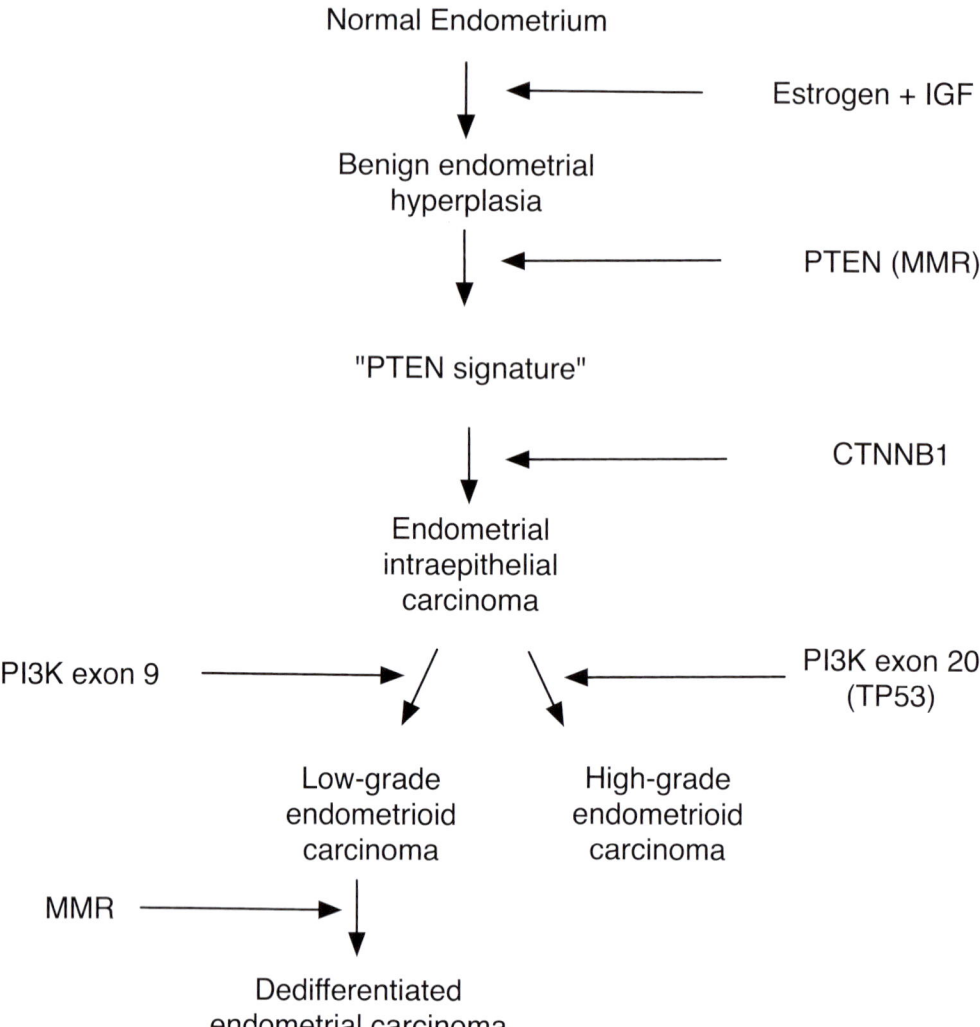

FIGURE 7-5: Proposed sequence of molecular changes during the pathogenesis of endometrioid carcinomas; see text. IGF, insulin-like growth factors.

to initiate and promote clonal growth and expand the neoplastic field. Notably, such oncogenic transformations mediate nuclear changes familiar to pathologists as nuclear atypia. For example, *KRAS* activation induces chromatin coarsening.[50] It seems that at least two alterations are necessary to cause endometrioid carcinomas, although it cannot be ruled out at this point that perhaps all of the previously mentioned pathways are somehow disturbed in endometrioid carcinogenesis (Fig. 7-5).

However, we are left with fragmented knowledge from reductive studies on several candidate genes. System analytic, comprehensive pathway analyses are required to illuminate further the complex functional interactions of those gene products and pathways. All the numbers presented likely represent underestimation due to the limited sensitivity of analytic techniques. Little is known about the events involved in progression of endometrioid carcinomas. Many open questions remain to be answered; for example, what causes the distinct patterns of progression or invasion of endometrioid carcinomas?

MOLECULAR PROGNOSTIC MARKERS

The ability to predict survival is of crucial importance in triaging women with endometrial carcinomas to therapy. There have been several hundred biomarker studies on prognostic associations with not a single marker introduced into clinical practice. There are several problems with these studies. The vast majority of studies included endometrial carcinomas of all types with confounding effects. Ignoring the biologic diversity of morphologically recognizable tumor types leads to findings such as the association of *TP53* expression with unfavorable outcome. The knowledge that *TP53* alterations are associated with an unfavorable type of endometrial carcinomas (serous) could therefore be predicted to be associated with unfavorable outcome. *TP53* alterations might be viewed as diagnostic markers to determine type, rather than an independent prognostic marker.

Despite some studies attempting to select a homogenous group of endometrioid carcinomas, none of the findings have been repeated in an independent set of endometrioid carcinomas so far. MMR-deficient tumors have been linked to unfavorable outcome.[51] This might not be surprising given the propensity to tumor progression of these highly mutating tumors. In contrast, tumors with $CD8^+$ tumor-infiltrating lymphocytes, a phenotypic hallmark of MMR deficiency, are associated with a favorable prognosis.[52] It remains to be seen whether these findings can be independently validated.

PIK3CA mutations, especially in the kinase domain (exon 20), have been associated with adverse prognostic parameters.[12] However, this mutation has also been associated with grade 3 endometrioid carcinomas, and therefore, the prognostic information is already available by light microscopy alone. It would be of outmost interest to develop surrogate markers whose expression would act as a sensor to the activation of the *PI3K* pathway. For example, EZR acts as a member of the NHERF1/PODXL family, which act as scaffold proteins for the *PTEN/PI3K* pathway components.[53] A study restricted to only endometrioid types of endometrial carcinomas demonstrated that EZR overexpression is an unfavorable prognostic marker for stage I carcinomas independent of grade.[54]

An unbiased approach to stratify endometrial carcinomas according to prognostic risk has been performed using genome-wide mRNA expression profiling.[55] Although the study consisted predominantly of endometrioid types, 15% of cases had nonendometrioid histology. Whether such a gene signature can be used to predict a given patient's prognostic outcome warrants further validation. Microarray platforms are still expensive and require additional setup; however, findings from these studies could translate into diagnostic tests using immunohistochemical marker panels as shown in a proof of principle study.[56] These specific marker panels reproduced morphologic recognizable types of endometrial carcinoma.

These examples highlight the importance of biomarker studies among and across specific tumor types. Studies between types can yield diagnostic markers that are highly correlated with a morphologic recognizable type. Diagnostic markers can be used to improve diagnostic reproducibility with respect to tumor type. It will be possible to move forward and understand the critical alterations of special cancer types through studies of case series where there is contemporary pathologic diagnosis and accompanying immunohistochemical typing. The chance to detect recurrent alterations is higher in homogeneous sets of tumors rather than in mixed cohorts of biologically diverse tumors. Studies among contemporary classified types might then yield prognostic markers beyond what is recognizable at the microscopic level.

In cases of synchronous ovarian tumors, the assessment of two independent primaries or clonal metastatic disease would impact significantly on outcome and management. Molecular studies using clonality analysis such as a combination of MSI and loss of heterozygosity or targeted approach (*PTEN* sequencing) have shown to improve the accuracy of such testing compared to the clinicopathologic decision alone.[57,58] Yet the analytic and interpretable complexities of such assays preclude routine diagnostic operation. A problem with those analyses is the intrinsic level of intratumoral heterogeneity caused by passenger alteration acquired during tumor progression. Even comprehensive genotyping by techniques such as new-generation sequencing that might be economically feasible in the near future would classify the tumors based on a few recurrent driver events and therefore likely represent a discovery tool.

TARGETED THERAPY

Unopposed estrogen provides the hormonal effect that results in endometrial hyperplasia and the background in which a monoclonal neoplasia can arise.[59] Empiric treatment of intraepithelial and invasive low-grade endometrioid neoplasias with antiestrogenic treatment such as progestin has resulted in regression in a significant portion of such lesions and is a clinical management consideration when preservation of fertilization is desired.[60] To date there are no reliable criteria that would allow prediction of treatment efficiency. The rational candidate progesterone receptor (PGR) is expressed in 92% of low-grade endometrioid carcinomas, but only up to 60% of low-grade endometrioid carcinomas respond to progestin.[60] This discrepancy raises the question of whether other mechanisms explain refraction to progestin in these cases or whether a quantitative assessment of PR expression using techniques such as automated quantitative analysis immunofluorescence[61] might identify a cutoff at which PR expression level predicts progestin response. A study on 16 endometrial endometrioid carcinomas treated with medroxyprogesterone acetate showed that PR, especially PRB, could predict the possible response of patients with endometrial carcinoma to progestin treatment.[62]

Tamoxifen and related substances are widely used in the adjuvant therapy of breast carcinomas based on their antiestrogenic function. But tamoxifen is also thought to have a dual estrogenic function, which might cause estrogen-related endometrial pathology. However, in a series of 700 patients treated with tamoxifen, 4.5% had endometrial carcinomas, of which 40% were of nonendometrioid type and not estrogen related. In comparison, endometrial polyps developed in 23% of these patients.[63] Another study followed 111 patients who were treated for breast cancer with tamoxifen for 3 years, and no atypical endometrial hyperplasia or endometrioid adenocarcinoma was found.[64] These authors even noted a decidual-type reaction in the absence of concomitant progestin treatment in a small number of the study patients. In other studies, some of the described pathology findings may have been underlying and already present before the study treatment was started.[65] These data challenge the widely accepted view that tamoxifen therapy might be associated with endometrioid type of endometrial carcinomas. Selective estrogen receptor modulators are currently being investigated in clinical trials of recurrent endometrial cancer.[66]

Given the high frequency of alterations in the *PI3K/AKT* pathway, it seems reasonable and rational to target this pathway in endometrioid carcinomas. The *PI3K/AKT* pathway, however, plays fundamental roles in homeostasis such as glucose metabolism. The downstream mTOR complex has pleiotropic and essential functions in protein translation. By interfering with this pathway for cancer therapy, significant challenges may arise in avoiding the effects of therapy competing with and complicating normal functions. For example, *PI3K* inhibition and resulting *AKT* inhibition cause toxicity such as hyperglycemia. XL765, as another example, is an oral dual PI3K and mTOR inhibitor with clinical phase I results in various solid tumors. In 26% of patients with advanced cancers treated with this drug, stable disease was achieved, but adverse effects were dose limiting.[67]

Rapamycin inhibits the activity of mTOR and has been used as an immunosuppressant for years. Three rapamycin analogs have been tested in clinical phase II studies in women with recurrent or metastatic endometrial carcinomas. Of 91 patients, 56% had some clinical benefit, defined as partial response or stable disease.[68] Assessment of pAKT, p-S6,[69] and p-mTOR was not correlated with response (keeping in mind the current reliability of phospho-specific antibodies for tissue-based analysis). Because all histologic types were included, these studies illustrates how widely histologic type is ignored with respect to targeted therapy in clinical trials.

Histone deacetylation and acetylation act as global epigenetic controls of gene expression in addition to actions as promoters of hypermethylation. Altered histone acetylation patterns have been reported in several tumor entities. Class I histone deacytelases are expressed in the majority of low-grade endometrioid carcinomas and associated with outcome, indicating biologic significance.[70] Preclinical studies using drugs that act as histone deacetylase inhibitors have shown increased induction of apoptosis in endometrial cancer cell lines and reduction of tumor size in nude mouse models.[71]

An overview of current clinical trials is beyond the scope of this chapter, but the reader is referred to an excellent article by Engelsen et al.[66] For some targets such as epidermal growth factor receptor or vascular endothelial growth factor, the molecular rationale is not well established for specific use in low-grade endometrioid carcinomas. By the time of this publication, new information on these types of trials may be available; however, it would not be surprising if many of these trials failed because most are based on empiric crossover from distinct tumor entities.

References

1. Zorn KK. Advancing our understanding of endometrial cancer histologic subtypes: should we lump or split? *Gynecol Oncol.* 2007;106:6–7.
2. Lax SF. Molecular genetic pathways in various types of endometrial carcinoma: from a phenotypical to a molecular-based classification. *Virchows Arch.* 2004;444:213–223.
3. Kohler MF, Berchuck A, Davidoff AM, et al. Overexpression and mutation of p53 in endometrial carcinoma. *Cancer Res.* 1992;52:1622–1627.
4. Risinger JI, Berchuck A, Kohler MF, et al. Genetic instability of microsatellites in endometrial carcinoma. *Cancer Res.* 1993;53:5100–5103.
5. Kong D, Suzuki A, Zou TT, et al. PTEN1 is frequently mutated in primary endometrial carcinomas. *Nat Genet.* 1997;17:143–144.
6. Risinger JI, Hayes AK, Berchuck A, et al. PTEN/MMAC1 mutations in endometrial cancers. *Cancer Res.* 1997;57:4736–4738.
7. Fukuchi T, Sakamoto M, Tsuda H, et al. Beta-catenin mutation in carcinoma of the uterine endometrium. *Cancer Res.* 1998;58:3526–3528.
8. Bokhman JV. Two pathogenetic types of endometrial carcinoma. *Gynecol Oncol.* 1983;15:10–17.
9. Lax SF, Kurman RJ. A dualistic model for endometrial carcinogenesis based on immunohistochemical and molecular genetic analyses. *Verh Dtsch Ges Pathol.* 1997;81:228–232.
10. Catasus L, Gallardo A, Cuatrecasas M, et al. Concomitant PI3K-AKT and p53 alterations in endometrial carcinomas are associated with poor prognosis. *Mod Pathol.* 2009;22:522–529.

11. An HJ, Logani S, Isacson C, et al. Molecular characterization of uterine clear cell carcinoma. *Mod Pathol.* 2004;17:530–537.
12. Catasus L, Gallardo A, Cuatrecasas M, et al. PIK3CA mutations in the kinase domain (exon 20) of uterine endometrial adenocarcinomas are associated with adverse prognostic parameters. *Mod Pathol.* 2008;21:131–139.
13. Saegusa M, Okayasu I. Frequent nuclear beta-catenin accumulation and associated mutations in endometrioid-type endometrial and ovarian carcinomas with squamous differentiation. *J Pathol.* 2001;194:59–67.
14. Llobet D, Pallares J, Yeramian A, et al. Molecular pathology of endometrial carcinoma: practical aspects from the diagnostic and therapeutic viewpoints. *J Clin Pathol.* 2009;62:777–785.
15. Hampel H, Frankel W, Panescu J, et al. Screening for Lynch syndrome (hereditary nonpolyposis colorectal cancer) among endometrial cancer patients. *Cancer Res.* 2006;66:7810–7817.
16. Lax SF, Kendall B, Tashiro H, et al. The frequency of p53, k-ras mutations, and microsatellite instability differs in uterine endometrioid and serous carcinoma: evidence of distinct molecular genetic pathways. *Cancer.* 2000;88:814–824.
17. Risinger JI, Maxwell GL, Chandramouli GV, et al. Microarray analysis reveals distinct gene expression profiles among different histologic types of endometrial cancer. *Cancer Res.* 2003;63:6–11.
18. Cao QJ, Belbin T, Socci N, et al. Distinctive gene expression profiles by cDNA microarrays in endometrioid and serous carcinomas of the endometrium. *Int J Gynecol Pathol.* 2004;23:321–329.
19. Moreno-Bueno G, Sánchez-Estévez C, Cassia R, et al. Differential gene expression profile in endometrioid and nonendometrioid endometrial carcinoma: STK15 is frequently overexpressed and amplified in nonendometrioid carcinomas. *Cancer Res.* 2003;63:5697–5702.
20. Shedden KA, Kshirsagar MP, Schwartz DR, et al. Histologic type, organ of origin, and wnt pathway status: effect on gene expression in ovarian and uterine carcinomas. *Clin Cancer Res.* 2005;11:2123–2131.
21. Mutter GL, Lin MC, Fitzgerald JT, et al. Altered PTEN expression as a diagnostic marker for the earliest endometrial precancers. *J Natl Cancer Inst.* 2000;92:924–930.
22. Chalhoub N, Baker SJ. PTEN and the pi3-kinase pathway in cancer. *Annu Rev Pathol.* 2009;4:127–150.
23. Stambolic V, Tsao MS, Macpherson D, et al. High incidence of breast and endometrial neoplasia resembling human Cowden syndrome in PTEN+/− mice. *Cancer Res.* 2000;60:3605–3611.
24. Zbuk KM, Eng C. Cancer phenomics: RET and PTEN as illustrative models. *Nat Rev Cancer.* 2007;7:35–45.
25. Black D, Bogomolniy F, Robson ME, et al. Evaluation of germline PTEN mutations in endometrial cancer patients. *Gynecol Oncol.* 2005;96:21–24.
26. Lacey JV, Mutter GL, Ronnett BM, et al. PTEN expression in endometrial biopsies as a marker of progression to endometrial carcinoma. *Cancer Res.* 2008;68:6014–6020.
27. Oda K, Stokoe D, Taketani Y, et al. High frequency of coexistent mutations of PIK3CA and PTEN genes in endometrial carcinoma. *Cancer Res.* 2005;65:10669–10673.
28. Hayes MP, Wang H, Espinal-Witter R, et al. PIK3CA and PTEN mutations in uterine endometrioid carcinoma and complex atypical hyperplasia. *Clin Cancer Res.* 2006;12:5932–5935.
29. Mirabelli-Primdahl L, Gryfe R, Kim H, et al. Beta-catenin mutations are specific for colorectal carcinomas with microsatellite instability but occur in endometrial carcinomas irrespective of mutator pathway. *Cancer Res.* 1999;59:3346–3351.
30. Ni Z, Anini Y, Fang X, et al. Transcriptional activation of the proglucagon gene by lithium and beta-catenin in intestinal endocrine L cells. *J Biol Chem.* 2003;278:1380–1387.
31. Matono H, Oda Y, Nakamori M, et al. Correlation between beta-catenin widespread nuclear expression and matrix metalloproteinase-7 overexpression in sporadic desmoid tumors. *Hum Pathol.* 2008;39:1802–1808.
32. González-Sancho JM, Aguilera O, García JM, et al. The wnt antagonist DICKKOPF-1 gene is a downstream target of beta-catenin/TCF and is downregulated in human colon cancer. *Oncogene.* 2005;24:1098–1103.

33. Jiang T, Wang S, Huang L, et al. Clinical significance of serum DKK-1 in patients with gynecological cancer. *Int J Gynecol Cancer.* 2009;19:1177–1181.
34. Backes FJ, Leon ME, Ivanov I, et al. Prospective evaluation of DNA mismatch repair protein expression in primary endometrial cancer. *Gynecol Oncol.* 2009;114:486–490.
35. Simpkins SB, Bocker T, Swisher EM, et al. MLH1 promoter methylation and gene silencing is the primary cause of microsatellite instability in sporadic endometrial cancers. *Hum Mol Genet.* 1999;8:661–666.
36. Esteller M, Levine R, Baylin SB, et al. MLH1 promoter hypermethylation is associated with the microsatellite instability phenotype in sporadic endometrial carcinomas. *Oncogene.* 1998;17:2413–2417.
37. Kawaguchi M, Banno K, Yanokura M, et al. Analysis of candidate target genes for mononucleotide repeat mutation in microsatellite instability-high (MSI-H) endometrial cancer. *Int J Oncol.* 2009;35:977–982.
38. Zighelboim I, Schmidt AP, Gao F, et al. ATR mutation in endometrioid endometrial cancer is associated with poor clinical outcomes. *J Clin Oncol.* 2009;27:3091–3096.
39. Konopka B, Janiec-Jankowska A, Czapczak D, et al. Molecular genetic defects in endometrial carcinomas: microsatellite instability, PTEN and beta-catenin (CTNNB1) genes mutations. *J Cancer Res Clin Oncol.* 2007;133:361–371.
40. Harfe BD, Jinks-Robertson S. Removal of frameshift intermediates by mismatch repair proteins in Saccharomyces cerevisiae. *Mol Cell Biol.* 1999;19:4766–4773.
41. Catasus L, Matias-Guiu X, Machin P, et al. Frameshift mutations at coding mononucleotide repeat microsatellites in endometrial carcinoma with microsatellite instability. *Cancer.* 2000;88:2290–2297.
42. Silva EG, Deavers MT, Bodurka DC, et al. Association of low-grade endometrioid carcinoma of the uterus and ovary with undifferentiated carcinoma: a new type of dedifferentiated carcinoma? *Int J Gynecol Pathol.* 2006;25:52–58.
43. Stoffel E, Mukherjee B, Raymond VM, et al. Calculation of risk of colorectal and endometrial cancer among patients with Lynch syndrome. *Gastroenterology.* 2009;137:1621–1627.
44. Hampel H, Frankel WL, Martin E, et al. Screening for the Lynch syndrome (hereditary nonpolyposis colorectal cancer). *N Engl J Med.* 2005;352:1851–1860.
45. Garg K, Soslow RA. Lynch syndrome (hereditary non-polyposis colorectal cancer) and endometrial carcinoma. *J Clin Pathol.* 2009;62:679–684.
46. Shia J, Tang LH, Vakiani E, et al. Immunohistochemistry as first-line screening for detecting colorectal cancer patients at risk for hereditary nonpolyposis colorectal cancer syndrome: a 2-antibody panel may be as predictive as a 4-antibody panel. *Am J Surg Pathol.* 2009;33:1639–1645.
47. Kang S, Lee JM, Jeon ES, et al. RASSF1A hypermethylation and its inverse correlation with BRAF and/or KRAS mutations in MSI-associated endometrial carcinoma. *Int J Cancer.* 2006;119:1316–1321.
48. Mutter GL, Ince TA, Baak JP, et al. Molecular identification of latent precancers in histologically normal endometrium. *Cancer Res.* 2001;61:4311–4314.
49. Maxwell GL, Risinger JI, Gumbs C, et al. Mutation of the PTEN tumor suppressor gene in endometrial hyperplasias. *Cancer Res.* 1998;58:2500–2503.
50. Fischer AH, Chadee DN, Wright JA, et al. Ras-associated nuclear structural change appears functionally significant and independent of the mitotic signaling pathway. *J Cell Biochem.* 1998;70:130–140.
51. An HJ, Kim KI, Kim JY, et al. Microsatellite instability in endometrioid type endometrial adenocarcinoma is associated with poor prognostic indicators. *Am J Surg Pathol.* 2007;31:846–853.
52. de Jong RA, Leffers N, Boezen HM, et al. Presence of tumor-infiltrating lymphocytes is an independent prognostic factor in type I and II endometrial cancer. *Gynecol Oncol.* 2009;114:105–110.
53. Georgescu MM. NHERF1: molecular brake on the PI3K pathway in breast cancer. *Breast Cancer Res.* 2008;10:106.

54. Köbel M, Langhammer T, Hüttelmaier S, et al. Ezrin expression is related to poor prognosis in FIGO stage I endometrioid carcinomas. *Mod Pathol.* 2006;19:581–587.
55. Ferguson SE, Olshen AB, Viale A, et al. Stratification of intermediate-risk endometrial cancer patients into groups at high risk or low risk for recurrence based on tumor gene expression profiles. *Clin Cancer Res.* 2005;11:2252–2257.
56. Alkushi A, Clarke BA, Akbari M, et al. Identification of prognostically relevant and reproducible subsets of endometrial adenocarcinoma based on clustering analysis of immunostaining data. *Mod Pathol.* 2007;20:1156–1165.
57. Irving JA, Catasús L, Gallardo A, et al. Synchronous endometrioid carcinomas of the uterine corpus and ovary: alterations in the beta-catenin (CTNNB1) pathway are associated with independent primary tumors and favorable prognosis. *Hum Pathol.* 2005;36:605–619.
58. Ramus SJ, Elmasry K, Luo Z, et al. Predicting clinical outcome in patients diagnosed with synchronous ovarian and endometrial cancer. *Clin Cancer Res.* 2008;14:5840–5848.
59. Hecht JL, Mutter GL. Molecular and pathologic aspects of endometrial carcinogenesis. *J Clin Oncol.* 2006;24:4783–4791.
60. Wheeler DT, Bristow RE, Kurman RJ. Histologic alterations in endometrial hyperplasia and well-differentiated carcinoma treated with progestins. *Am J Surg Pathol.* 2007;31:988–998.
61. Camp RL, Chung GG, Rimm DL. Automated subcellular localization and quantification of protein expression in tissue microarrays. *Nat Med.* 2002;8:1323–1327.
62. Utsunomiya H, Suzuki T, Ito K, et al. The correlation between the response to progestogen treatment and the expression of progesterone receptor B and 17beta-hydroxysteroid dehydrogenase type 2 in human endometrial carcinoma. *Clin Endocrinol (Oxf).* 2003;58:696–703.
63. Deligdisch L, Kalir T, Cohen CJ, et al. Endometrial histopathology in 700 patients treated with tamoxifen for breast cancer. *Gynecol Oncol.* 2000;78:181–186.
64. Barakat RR, Gilewski TA, Almadrones L, et al. Effect of adjuvant tamoxifen on the endometrium in women with breast cancer: a prospective study using office endometrial biopsy. *J Clin Oncol.* 2000;18:3459–3463.
65. Berlière M, Charles A, Galant C, et al. Uterine side effects of tamoxifen: a need for systematic pretreatment screening. *Obstet Gynecol.* 1998;91:40–44.
66. Engelsen IB, Akslen LA, Salvesen HB. Biologic markers in endometrial cancer treatment. *APMIS.* 2009;117:693–707.
67. Molckovsky A, Siu LL. First-in-class, first-in-human phase I results of targeted agents: highlights of the 2008 American Society of Clinical Oncology meeting. *J Hematol Oncol.* 2008;1:20.
68. Delmonte A, Sessa C. Molecule-targeted agents in endometrial cancer. *Curr Opin Oncol.* 2008;20:554–559.
69. Iwenofu OH, Lackman RD, Staddon AP, et al. Phospho-S6 ribosomal protein: a potential new predictive sarcoma marker for targeted mTOR therapy. *Mod Pathol.* 2008;21:231–237.
70. Weichert W, Denkert C, Noske A, et al. Expression of class I histone deacetylases indicates poor prognosis in endometrioid subtypes of ovarian and endometrial carcinomas. *Neoplasia.* 2008;10:1021–1027.
71. Takai N, Desmond JC, Kumagai T, et al. Histone deacetylase inhibitors have a profound antigrowth activity in endometrial cancer cells. *Clin Cancer Res.* 2004;10:1141–1149.

High-Risk Endometrial Carcinoma

▸ Martin Köbel, MD

High-risk endometrial carcinomas are a heterogeneous group of tumors that include grade 3 endometrioid, serous, and clear cell carcinomas and other rare types of endometrial carcinoma. The term high risk can be used interchangeably with high grade. High risk is related to the putative outcome of women diagnosed with this disease and is assessed as a risk of tumor-related death of more than 30% to 40% within 5 to 10 years. Each of these tumor types as a group shows high risk, although disease stage–related differences exist.[1] There remain significant questions about the natural history of these tumor types. For example, the 5-year survival rate for grade 3 endometrioid carcinomas, all stages, varies from 45% to 77%,[1,2] and the rate for serous carcinomas, all stages, ranges from 29% to 55%.[1,3] A number of factors could have contributed to the differences in the 5-year survival rate observed in these studies (e.g., extent of surgical staging, use of adjuvant therapy). However, it is also possible that these discordant results with respect to prognosis might be due to differences in accurate classification regarding tumor histologic type of the high-grade endometrial carcinomas. These high-grade tumors particularly represent a clinical challenge because they are uncommon yet account for a disproportionate percentage of tumor-related deaths. Specific studies on molecular alterations in these tumor types have been limited in the past. Currently, these tumors are intensely being studied.

GRADE 3 ENDOMETRIOID CARCINOMAS

The distinction of grade 3 endometrioid carcinomas from low-grade endometrioid tumors as a separate tumor type is based on a distinct phenotype and the presentation at higher stage and high risk of recurrence. However, it is not yet supported by a unique molecular difference, although some differences have been identified. In fact, grade 3 (high-grade) endometrioid carcinomas share the most characteristic abnormalities with grade 1 or 2 (low-grade) endometrioid carcinomas such as similar frequencies of *PTEN* and *PIK3CA* mutation (see Table 7-1). Notably, the histologic grade varied according to location of the *PIK3CA* mutations. Exon 9 (helical domain) mutations were more often detected in low-grade endometrioid carcinomas compared with high-grade endometrioid carcinomas, which more often showed mutations in exon 20 (kinase domain).[4]

TP53 mutations, a hallmark of serous carcinomas (see below), have been found in 17% of grade 3 endometrioid carcinomas, and *TP53* overexpression is detectable in up to 40% of these tumors (Table 8-1).[3,5–8] This more than twofold discrepancy again illustrates the need for a more reproducible diagnosis of grade 3 endometrioid carcinomas. The separation of grade 3 endometrioid carcinoma as a unique biologic tumor type may be disputable based

Table 8-1 Biomarker Expression

Gene	EC-1/2	EC-3	SC	CCC
ESR1[3]	106/110; 97%	27/33; 82%	6/12; 50%	2/7; 29%
PGR[3]	72/78; 92%	21/31; 68%	5/11; 46%	1/7; 14%
SCGB2A2[5]	26/28; 93%	6/22; 27%		
TFF3[7]		20/25; 79%		
PTEN (loss of)[3]	45/96; 47%	12/31; 39%	0/10; 0%	1/6; 17%
CTNNB1 (nuclear)[8]	9/13; 69%		0/16; 0%	
TP53 (overexpression)[3]	3/108; 3%	13/33; 40%	9/13; 70%	2/8; 25%
CDKN2A (overexpression)[3]	1/109; 1%	6/31; 20%	9/10; 90%	1/6; 17%
IGF2BP3	5/70; 7%[6]	6/30; 20%[3]	48/51; 97%[6]	3/12; 25%[6]

CCC, clear cell carcinoma; EC-1/2, low-grade (grades 1 and 2) endometrioid carcinoma; EC-3, high-grade (grade 3) endometrioid carcinoma; SC, serous carcinoma.

on current knowledge. Yet it is the opinion of the author that understanding of this clinically relevant type will only evolve after adjusting study cohorts for clinical (cohort frequency, stage distribution, outcome) and pathologic criteria. This will allow the cases in different studies to be compared directly and ensure that differences are not related to differences in diagnostic criteria used for type assignment.

SEROUS CARCINOMA

Characteristics

Serous carcinomas display severe nuclear atypia, which is the result of chromosomal instability. The hallmark mutation of serous carcinomas is the somatic mutation of *TP53* in more than 90% of cases (see Table 7-1). There is a paucity of other recurrent alterations except the high level of genomic instability, which characterizes serous carcinomas and presents a tremendous challenge to identify further relevant alterations. It seems that *TP53* mutations are necessary to allow this level of chromosomal rearrangement and to escape the stability control of normal mammalian cells. This assumption is supported by evidence that *TP53* mutations are an early event found in precursor lesions of serous carcinomas and from genetically engineered mouse models that reflect serous carcinogenesis. Genetically engineered mouse models developed serous carcinomas exclusively in *TP53*-mutated background, but *TP53* mutation alone was insufficient to generate serous carcinomas. A second oncogenic mutation in a proliferation pathway such as *RB1* or *MYC* was required.[9,10] Together, these data suggest that *TP53* deficiency is a requirement for serous carcinogenesis (i.e., preventing apoptosis prior to chromosomal instability).

TP53 mutation has been detected in precursor lesions of serous carcinomas.[11] The earliest recognizable lesion with evidence of *TP53* mutation is the so-called p53 signature.[12] p53 signature can be detected by immunohistochemistry as a surrogate for direct sequencing with a minimal requirement of strong nuclear staining in greater than 12 consecutive epithelial cells. p53 signature displays normal morphology without increased proliferation rate, which delineates it from morphologically recognizable precursors. p53 signatures have been found in the epithelium of 4% of 137 investigated endometrial polyps.[13] The significance of p53 signatures remains to be clarified because it is not clear whether these p53 signatures already represent a risk factor or whether p53 signatures represent a lesion with only a minimal risk of progression unless an additional oncogenic hit initiates carcinogenesis.

The earliest morphologic recognizable precursor lesions are endometrial glandular dysplasia (EmGD) and endometrial intraepithelial carcinoma (EIC), which are both associated with *TP53* mutations. EmGD is defined as glands or surface epithelium displaying a single layer or occasionally two layers of pseudostratification of cells with increased nuclear size (two to three times larger compared with background endometrium but less than four to five times the enlargement seen in EIC).[14] *TP53* mutations have been detected in 43% of EmGD and 72% of EIC.[11] With the assumption that *TP53* mutation is a necessity for serous carcinogenesis, the absence of *TP53* mutation in a significant portion of precursor lesions needs further elucidation but might be explained by limited sensitivity of direct sequencing, giving the small size of some of those lesions. Although direct sequencing remains the gold standard to detect *TP53* mutations, mutational analyses are time consuming and expensive. Therefore, immunohistochemistry has been frequently used as a surrogate marker under the assumption that missense *TP53* mutations are associated with nonfunctional protein accumulation, which can be detected by immunohistochemistry with strong staining in more than 50% of tumor cell nuclei.[15]

A minority of *TP53* mutations are nonsense mutations. Nonsense mutations result in a nonsense or premature stop codon, which theoretically translates into a nonfunctional or truncated protein. Yet such nonfunctional proteins do not occur due to the nonsense-mediated mRNA decay pathway, which degrades mRNAs containing nonsense mutation before they are translated. As a result, no protein should be present. It remains to be validated whether based on this theoretical framework, *TP53* immunohistochemistry can reliably be used as a surrogate marker for the *TP53* mutation status. Aberrant *TP53* expression would be defined as an overexpression, with more than 50% of tumor cell nuclei expressing the missense mutation, or as completely negative, correlating with the nonsense mutation. In contrast, any expression from single cell to patchy expression would indicate *TP53* wild type.

These precursor lesions categorize a morphologic continuum from p53 signature to EmGD to EIC to invasive serous carcinoma (Fig. 8-1). All are characterized by *TP53* mutation but differ with respect to the accumulation of additional chromosomal instability reflected by increasing nuclear atypia and proliferation.[12] There is a need for further objective criteria that would assign these lesions into meaningful categories for clinical management. For example, EIC is defined as an intraepithelial noninvasive growth pattern but might be already associated with extrauterine disease, although a minority of these cases may actually arise within the distal fallopian tube.[16]

Compared with other types, serous carcinomas display a high level of chromosomal instability seen as severe nuclear atypia under the microscope or shown by DNA copy number analysis.[17,18] As previously mentioned, *TP53* mutations do not directly cause chromosomal instability but rather provide the background for the acquisition of such changes by preventing apoptosis. Hence, additional alterations affecting DNA repair, preferentially double-stranded, have been suggested. Ovarian high-grade serous carcinoma is the typical tumor type associated with *BRCA1* or *BRCA2* mutations.[19] Despite some case reports on endometrial serous carcinomas associated with *BRCA* mutation, the most comprehensive series on 56 cases of endometrial serous carcinomas failed to show any *BRCA1* or *BRCA2* mutations using tests that would detect approximately 70% of those mutations.[20] However,

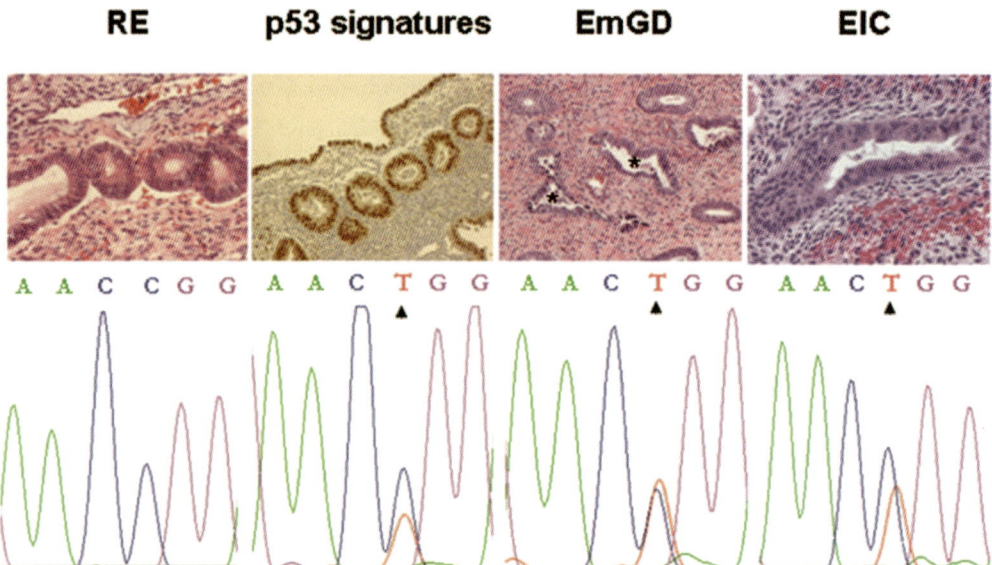

FIGURE 8-1: Proposed sequence of serous carcinogenesis. **Top row** shows representative images of hematoxylin and eosin staining of resting endometrium (RE), *TP53* immunohistochemical staining (p53 signatures), endometrial glandular dysplasia (EmGD), and serous endometrial intraepithelial carcinoma (EIC). Original magnification, ×200. Noticeable degree of nuclear atypia in EmGD (*asterisks*) clearly exceeds the RE but falls short of EIC. **Bottom row** shows corresponding DNA sequence analyses that showed identical *TP53* gene mutations of exon 7 at codon 248 from CGG to TGG (Arg to Trp), whereas no mutation was found in the corresponding RE sample; results derived from laser capture microdissected samples. These samples were obtained from the same case. Identical mutation was also observed in endometrial serous carcinoma area (not shown) in the same uterus. (With permission from Jarboe EA, Miron A, Carlson JW, et al. Coexisting intraepithelial serous carcinomas of the endometrium and fallopian tube: frequency and potential significance. *Int J Gynecol Pathol.* 2009;28:308–315.)

a recent analysis identified three cases of uterine serous carcinomas associated with *BRCA* mutation in a population-based series.[21]

Random chromosomal rearrangements detectable as DNA copy number gains and losses likely activate oncogenes involved in regulating proliferation. Endometrial serous carcinomas are characterized by a high proliferation rate that is already present in its precursor lesions. The Ki-67 labeling index of endometrial serous carcinoma is usually between 50% and 90% of tumor cells. DNA copy number analyses have detected frequent gains at several recurrent chromosomal regions including 8q[17,18] containing candidate oncogenes such as *MYC*.[22] Multiple different genetic abnormalities can contribute to a pro-proliferative state by abrogating cell cycle checkpoints, leading to uncontrolled cell cycle progression through G_1 and S phases. This further contributes to missegregation of chromosomes during mitosis and fortifying genomic instability. Because a high proliferative rate is characteristic of all serous carcinomas, it is conceivable that all serous carcinomas carry defects in one or more oncogenes regulating proliferation (e.g., cases with amplification of *MYC*, *CCND1*, or *CCNE1* may be functionally equivalent or synergistic). There has not been a comprehensive survey of all of these alterations in serous carcinoma, and we are left with fragmentary information, typically consisting of data for one or two markers in any given study. We are far from understanding how these abnormalities co-operate during tumor genesis and how such perturbations in cell cycle control could be used clinically.

CDKN2A (p16) seems to be a useful surrogate marker of underlying increased proliferation that characterizes endometrial serous carcinomas. *CDKN2A* is overexpressed in 90% to 100% of endometrial serous carcinomas using a high cutoff with greater than 80% of tumor cells showing either nuclear or cytoplasmic positive staining.[23,24] In contrast to carcinomas of the cervix uteri, endometrial serous carcinomas are not related to human papillomavirus infection. The specific cause for *CDKN2A* overexpression remains elusive and might represent a futile attempt to stop cell cycle progression, which may be caused by alterations in different cell cycle regulating proteins. This assumption is supported by the concordant overexpression of *CDKN2A* with *CDK2AP2* (p14).

Molecular Prognostic Markers

Prognostic marker studies for endometrial serous carcinomas are hampered by the rarity of this tumor type in a single institution. The favorable prognostic significance of the host immune response, as defined by the presence of tumor-infiltrating lymphocytes (i.e., intraepithelial lymphocytes), has been reported in 186 advanced-stage ovarian cancers, likely predominantly high-grade serous carcinomas.[25] Tumor-infiltrating lymphocytes are also associated with favorable outcome in endometrial serous carcinomas.[26]

To date, no specific therapeutic target is emerging. Candidate alterations seen in other tumor entities such as *EGFR* mutations have not been detected in serous carcinomas.[27] Similarly, ERBB2 amplification has only been found in 2 (3%) of 64 of endometrial serous carcinomas,[28] limiting its potential clinical utility.

The high level of chromosomal instability and the paucity of recurrent mutation other than *TP53* present a tremendous challenge in attempts to subclassify serous carcinomas for novel treatment strategies that target specific molecular defects. As a corollary, serous carcinomas display a myriad of passenger molecular alterations, and a comprehensive analysis is needed to delineate major molecular differences. Another consequence of chromosomal instability is the high degree of intratumoral heterogeneity indicating that the study of multiple tumor foci might be needed to filter for passenger events. However, evolution of subclones might cause therapy resistance.

CLEAR CELL CARCINOMAS

Clear cell carcinomas are classified along with serous carcinoma as type 2 due to their clinicopathologic similarities. Clear cell carcinomas have only rarely been studied as a defined group using molecular techniques. Eleven pure clear cell carcinomas in one study were evaluated with respect to their *TP53* and *PTEN* mutational status and for microsatellite instability.[29] Only a single case showed *TP53* mutation, and it had been recognized earlier that *TP53* overexpression is not a characteristic feature of clear cell carcinoma.[30] Two (22%) of nine cases revealed a *PTEN* mutation.[29] In a different study, 6 (46%) of 13 clear cell carcinomas showed *PIK3CA* mutations,[31] the highest frequency among all types (Fig. 8-2). From a molecular perspective, clear cell carcinomas seem to share alterations within the *PTEN/PI3K* pathway with endometrioid carcinomas, which challenge their classification as type 2 cancer in the binary system. Endometrioid and clear cell carcinomas differ across abnormalities affecting the *Wnt/CTNNB1* pathway, which is so far specific for endometrioid types.

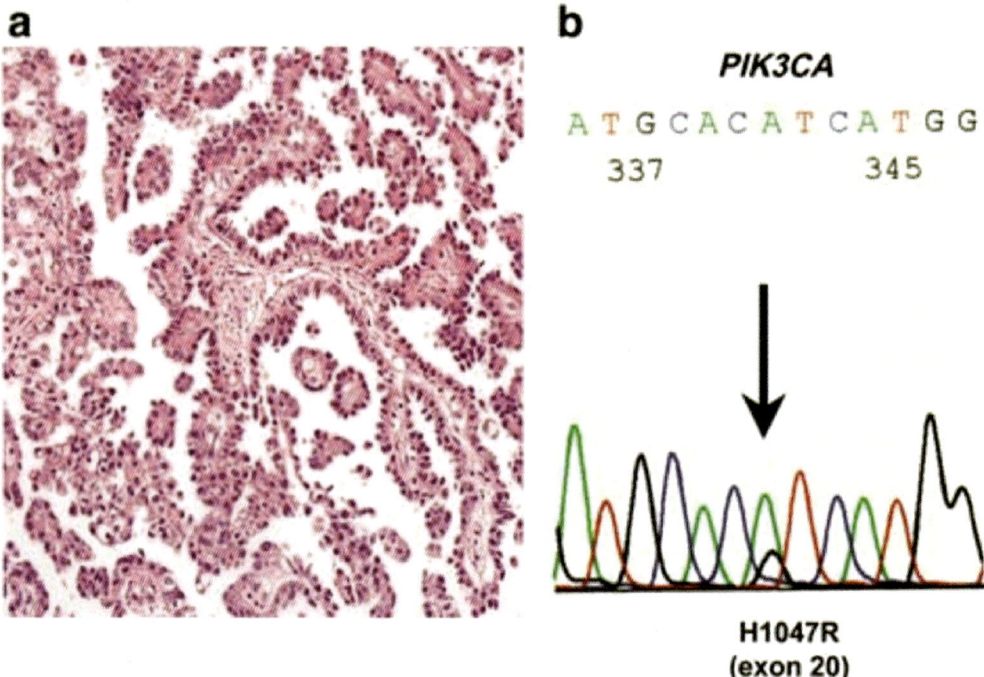

FIGURE 8-2: **a:** Clear cell carcinoma. **b:** Sequence analysis of exon 20 of *PIK3CA* reveals a missense mutation (H1047R). (With permission from Catasus L, Gallardo A, Cuatrecasas M, et al. Concomitant PI3K-AKT and p53 alterations in endometrial carcinomas are associated with poor prognosis. *Mod Pathol.* 2009;22:522–529.)

These studies, although small, raise some important questions regarding the pathogenesis of endometrial clear cell carcinoma and indicate the need to study pure, expertly classified clear cell carcinomas in the future. As more studies using new comprehensive techniques on the molecular mechanisms underlying this tumor are revealed, we may be able to better understand the pathogenesis of this enigmatic tumor that represents a particular therapeutic challenge. This goal should be approached by a multi-institutional consortium of researchers interested in this unique disease.

DIAGNOSTIC MARKERS

There is a paradigm in cancer research that the identification of molecular alterations defining entities follows, in most instances, an accurate description by pathologists of the entity based on morphologic and immunophenotypic parameters. Therefore, the importance of accurate classification for research and clinical studies cannot be overemphasized. It will only be possible to resolve outstanding research questions if there is highly reproducible diagnosis of tumor type. Application of reproducible morphologic criteria is the first step, but in a minority of cases, use of immunohistochemistry (or other molecular markers) might be required in order to obtain diagnostic accuracy and reproducibility. Ultimately, our ability to develop and implement type-specific ("personalized") treatment will depend on making reproducible diagnoses. Studies to determine whether such tests, as an adjunct to routine histopathologic examination, can enhance diagnostic reproducibility are needed.

A diagnostic marker might be defined as a tool that enables the distinction of entities, diseases, or conditions that are characterized by distinct molecular alterations, phenotypes, and clinical behavior. In contrast, a prognostic marker might allow stratification within such an entity. Such markers may be derived from the cell lineage or associated with the underlying oncogenic pathways.

Examples of endometrioid cell lineage markers that have not been implicated in oncogenic pathways but are present in corresponding normal tissue are hormone receptors and SCGB2A2 (mammaglobin B).[5] There is no marker of cell lineage for serous carcinoma with sufficient sensitivity. WT1, which is a good marker for other pelvic high-grade serous carcinomas and is expressed in the normal fallopian tube, has been reported to have significantly lower expression in endometrial serous carcinomas (29% versus 90% for other pelvic high-grade serous carcinomas).[32] IGF2BP3 (IMP3), an oncofetal protein involved in IGF2 mRNA stabilization, has recently been reported as being reexpressed in endometrial serous carcinomas[6] and might be useful for the distinction from low-grade endometrioid carcinomas. However, IGF2BP3 is also expressed in approximately half of ovarian clear cell carcinomas[33]; hence, the use for the differential diagnosis versus clear cell carcinomas may be limited.

The biomarker expression profiles of the four major tumor types are shown in Table 8-1. In the optimal scenario, a low-grade endometrioid carcinoma is characterized by the expression of ESR1 (estrogen receptor)/PGR (progesterone receptor) and SCGB2A2; *PTEN* or nuclear *CTNNB1* may or may not be present, but there is no aberrant *TP53* expression, *CDKN2A* overexpression, or IGF2BP3 expression. In contrast, serous carcinomas show an inverse pattern with respect to *TP53*, *CDKN2A*, and IGF2BP3, and hormone receptors may or may not be expressed, but *PTEN* is certainly present, and nuclear *CTNNB1* is not observed (Fig. 8-3). Clear cell carcinomas show IGF2BP3 expression or loss of *PTEN* expression in some cases. In analogy to ovarian clear cell carcinomas, HNF1B expression has been suggested as a sensitive marker for endometrial clear cell carcinomas as well. However, specificity needs further validation in larger series.

For practical considerations, the complexity shown in Table 8-1 may be translated into a type-to-type comparison (Fig. 8-4) because most diagnostic problems that arise when based on morphology occur when the differential diagnosis has been narrowed to a decision between two of those types. For challenging diagnoses such as grade 2 endometrioid carcinomas with small nonvillous papillae versus serous carcinomas, immunohistochemistry has been advocated (Table 8-2).

Given that the distinction between low-grade endometrioid carcinoma and serous carcinomas is important because of the significant therapeutic implications, a table like Table 8-2 can guide the selection of markers for a specific diagnostic question (i.e., using a two-marker panel of *CDKN2A* and IGF2BP3 likely resolves diagnostic uncertainties in >95% of cases). Another example is given in Figure 8-5 for the distinction between serous carcinoma and grade 3 endometrioid carcinomas; the combination of *CDKN2A* and *PTEN* immunohistochemistry is able to distinguish between these two with a sensitivity of 90% and specificity of 96%.

The genotype–phenotype correlation is mediated by differential expression of a minority (the exact number is unknown) of genes. Microarray studies on the mRNA profile of specific cancer types used several hundreds of differentially expressed genes for classification. It is possible that further studies will reveal some more useful diagnostic markers, but it is unlikely that there will be a single prefect marker for each type (i.e., a single marker with the desired sensitivity or specificity >95%). Therefore, refinement of our current tools has the potential to yield a tool consisting of an immunohistochemical

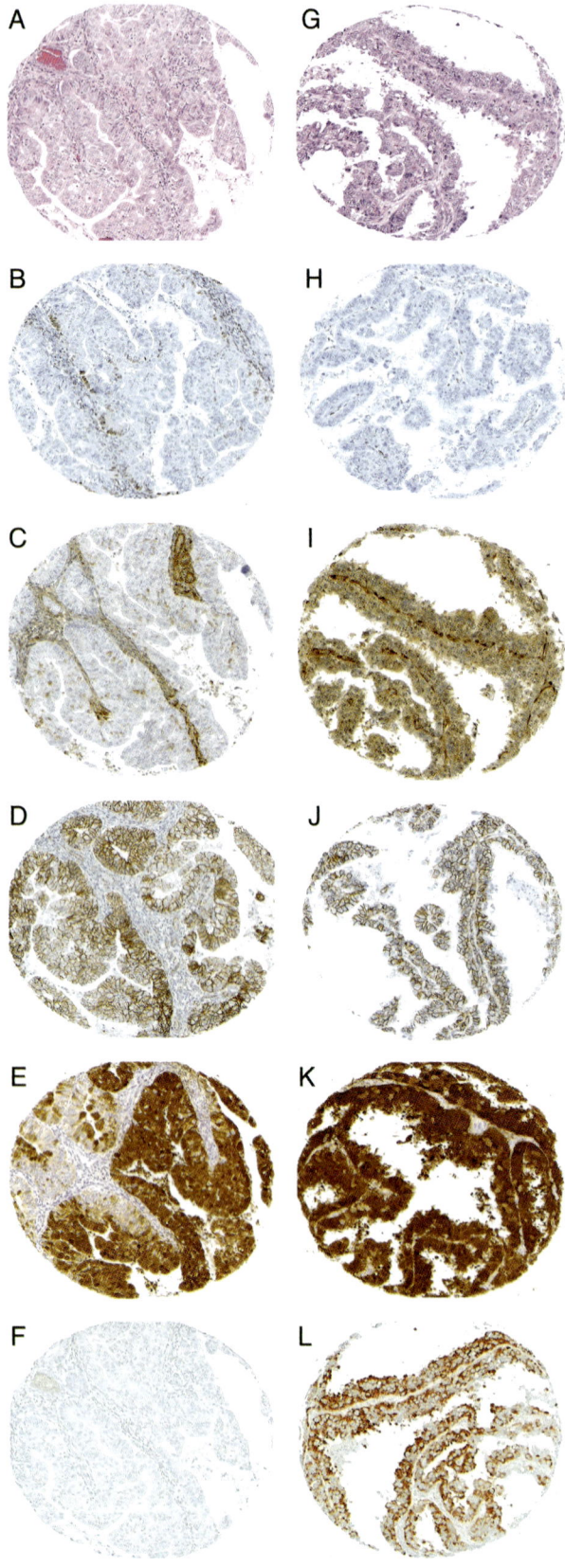

FIGURE 8-3: Biomarker expression with one low-grade endometrioid carcinomas (**left column**) versus one serous carcinoma (**right column**): (**A, E**) hematoxylin and eosin; (**B, F**) PGR (PR); (**C, G**) *PTEN*; (**D, G**) *CTNNB1* (β-catenin); (**E, K**) *CDKN2A* (p16); and (**F, L**) IGF2BP3 (IMP3). The endometrioid carcinoma in the left column panel shows focal PGR expression (the majority of low-grade endometrioid carcinomas would show diffuse PGR expression), loss of *PTEN* expression (note retained expression within the stroma and intraepithelial inflammatory cells), and membranous *CTNNB1* expression (a significant minority of low-grade endometrioid carcinomas would show aberrant *CTNNB1* expression with protein localized in the nucleus and cytoplasm). Note that p16 expression in low-grade endometrioid carcinomas can be high but should still present as a mosaic pattern (in contrast to the diffuse expression of all tumor cells in an endometrial serous carcinoma), and IGF2BP3 is negative.

Chapter 8 • High-Risk Endometrial Carcinoma

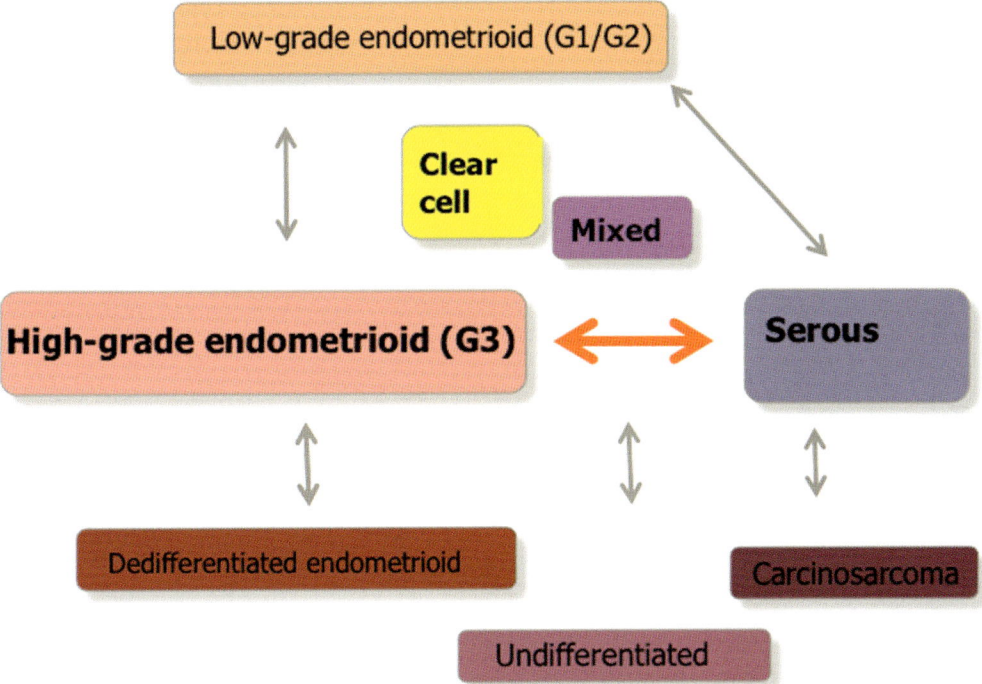

FIGURE 8-4: Differential diagnostic problem areas. Endometrial carcinomas can also be broadly divided into morphologically homogeneous versus heterogeneous tumors. The latter may cause a tremendous challenge with respect to correct typing, particularly when the nuclear atypia is or borders on high grade. The refined use of markers we currently know and the translation of new markers (ARID1A, PPP2R1A) into diagnostic practice should enable us in the future to achieve a similar high level of concordance with respect to typing of endometrial carcinomas compared to their ovarian counterparts.

Table 8-2	Sensitivity and Specificity of Immunohistochemical Markers for the Discrimination between Low-Grade Endometrioid Carcinoma (EC-1/2) and Serous Carcinoma (SC)		
Gene	Sensitivity (%)	EC-3 Specificity (%)	Positive Level
ESR1	97	50	EC-1/2
PGR	92	54	EC-1/2
PTEN (loss of)	47	100	EC-1/2
CTNNB1 (nuclear)	69	100	EC-1/2
TP53 (overexpression)	70	97	SC
CDKN2A (overexpression)	90	99	SC
IMP3	97	93	SC

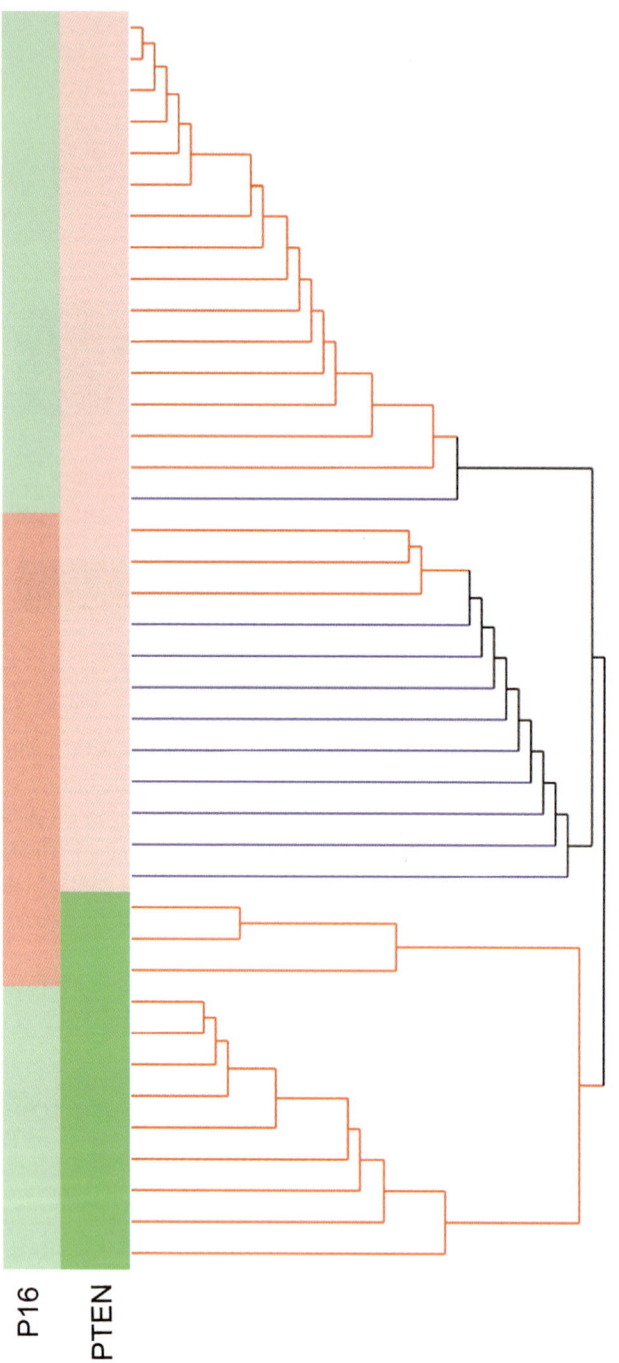

FIGURE 8-5: Heat map representing the combination of *CDKN2A*/p16 and *PTEN* expression (*green* = negative, *red* = positive) for 30 grade 3 endometrioid (EC3) and 10 serous carcinomas (SC). Each EC3 is represented by a *red line*, and each SC is represented by a *blue line*. Nine of 10 SCs showed diffuse *CDKN2A* overexpression and retained *PTEN* expression.

marker panel that is similar or superior in performance when compared to conventional morphology. Interpretation of marker panels easily overstrains pathologists in routine practice. For example, a panel of two markers all with two degrees of possible outcome (negative/positive) results in four possible combinations. A panel of nine markers scored in two categories results in 512 combinations, and this panel scored in a three-tier system results in 19,683 permutations. Hierarchical regression is usually used to circumvent this complexity; however, other models such as the nominal logistic regression model would be useful statistical tools because these models calculate probabilities for a given type. The interpretation of probabilities in the morphologic context embraces conventional morphology with objective molecular markers and avoids reporting of conflicting results from standard histopathology and independent molecular tests. Before such a marker panel may be used routinely, the main challenges to overcome would be in terms of tissue handling (fixation times), standardization of immunohistochemistry, and interpretation (i.e., cutoffs). As with any other laboratory test, external quality assurance programs should monitor immunohistochemistry.

MIXED ENDOMETRIAL CARCINOMAS

The World Health Organization defines mixed endometrial carcinomas as a combined tumor consisting of at least 10% of both a type 1 (endometrioid/rarely mucinous) and a type 2 (mostly serous/occasionally clear cell) component. Mixed endometrial carcinomas are biologically interesting because they represent a possible transition between types, but they are also diagnostically challenging because in some cases, tumors with ambiguous but homogeneous features (i.e., inconclusive whether serous or endometrioid) are included within this category. Clinically, these tumors are managed as serous carcinomas because the threshold of the serous component that accounts for adverse outcome has been continuously lowered over the years and is now at 10%.[34] Therefore, there is a controversy about the use of an additional category of mixed endometrial carcinomas. Given the unique morphologic features and the potential biologic implication, it is believed that these tumors should be separately classified with specific reference to the combination (e.g., serous/endometrioid, clear cell/endometrioid). For clinical purposes and at the present time, mixed tumors are considered based on their highest grade component (i.e., serous or clear cell), rather than viewing this heterogeneous group as a separate tumor type (mixed).

With emergence of knowledge on molecular alterations in pure types, these markers can be used to study and diagnose mixed endometrial carcinomas. For example, if in doubt whether there is a morphologically identifiable second component, the aforementioned diagnostic markers should be applied, and the differential expression of at least one marker in the suspected components should be seen. The rare tumor with homogeneous intermediate features that cannot be resolved by immunohistochemistry may be left as "unclassifiable." A stricter definition of mixed endometrial carcinomas by the use of ancillary techniques may reduce the frequency of cases within this category, resulting in restriction of cases to those of special biologic interest and in the question of whether these tumors are the result of progression or collision. Based on unpublished personal observations, two cases of mixed endometrial carcinomas (clear cell/endometrioid) were noted that were small and physically separated, indicating independent synchronous primary. In both cases, both components showed a loss of *PTEN* expression, indicating the origin from a common precancerous field, but they differed with respect to their hormone receptor expression (Fig. 8-6). These cases have not been tested for mismatch repair (MMR) deficiency. Endometrioid carcinomas occasionally show small superficial papillary projections ("sloughing") that should not be overdiagnosed as serous carcinomas. However, there are well-documented cases of endometrioid carcinomas with abrupt bordering of serous carcinomas supported by *TP53* or *CDKN2A* expression differences.[35]

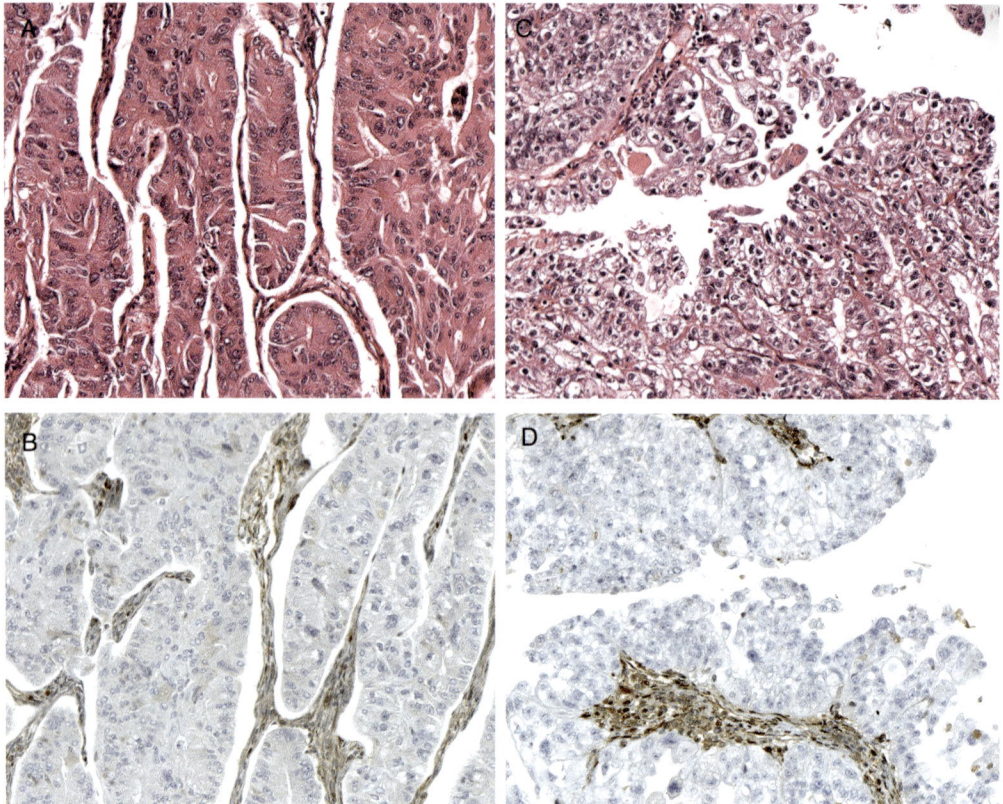

FIGURE 8-6: Mixed clear cell/endometrioid carcinomas, with loss of *PTEN* expression in both components.

RARE TUMOR TYPES

Rare tumors as a group account for less than 5% of endometrial carcinomas and include dedifferentiated, undifferentiated, neuroendocrine, and squamous carcinomas. The morphologic features of these tumors are clearly described, yet their association with molecular markers needs further definition.

Occasionally, low-grade endometrioid carcinomas show an admixture with undifferentiated carcinomas.[36] Given the unique morphologic combination, potential aggressive behavior, and association with MMR deficiency, these tumors should be separately classified as dedifferentiated endometrial carcinomas.

Undifferentiated carcinoma has been diagnosed with a frequency of 1.6% among 1,985 uterine carcinomas[37] and is associated with a particular adverse outcome.[38] Undifferentiated carcinomas should only be diagnosed after careful exclusion of other malignancies, including high-grade carcinomas. Any glandular (grade 3 endometrioid), serous, or neuroendocrine component should be sufficient to diagnose a more specific type. Undifferentiated carcinomas might be classified in the future solely based on molecular markers.

The diagnosis of neuroendocrine carcinomas might affect adjuvant therapy because some centers use etoposide/cisplatin chemotherapy for neuroendocrine carcinomas instead of paclitaxel/cisplatin. This diagnosis is usually based on positivity of at least one of the neuroendocrine markers (chromogranin A, synaptophysin, CD56), although expression of these markers did not correlate with outcome when undifferentiated endometrial carcinomas with or without neuroendocrine marker expression were compared.[39]

The significance of squamous differentiation within endometrial carcinomas has been disputed for years, and the present consensus is to diagnose these tumors as endometrioid carcinomas with squamous differentiation. It remains to be seen whether a separate group of endometrial squamous or adenosquamous (i.e., such tumors with a malignant squamous component) can be defined and separated from the much more common endocervical squamous cell carcinomas. To date, less than 100 cases of primary squamous cell carcinomas of the endometrium have been reported in the literature. The pathogenesis of primary squamous cell carcinomas of the endometrium is poorly characterized. Review of the literature has shown that there are many postulated risk factors, including pyometra, cervical stenosis, hypovitaminosis A, senile involution of the endometrium with squamous metaplasia, chronic irritation due to an intrauterine device, prolapse, and previous irradiation. The pathogenetic mechanisms that have also been proposed include malignant transformation of squamous epithelium arising from either heterotopic cervical tissue or squamous differentiation of a pluripotent endometrial precursor cell.[40] The human papillomavirus does not appear to be associated with primary squamous cell carcinomas of the endometrium, and recent studies have looked at some of the cell cycle pathways involved with these lesions. The literature suggests that primary squamous cell carcinomas of the endometrium may have alterations of *CDKN2A* and *CCND1* but not *TP53*, indicating alterations to the *RB1* pathway independent of human papillomavirus.[41]

A better understanding of the major pure types will reveal potential links but may also yield a more precise separation of these rare special types.

CARCINOSARCOMAS/MALIGNANT MÜLLERIAN MIXED TUMORS

Malignant müllerian mixed tumors (MMMTs) contain admixed carcinomatous and sarcomatoid components with clear demarcation of the components (without extensive merging of the two).[42] Because *TP53* alterations are frequently found and are concordant between the carcinomatous and sarcomatous components, MMMTs are thought of as being monoclonal in origin.[43–45] These tumors have also been referred to as sarcomatoid carcinomas or carcinosarcomas.

MMMT could be considered as the prototype for mesenchymal-epithelial transition, in which a subpopulation of carcinomatous tumor cells have lost epithelial characteristics and acquired a mesenchymal phenotype. These phenotypic changes are associated with global modifications of gene expression and lead to an increased expression of mesenchymal markers such as VIM, SPARC, and CDH3 (P-cadherin), together with a reduction in epithelial markers such as CDH1 (E-cadherin) and cytokeratins. The cadherin switching results in reorganization of the cytoskeleton and mesenchymal appearance. Transcription factors that induce mesenchymal-epithelial transition (*MET*) are SNAIL1/2, which are controlled by TGFB1.[46]

In the carcinomatous and sarcomatous component, MMMTs display a similar expression frequency of *TP53* and *CDKN2A* compared to pure serous carcinomas.[47] Approximately 80% of MMMTs express WT1 in both components.[48] This frequency is similar to what is seen in pelvic high-grade serous carcinomas and higher than endometrial serous carcinomas, raising the question for a potential association with pelvic serous carcinomas.[49] The subcellular localization for WT1 is nuclear in the carcinomatous component and cytoplasmic in the mesenchymal component, suggesting alternative splice products in the sarcomatoid component. Notably, VIM shows diffuse cytoplasmic expression in the sarcomatoid components of MMMTs. VIM is also often expressed in endometrioid carcinomas, although the cellular localization differs with membranous staining.

The group of MMMTs is heterogeneous. The carcinomatous component is frequently serous or occasionally endometrioid, and the sarcomatoid component is equally frequently homologous or heterologous, resulting in four major combinations. If the current assumption holds true that MMMTs are sarcomatoid carcinomas, then these tumors may follow oncogenic pathways of their pure carcinomatous counterparts, although it has been suggested that the character of the sarcomatoid component is associated with outcome.[42] Further progress in the knowledge of outcome in these tumors would need separate recognition of the major four combinations (serous/heterologous, serous/homologous, endometrioid/heterologous, and endometrioid/homologous).

OUTLOOK

The practice of medicine often changes slowly in face of scientific discovery. Clinicopathologic correlation used to manage endometrial carcinomas has evolved over decades. Rigorous standards are in place, and classification is based on morphology as the primary discriminator. New molecular classifiers have to significantly impact clinical practice beyond the current standard. Examples exist in other tumor entities such as breast cancers. With the discovery of ERBB2 as a molecular predictive marker for targeted therapy that is superior to the conventional approach, the primary discriminator may change to a purely molecular parameter. Yet in most instances, the discovery phase of characteristic molecular alteration requires an accurate description of the disease by a pathologist based on morphologic, immunohistochemical, and clinical parameters.[50] The partnership of the pathologist and cancer geneticist is crucial in the classification of cancers. It will only be possible to resolve outstanding questions if there are highly reproducible diagnoses of tumor types. Use of immunohistochemistry or other molecular markers to improve accuracy and reproducibility of diagnoses is promising, and studies to determine whether such tests as an adjunct to routine histopathologic examination can enhance diagnostic reproducibility are needed. If there are differences in how the diagnoses of types of high-grade endometrial carcinoma are being made, it will only be possible to move forward and understand the natural history and clinical significance of these subtypes through studies of case series where there is accompanying immunophenotypic or molecular data. This will allow the cases in different studies to be directly compared and will ensure that differences are not related to variations in diagnostic criteria used for cell type assignment (i.e., if tumors of a given subtype are immunophenotypically dissimilar in different studies, the implication is that they are fundamentally dissimilar and not comparable). Ultimately, our ability to develop and implement type-specific treatment will depend on making reproducible diagnoses.

We now witness the next technologic revolution, namely the advent of achievable massively parallel DNA sequencing technology. Within the next 5 years, the costs are expected to decrease to about $1,000 per genome, making this technology readily available despite significant bioinformatic challenges.[51] Such comprehensive techniques in assessing the whole genome, epigenome, or transcriptome have already been proven to revolutionize some aspects of cancer. Particularly, monomorphic, low-grade, genomically stable cancers will likely reveal recurrent somatic driver mutations. For example, the initial discovery of the C134Y *FOXL2* mutation in ovarian granulosa cell tumors was made from the transcriptome of four cases.[50] Low-grade endometrioid and clear cell carcinomas, at least in cases without MMR deficiency, are considered as relatively stable, and new-generation sequencing will likely yield a more accurate picture of the mutational landscape as shown in Table 7-1. Because of the massive parallel generation of short reads depending on the depth of coverage of a specific target, sensitivity of new-generation sequencing is much higher compared with conventional Sanger sequencing, likely revealing current numbers as an underestimate. Next-generation sequencing also offers the prospect of interrogating intratumoral heterogeneity by capturing the mutational landscape in a comprehensive manner. It is also possible that the variable responses of high-risk endometrial carcinomas to chemotherapy could be related to differing proportions of subpopulations of cancer cells with stem cell–like features. It has been suggested that such subpopulations could exist; more research is required to determine whether cancer stem cell–like subclones can be reproducibly identified within endometrial carcinomas and whether they could be used as prognostic tools or targeted as a therapeutic strategy to prevent relapses.[52] The interrogation of intratumoral heterogeneity will also help to determine the biologic relationship of mixed endometrial carcinomas and MMMTs to the major types of endometrial carcinomas.

However, it is conceivable that for some tumor types, other recurrent alterations will never appear. For example, genomic chaos might be the defining feature of serous carcinomas arising in a background of *TP53* mutations, with these being the only recurrent alterations found. Therapeutic approaches restoring *TP53* function might be counterproductive with conventional chemotherapy (i.e., platinum-based chemotherapy induces double-stranded DNA breaks, which lead to cellular crisis and death in a *TP53*-deficient state but might be repaired in a *TP53*-functional state). However, such comprehensive technologies might be the only way to determine the complexity of these tumors and might reveal—in concert with DNA copy number assays such as high-density, single-nucleotide polymorphism array—reproducible subgroups.

The new catalogue of the mutational landscape for endometrial carcinomas will yield many novel hypotheses with respect to potential predictive markers. The combination of targeted therapies and predictive markers needs testing in prospective randomized trials, but some information might be obtained by carefully designed retrospective studies. Through such research and the application of other technologies such as high-content screening of novel drug combinations and proteomics, the knowledge base required to develop more type-specific/targeted and effective treatments, especially for women with high-risk endometrial carcinomas, could be obtained within the next few years. Improved and more robust classification with molecular markers embracing morphology will also prevent unnecessary ineffective treatment of women with low-risk tumors. The translation of such knowledge into improved outcomes for women with endometrial carcinomas will be an exciting challenge for the endometrial cancer research community.

References

1. Hamilton CA, Cheung MK, Osann K, et al. Uterine papillary serous and clear cell carcinomas predict for poorer survival compared to grade 3 endometrioid corpus cancers. *Br J Cancer*. 2006;94:642–646.
2. Soslow RA, Bissonnette JP, Wilton A, et al. Clinicopathologic analysis of 187 high-grade endometrial carcinomas of different histologic subtypes: similar outcomes belie distinctive biologic differences. *Am J Surg Pathol*. 2007;31:979–987.

3. Alkushi A, Kobel M, Kalloger SE, et al. High grade endometrial carcinoma: serous and grade 3 endometrioid carcinomas have different immunophenotypes and outcomes. *Int J Gynecol Pathol.* 2010;29:343–350.
4. Catasus L, Gallardo A, Cuatrecasas M, et al. PIK3CA mutations in the kinase domain (exon 20) of uterine endometrial adenocarcinomas are associated with adverse prognostic parameters. *Mod Pathol.* 2008;21:131–139.
5. Tassi RA, Bignotti E, Falchetti M, et al. Mammaglobin B expression in human endometrial cancer. *Int J Gynecol Cancer.* 2008;18:1090–1096.
6. Zheng W, Yi X, Fadare O, et al. The oncofetal protein IMP3: a novel biomarker for endometrial serous carcinoma. *Am J Surg Pathol.* 2008;32:304–315.
7. Bignotti E, Ravaggi A, Tassi RA, et al. Trefoil factor 3: a novel serum marker identified by gene expression profiling in high-grade endometrial carcinomas. *Br J Cancer.* 2008;99:768–773.
8. Darvishian F, Hummer AJ, Thaler HT, et al. Serous endometrial cancers that mimic endometrioid adenocarcinomas: a clinicopathologic and immunohistochemical study of a group of problematic cases. *Am J Surg Pathol.* 2004;28:1568–1568.
9. Xing D, Orsulic S. A mouse model for the molecular characterization of BRCA1-associated ovarian carcinoma. *Cancer Res.* 2006;66:8949–8953.
10. Flesken-Nikitin A, Choi KC, Eng JP, et al. Induction of carcinogenesis by concurrent inactivation of p53 and rb1 in the mouse ovarian surface epithelium. *Cancer Res.* 2003;63:3459–3463.
11. Jia L, Liu Y, Yi X, et al. Endometrial glandular dysplasia with frequent p53 gene mutation: genetic evidence supporting its precancer nature for endometrial serous carcinoma. *Clin Cancer Res.* 2008;14:2263–2269.
12. Zhang X, Liang SX, Jia L, et al. Molecular identification of "latent precancers" for endometrial serous carcinoma in benign-appearing endometrium. *Am J Pathol.* 2009;174:2000–2006.
13. Jarboe EA, Miron A, Carlson JW, et al. Coexisting intraepithelial serous carcinomas of the endometrium and fallopian tube: frequency and potential significance. *Int J Gynecol Pathol.* 2009;28:308–315.
14. Zheng W, Baker HE, Mutter GL. Involution of PTEN-null endometrial glands with progestin therapy. *Gynecol Oncol.* 2004;92:1008–1013.
15. Alkushi A, Lim P, Coldman A, et al. Interpretation of p53 immunoreactivity in endometrial carcinoma: establishing a clinically relevant cut-off level. *Int J Gynecol Pathol.* 2004;23:129–137.
16. Jarboe EA, Pizer ES, Miron A, et al. Evidence for a latent precursor (p53 signature) that may precede serous endometrial intraepithelial carcinoma. *Mod Pathol.* 2009;22:345–350.
17. Pere H, Tapper J, Wahlström T, et al. Distinct chromosomal imbalances in uterine serous and endometrioid carcinomas. *Cancer Res.* 1998;58:892–895.
18. Micci F, Teixeira MR, Haugom L, et al. Genomic aberrations in carcinomas of the uterine corpus. *Genes Chromosomes Cancer.* 2004;40:229–246.
19. Press JZ, De Luca A, Boyd N, et al. Ovarian carcinomas with genetic and epigenetic BRCA1 loss have distinct molecular abnormalities. *BMC Cancer.* 2008;8:17.
20. Goshen R, Chu W, Elit L, et al. Is uterine papillary serous adenocarcinoma a manifestation of the hereditary breast-ovarian cancer syndrome? *Gynecol Oncol.* 2000;79:477–481.
21. Kwon JS, Lenehan J, Carey M, et al. Prolonged survival among women with BRCA germline mutations and advanced endometrial cancer: a case series. *Int J Gynecol Cancer.* 2008;18:546–549.
22. Sasano H, Comerford J, Wilkinson DS, et al. Serous papillary adenocarcinoma of the endometrium. Analysis of proto-oncogene amplification, flow cytometry, estrogen and progesterone receptors, and immunohistochemistry. *Cancer.* 1990;65:1545–1551.
23. Reid-Nicholson M, Iyengar P, Hummer AJ, et al. Immunophenotypic diversity of endometrial adenocarcinomas: implications for differential diagnosis. *Mod Pathol.* 2006;19:1091–1100.
24. Yemelyanova A, Ji H, Shih IM, et al. Utility of p16 expression for distinction of uterine serous carcinomas from endometrial endometrioid and endocervical adenocarcinomas: immunohistochemical analysis of 201 cases. *Am J Surg Pathol.* 2009;33:1504–1514.

25. Zhang L, Conejo-Garcia JR, Katsaros D, et al. Intratumoral T cells, recurrence, and survival in epithelial ovarian cancer. *N Engl J Med*. 2003;348:203–213.
26. de Jong RA, Leffers N, Boezen HM, et al. Presence of tumor-infiltrating lymphocytes is an independent prognostic factor in type I and II endometrial cancer. *Gynecol Oncol*. 2009;114:105–110.
27. Hayes MP, Douglas W, Ellenson LH. Molecular alterations of EGFR and PIK3CA in uterine serous carcinoma. *Gynecol Oncol*. 2009;113:370–373.
28. Slomovitz BM, Broaddus RR, Burke TW, et al. Her-2/neu overexpression and amplification in uterine papillary serous carcinoma. *J Clin Oncol*. 2004;22:3126–3132.
29. An HJ, Logani S, Isacson C, et al. Molecular characterization of uterine clear cell carcinoma. *Mod Pathol*. 2004;17:530–537.
30. Lax SF, Pizer ES, Ronnett BM, et al. Clear cell carcinoma of the endometrium is characterized by a distinctive profile of p53, ki-67, estrogen, and progesterone receptor expression. *Hum Pathol*. 1998;29:551–558.
31. Catasus L, Gallardo A, Cuatrecasas M, et al. Concomitant PI3K-AKT and p53 alterations in endometrial carcinomas are associated with poor prognosis. *Mod Pathol*. 2009;22:522–529.
32. Heatley MK. WT-1 in ovarian and endometrioid serous carcinoma: a meta-analysis. *Histopathology*. 2005;46:468.
33. Köbel M, Xu H, Bourne PA, et al. IGF2BP3 (IMP3) expression is a marker of unfavorable prognosis in ovarian carcinoma of clear cell subtype. *Mod Pathol*. 2009;22:469–475.
34. Lim P, Al Kushi A, Gilks B, et al. Early stage uterine papillary serous carcinoma of the endometrium: effect of adjuvant whole abdominal radiotherapy and pathologic parameters on outcome. *Cancer*. 2001;91:752–757.
35. Matias-Guiu X, Catasus L, Bussaglia E, et al. Molecular pathology of endometrial hyperplasia and carcinoma. *Hum Pathol*. 2001;32:569–577.
36. Silva EG, Deavers MT, Bodurka DC, et al. Association of low-grade endometrioid carcinoma of the uterus and ovary with undifferentiated carcinoma: a new type of dedifferentiated carcinoma? *Int J Gynecol Pathol*. 2006;25:52–58.
37. Abeler VM, Kjørstad KE, Nesland JM. Undifferentiated carcinoma of the endometrium. A histopathologic and clinical study of 31 cases. *Cancer*. 1991;68:98–105.
38. Huntsman DG, Clement PB, Gilks CB, et al. Small-cell carcinoma of the endometrium. A clinicopathological study of sixteen cases. *Am J Surg Pathol*. 1994;18:364–375.
39. Taraif SH, Deavers MT, Malpica A, et al. The significance of neuroendocrine expression in undifferentiated carcinoma of the endometrium. *Int J Gynecol Pathol*. 2009;28:142–147.
40. Baggish MS, Woodruff JD. The occurrence of squamous epithelium in the endometrium. *Obstet Gynecol Surv*. 1967;22:69–115.
41. Horn LC, Richter CE, Einenkel J, et al. P16, p14, p53, cyclin D1, and steroid hormone receptor expression and human papillomaviruses analysis in primary squamous cell carcinoma of the endometrium. *Ann Diagn Pathol*. 2006;10:193–196.
42. Ferguson SE, Tornos C, Hummer A, et al. Prognostic features of surgical stage I uterine carcinosarcoma. *Am J Surg Pathol*. 2007;31:1653–1661.
43. Jin Z, Ogata S, Tamura G, et al. Carcinosarcomas (malignant mullerian mixed tumors) of the uterus and ovary: a genetic study with special reference to histogenesis. *Int J Gynecol Pathol*. 2003;22:368–373.
44. Kounelis S, Jones MW, Papadaki H, et al. Carcinosarcomas (malignant mixed mullerian tumors) of the female genital tract: comparative molecular analysis of epithelial and mesenchymal components. *Hum Pathol*. 1998;29:82–87.
45. Taylor NP, Zighelboim I, Huettner PC, et al. DNA mismatch repair and TP53 defects are early events in uterine carcinosarcoma tumorigenesis. *Mod Pathol*. 2006;19:1333–1338.
46. Medici D, Hay ED, Goodenough DA. Cooperation between snail and LEF-1 transcription factors is essential for tgf-beta1-induced epithelial-mesenchymal transition. *Mol Biol Cell*. 2006;17:1871–1879.

47. Buza N, Tavassoli FA. Comparative analysis of P16 and P53 expression in uterine malignant mixed mullerian tumors. *Int J Gynecol Pathol*. 2009;28:514–521.
48. Franko A, Duggan MA. WT1 expression in MMMT. *Int J Gynecol Pathol*. 2010;29:452–458.
49. Gagner JP, Mittal K. Malignant mixed mullerian tumor of the fimbriated end of the fallopian tube: origin as an intraepithelial carcinoma. *Gynecol Oncol*. 2005;97:219–222.
50. Shah SP, Köbel M, Senz J, et al. Mutation of FOXL2 in granulosa-cell tumors of the ovary. *N Engl J Med*. 2009;360:2719–2729.
51. Aparicio SA, Huntsman DG. Does massively parallel DNA resequencing signify the end of histopathology as we know it? *J Pathol*. 2009;220:307–315.
52. Gupta PB, Chaffer CL, Weinberg RA. Cancer stem cells: mirage or reality? *Nat Med*. 2009;15: 1010–1012.

Endometrial Sarcomas

▶ Cheng-Han Lee, MD

The molecular alterations of uterine mesenchymal tumors have attracted more attention in recent decades because of the findings of recurrent genetic aberrations in a subset of these tumors. Although some of these genetic alterations show overlap between epithelial and mesenchymal malignancies in the uterus, there are some aberrations that are unique to uterine sarcomas. As a group, uterine sarcomas account for approximately 2% of all uterine malignancies if epithelial tumors with sarcomatous differentiation (carcinosarcomas/malignant müllerian mixed tumors and adenosarcomas) are excluded. Uterine sarcomas can be broadly classified into three major groups based on their line of cellular differentiation: endometrial stromal sarcomas (ESSs), uterine leiomyosarcomas (ULMSs), and undifferentiated endometrial/uterine sarcomas (UESs) (Table 9-1). Although a number of other sarcoma types that occur more frequently in extrauterine locations have been reported to occur in the uterus, embryonal rhabdomyosarcoma (RMS) forms the bulk of this remaining miscellaneous group of uterine sarcomas. This classification scheme also reflects our current understanding of the molecular biology of these tumors. With the exception of RMS, which tends to develop in younger age patients, the other uterine sarcomas typically occur in middle to older age women. This chapter will review briefly the molecular biology of the more common uterine sarcomas and the implication in disease classification, pathologic diagnosis, and therapy.

ENDOMETRIAL STROMAL SARCOMA

ESS is a histologically low-grade sarcoma that exhibits a histology and immunophenotype akin to that of endometrial stromal cells.[1] Even though some cases can display foci of convincing smooth muscle differentiation by histology and immunohistochemistry, most cases of ESS typically have admixed areas that demonstrate more classic histology and immunophenotype.[2] Although the risk of metastases is low, ESS is associated with a significant risk of local recurrence. Over time, a subset of ESS can progress, displaying a higher grade histology and eventually dedifferentiating to an apparently undifferentiated sarcoma while still possessing the same genetic aberration typical of usual low-grade ESS.[3]

Molecular Genetics and Biology

The published karyotypes on ESS are variable, but the majority exhibit a relatively simple karyotype.[4–9] Even though cases with more complex karyotype have been reported, it is likely that some of these tumors previously classified as ESS would now be reclassified

Table 9-1 Classification of Uterine Sarcomas

	Genetic Aberrations	Genes of Interest	Frequency	Specificity
Uterine leiomyosarcomas (ULMSs)	Complex karyotype; frequent random structural and numerical aberrations and frequent imbalances in 1, loss in 14q and 22q, gains in 8, 17, X	Frequent *TP53* mutation	Majority	No tumor-specific recurrent aberrations
Endometrial stromal sarcoma (ESS)	t(7;17)(p15;q21)	*JAZF1-JJAZ1*	~50%	Specific for ESN and ESS*
	t(6;7)(p21;p15)	*JAZF1-PHF1*	~5%	Specific for ESS
	Other types of 6p21 rearrangement: t(6;10;10)(p21;q22;p11), t(3;6)(q29;p21.1)	*PHF1* rearrangement; partner gene *EPC1* in 10p11	<5%	Unknown
	Other undefined translocation: t(10;17)(q22;p13), t(X;17)(p11;q23)	Genes unknown	~5%	Unknown
Undifferentiated endometrial/uterine sarcoma (UES)	Complex karyotype; multiple numerical and structural aberrations	Frequent *TP53* mutation	Majority	No tumor-specific recurrent aberrations*
Embryonal rhabdomyosarcoma (ERMS)	Frequent allelic loss in 11p15; some show complex karyotype		Majority	No tumor-specific recurrent aberrations

*One case of UES with uniform nuclear feature was reported to express *JAZF1-JJAZ1* fusion gene transcript.
ESN, endometrial stromal nodule.

under UES. Overall, rearrangements of chromosome 6p21, 7p15, and 17q21 are frequent in ESS.[7,8] By cytogenetic, polymerase chain reaction, and/or fluorescence in situ hybridization (FISH) analysis (Fig. 9-1), approximately half of ESSs carry a characteristic t(7;17)(p15;q21), resulting in gene fusion between *JAZF1* and *SUZ12*.[10] The same t(7;17) and gene fusion is also present in all endometrial stromal nodules examined to date.[10,11] Normal unrearranged *SUZ12* allele is also expressed in endometrial stromal nodules not expressed in ESS with t(7;17).[12] Additionally, a small subset of cases lacking t(7;17) show 6p21 rearrangement, most often in the form of der(7)t(6;7)(p21;p22)[5,10] with the rearrangement of 6p21 leading to the fusion of *PHF1* with partner genes such as *JAZF1* or *EPC1*.[5,13] One case of ESS with t(X;17) involving rearrangement of *SUZ12* was recently described.[9] *SUZ12* and *PHF1* are both members of Polycomb group proteins, which participate in transcriptional silencing through chromatin remodeling, a mechanism that is crucial in cellular development.[14] In ESS, the gene fusion likely results in the formation of functionally aberrant Polycomb complexes. Furthermore, although both endometrial stromal nodules and ESS carry t(7;17),

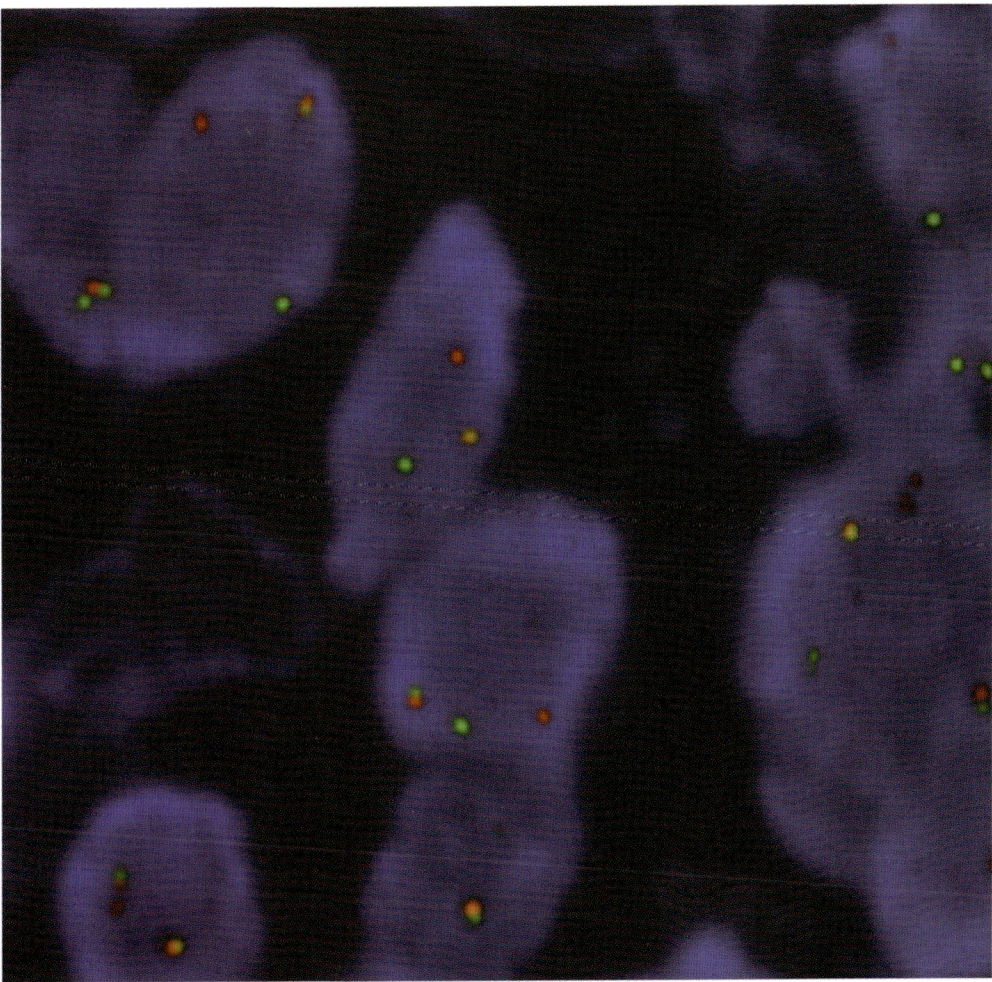

FIGURE 9-1: A case of endometrial stromal sarcoma positive for *JAZF1* rearrangement, as demonstrated by the break-apart fluorescence in situ hybridization assay (*red signal*: centromeric *JAZF1* probe; *green signal*: telomeric *JAZF1* probe).

only ESS exhibits concurrent silencing of the unrearranged *SUZ12* allele and would result in the complete abrogation of normal *SUZ12* protein function. Although the precise oncogenic mechanism has not been elucidated, it would appear that abnormal transcriptional repression is central to oncogenesis of ESS. Even though abnormal expressions of Polycomb genes are commonly seen in other malignancies,[14] genetic fusion/rearrangement of these Polycomb group members as demonstrated by cytogenetic and/or FISH analysis using, for example, the *JAZF1* break-apart probe set (Fig. 9-1) has only been described for endometrial stromal nodules, ESS, and a subset of UES (suspected dedifferentiated ESS) to date. Therefore, this series of genetic aberrations represents a highly specific molecular diagnostic feature for the family of endometrial stromal tumors, even in cases with smooth muscle differentiation.[2,11,15,16] However, the sensitivity of such molecular testing is inadequate because 40% to 50% of ESSs can lack these changes. There is currently also no diagnostic immunomarker that can be used to reliably distinguish ESS from other uterine sarcomas like ULMS. Further characterization of the full molecular/genetic spectrum of this disease perhaps using a next-generation sequencing approach is needed to improve the sensitivity of these diagnostic molecular tests.

Potential Biologically Oriented Therapies

A notable feature of ESS is its expression of estrogen receptor (ER) and progesterone receptor (PR).[3,17] The consistent expression of these hormone receptors in ESS has led to the consideration of hormonal therapy for ESS, particularly in advanced-stage disease, and the results appear promising.[18–21] The *Wnt/β-catenin* pathway has also been implicated in ESS because of nuclear *β-catenin* expression observed in 40% to 92% of ESS examined to date[3,22–24] and represents another potentially targetable pathway. Another gene of therapeutic relevance is the family of histone deacetylase (HDAC) because *HDAC2* expression was found to be increased in ESS.[25] *HDAC2* and other HDAC family genes are important in regulating chromatin structure. Given that the fundamental abnormalities in most ESS likely relate to abnormal chromatin remodeling and transcriptional dysregulation, the observed upregulation of *HDAC2* may be etiologically related. In support of this idea, experimental inhibition of HDAC in ESS cell lines has resulted in decreased cell proliferation,[25,26] suggesting that HDAC inhibition may be an effective therapeutic strategy in the treatment of ESS.

UTERINE LEIOMYOSARCOMA

ULMS is the most common type of uterine sarcoma and is characterized by tumor cells with diffuse morphologic and/or immunophenotypic evidence of smooth muscle differentiation. Although there are some speculated syndromic associations,[27,28] the vast majority of ULMSs occur sporadically. Most ULMSs appear to arise de novo, but there are a number of reports in the literature that describe apparent malignant transformation of ULMS from preexisting/coexisting uterine leiomyoma.[29,30] Mittal et al.[31] recently examined a series of such cases by array comparative genomic hybridization (CGH) analysis and observed overlapping patterns of gene copy number aberrations between corresponding leiomyoma and ULMS regions, thus providing further support for the phenomenon of step-wise malignant progression of uterine smooth muscle tumors in a subset of ULMS.[31]

Molecular Genetics and Biology

Cytogenetically, ULMSs are karyotypically complex with structural changes involving a large number of chromosomes.[32] Both conventional and array-based CGH analyses have identified chromosomal imbalances in nearly all ULMS examined.[33–37] The imbalances typically involve several chromosomes with comparable numbers of gains and losses present, and no consistent patterns have been observed. In comparison to uterine leiomyomas, ULMS consistently showed greater number and greater complexity of chromosomal aberrations overall, such that uterine smooth muscle tumors with complex cytogenetic or CGH abnormalities are very likely malignant; however, no single change is sufficiently sensitive or specific to be diagnostically useful.

Gene expression profiling analysis has identified several differentially expressed genes in ULMS when compared with normal myometrium and/or leiomyomas.[38–40] Compared with normal myometrium or uterine leiomyoma, ULMS shows upregulation of several cell proliferation–associated genes including *TOP2A*, *PTTG1*, *CDKN2A*, *UBE2C*, *MCM2*, and *FOXM1*, indicating presence of greater degree of disruption in cell proliferation/cell cycle control in ULMS. Additionally, abnormalities in *RB1* and *TP53* in the form of missense mutation and/or loss of heterozygosity are common in ULMS.[41,42]

Diagnostic Markers

The observed genetic abnormalities found in ULMS have led to the speculation that a combination of biomarkers including p16, p53, and Ki-67 proliferation index immunostaining can help to distinguish malignant from benign uterine smooth muscle tumors and predict the behaviors of tumors currently classified as smooth muscle tumors of uncertain malignant potential. Although several studies have demonstrated promising staining patterns with these markers,[43–47] they are not perfectly sensitive or specific, and pathologists need to exercise caution when interpreting the results. For instance, for p16, homozygous deletion of *CDKN2A* that encodes p16 can occur in a subset of ULMS,[37,48] and therefore, absent p16 staining in these instances cannot be regarded as a sign of benignancy. However, if the biopsy of a uterine mass shows a smooth muscle tumor that exhibits diffuse p16 and p53 staining concurrently, one certainly needs to seriously entertain the likelihood of a ULMS.

Potential Biologically Oriented Therapies

Although a large number of genetic abnormalities have been uncovered, the oncogenic mechanisms underlying development of ULMS remain elusive. In general, ULMS is a genetically unstable tumor that demonstrates complex structural chromosomal abnormalities and highly disturbed gene expression, which likely reflect an end-stage state of the accumulation of multiple genetic defects during tumor development. In keeping with this notion, Xing et al.[49] have demonstrated epigenetic silencing of *BRCA1* in a subset of ULMS. Although further confirmation is needed, *BRCA1* aberration or analogous mechanism(s) may underlie the apparent genetic instability seen in the majority of ULMS.

UNDIFFERENTIATED ENDOMETRIAL/UTERINE SARCOMA

UES is an uncommon and poorly defined group of mesenchymal malignancies that, as its name suggests, lack histologic and immunophenotypic evidence of a specific line of cellular differentiation.

Molecular Genetics and Biology

Biologically, UES appears to represent a mixture of tumor types that encompasses dedifferentiated ESS, very poorly differentiated leiomyosarcoma, and sarcomatous overgrowth of carcinosarcomas (malignant müllerian mixed tumors) or adenosarcomas. In support of this notion, a recent study attempted to classify UES into tumors showing uniform nuclear features (UES-U) and tumors showing pleomorphic nuclear features (UES-P).[3] One case of UES-U was found to carry *JAZF1-SUZ12* fusion transcript, and about half of UES-Us show ER and PR immunoreactivity, similar to the frequency seen in ESS. In contrast, all of the UES-Ps lack either ER/PR immunoreactivity or evidence of *JAZF1-SUZ12* gene fusion. UES-U represents nearly half of the UESs in this series. p53 immunoreactivity and *TP53* mutations are present in a subset of UES-P. These findings show that a subset of UES represents a dedifferentiated form of ESS and suggests the importance of adjunct molecular and immunohistochemical analysis in the proper classification of these undifferentiated uterine mesenchymal malignancies, particularly in the era of emerging targeted therapy.

Biomarker Expression

Little is known regarding the genetics of UES because most studies to date are limited to immunohistochemical characterization of this rare and heterogeneous group of malignancies. Epidermal growth factor receptor (*EGFR*) expression has been described in three cases of UES.[50] Recently, *EGFR* amplification as assessed by FISH was reported in a case of *EGFR*-immunopositive UES, and this case showed partial treatment response to imatinib therapy.[51] Further study is needed to assess the frequency of *EGFR* expression and gene amplification in UES. Similar to ESS, a subset (40% to 75%) of UES can also exhibit nuclear b-catenin expression.[3,22–24] In contrast to ESS, ER and PR expression is rare in UES.[3,52]

RHABDOMYOSARCOMA

RMS is a malignant mesenchymal tumor that exhibits evidence of skeletal muscle differentiation. In the uterus, RMS most commonly involves the cervix in the form of botryoid embryonal RMS in young children. Less frequently, uterine RMS can occur in adults in the form of embryonal RMS or pleomorphic RMS.[53] Alveolar RMS, which is characterized by pathognomonic t(1;13) or t(2;13), is exceedingly rare in the uterus.[54] In contrast to alveolar RMS, the genetics of childhood botryoid or embryonal RMS of gynecologic tract is not well defined, and no characteristic genetic abnormalities have been identified. DNA analysis has shown that most childhood gynecologic tract RMSs are hyperdiploid,[55] and it appears that hyperdiploid RMS is associated with better overall survival than diploid or tetraploid RMS.[56] The diagnosis of childhood RMS is typically straightforward, and evidence of skeletal muscle differentiation can be confirmed with immunomarkers like myogenin. In older adults, the differential would include adenosarcoma or carcinosarcoma with heterologous rhabdomyosarcomatous differentiation, and there are currently no reliable genetic or immunohistochemical markers that can differentiate between these possibilities.

SUMMARY

Similar to endometrial carcinomas, uterine sarcomas are genetically heterogeneous, ranging from ESS, which is characterized by a simple karyotype and recurrent genetic fusion, to ULMS and some UES, which demonstrate highly complex karyotype and traits of genetic instability. In addition, ULMS and some UES bear some resemblance to serous carcinomas, based on their genetic instability, frequent *TP53* abnormalities, and aggressive behavior. As such, therapies that exploit the underlying genetic instability of ULMS, including the use of PARP inhibitors in *BRCA1*-deficient cases, may prove to be a more effective therapeutic strategy, leading to a similar management of high-risk epithelial and mesenchymal tumors.[57]

References

1. Chew I, Oliva E. Endometrial stromal sarcomas: a review of potential prognostic factors. *Adv Anat Pathol.* 2010;17:113–121.
2. Oliva E, de Leval L, Soslow RA, et al. High frequency of JAZF1-JJAZ1 gene fusion in endometrial stromal tumors with smooth muscle differentiation by interphase FISH detection. *Am J Surg Pathol.* 2007;31:1277–1284.
3. Kurihara S, Oda Y, Ohishi Y, et al. Endometrial stromal sarcomas and related high-grade sarcomas: immunohistochemical and molecular genetic study of 31 cases. *Am J Surg Pathol.* 2008;32:1228–1238.
4. Leunen K, Amant F, Debiec-Rychter M, et al. Endometrial stromal sarcoma presenting as postpartum haemorrhage: report of a case with a sole t(10;17)(q22;p13) translocation. *Gynecol Oncol.* 2003;91:265–271.
5. Micci F, Walter CU, Teixeira MR, et al. Cytogenetic and molecular genetic analyses of endometrial stromal sarcoma: nonrandom involvement of chromosome arms 6p and 7p and confirmation of JAZF1/JJAZ1 gene fusion in t(7;17). *Cancer Genet Cytogenet.* 2003;144:119–124.
6. Regauer S, Emberger W, Reich O, et al. Cytogenetic analyses of two new cases of endometrial stromal sarcoma—non-random reciprocal translocation t(10;17)(q22;p13) correlates with fibrous ESS. *Histopathology.* 2008;52:780–783.
7. Micci F, Panagopoulos I, Bjerkehagen B, et al. Consistent rearrangement of chromosomal band 6p21 with generation of fusion genes JAZF1/PHF1 and EPC1/PHF1 in endometrial stromal sarcoma. *Cancer Res.* 2006;66:107–112.
8. Dal Cin P, Aly MS, De Wever I, et al. Endometrial stromal sarcoma t(7;17)(p15–21;q12–21) is a nonrandom chromosome change. *Cancer Genet Cytogenet.* 1992;63:43–46.
9. Amant F, Moerman P, Cadron I, et al. Endometrial stromal sarcoma with a sole t(X;17) chromosome change: report of a case and review of the literature. *Gynecol Oncol.* 2003;88: 459–462.
10. Koontz JI, Soreng AL, Nucci M, et al. Frequent fusion of the JAZF1 and JJAZ1 genes in endometrial stromal tumors. *Proc Natl Acad Sci U S A.* 2001;98:6348–6353.
11. Nucci MR, Harburger D, Koontz J, et al. Molecular analysis of the JAZF1-JJAZ1 gene fusion by RT-PCR and fluorescence in situ hybridization in endometrial stromal neoplasms. *Am J Surg Pathol.* 2007;31:65–70.
12. Li H, Ma X, Wang J, et al. Effects of rearrangement and allelic exclusion of JJAZ1/SUZ12 on cell proliferation and survival. *Proc Natl Acad Sci U S A.* 2007;104:20001–20006.
13. Panagopoulos I, Mertens F, Griffin CA. An endometrial stromal sarcoma cell line with the JAZF1/PHF1 chimera. *Cancer Genet Cytogenet.* 2008;185:74–77.

14. Simon JA, Kingston RE. Mechanisms of polycomb gene silencing: knowns and unknowns. *Nat Rev Mol Cell Biol.* 2009;10:697–708.
15. Hrzenjak A, Moinfar F, Tavassoli FA, et al. JAZF1/JJAZ1 gene fusion in endometrial stromal sarcomas: molecular analysis by reverse transcriptase-polymerase chain reaction optimized for paraffin-embedded tissue. *J Mol Diagn.* 2005;7:388–395.
16. Huang HY, Ladanyi M, Soslow RA. Molecular detection of JAZF1-JJAZ1 gene fusion in endometrial stromal neoplasms with classic and variant histology: evidence for genetic heterogeneity. *Am J Surg Pathol.* 2004;28:224–232.
17. Balleine RL, Earls PJ, Webster LR, et al. Expression of progesterone receptor A and B isoforms in low-grade endometrial stromal sarcoma. *Int J Gynecol Pathol.* 2004;23:138–144.
18. Paillocher N, Lortholary A, Abadie-Lacourtoisie S, et al. Low-grade endometrial stromal sarcoma: contribution of hormone therapy and etoposide. *J Gynecol Obstet Biol Reprod (Paris).* 2005;34 (pt 1):41–46.
19. Reich O, Regauer S. Survey of adjuvant hormone therapy in patients after endometrial stromal sarcoma. *Eur J Gynaecol Oncol.* 2006;27:150–152.
20. Reich O, Regauer S. Hormonal therapy of endometrial stromal sarcoma. *Curr Opin Oncol.* 2007;19:347–352.
21. Amant F, Coosemans A, Debiec-Rychter M, et al. Clinical management of uterine sarcomas. *Lancet Oncol.* 2009;10:1188–1198.
22. Kildal W, Pradhan M, Abeler VM, et al. Beta-catenin expression in uterine sarcomas and its relation to clinicopathological parameters. *Eur J Cancer.* 2009;45:2412–2417.
23. Jung CK, Jung JH, Lee A, et al. Diagnostic use of nuclear beta-catenin expression for the assessment of endometrial stromal tumors. *Mod Pathol.* 2008;21:756–763.
24. Ng TL, Gown AM, Barry TS, et al. Nuclear beta-catenin in mesenchymal tumors. *Mod Pathol.* 2005;18:68–74.
25. Hrzenjak A, Moinfar F, Kremser ML, et al. Valproate inhibition of histone deacetylase 2 affects differentiation and decreases proliferation of endometrial stromal sarcoma cells. *Mol Cancer Ther.* 2006;5:2203–2210.
26. Hrzenjak A, Kremser ML, Strohmeier B, et al. SAHA induces caspase-independent, autophagic cell death of endometrial stromal sarcoma cells by influencing the mTOR pathway. *J Pathol.* 2008;216:495–504.
27. Lehtonen HJ, Kiuru M, Ylisaukko-Oja SK, et al. Increased risk of cancer in patients with fumarate hydratase germline mutation. *J Med Genet.* 2006;43:523–526.
28. Ylisaukko-oja SK, Kiuru M, Lehtonen HJ, et al. Analysis of fumarate hydratase mutations in a population-based series of early onset uterine leiomyosarcoma patients. *Int J Cancer.* 2006;119:283–287.
29. Indraccolo U, Luchetti G, Indraccolo SR. Malignant transformation of uterine leiomyomata. *Eur J Gynaecol Oncol.* 2008;29:543–544.
30. Hodge JC, Morton CC. Genetic heterogeneity among uterine leiomyomata: insights into malignant progression. *Hum Mol Genet.* 2007;16:R7–R13.
31. Mittal KR, Chen F, Wei JJ, et al. Molecular and immunohistochemical evidence for the origin of uterine leiomyosarcomas from associated leiomyoma and symplastic leiomyoma-like areas. *Mod Pathol.* 2009;22:1303–1311.
32. Sandberg AA. Updates on the cytogenetics and molecular genetics of bone and soft tissue tumors: leiomyosarcoma. *Cancer Genet Cytogenet.* 2005;161:1–19.
33. Hu J, Khanna V, Jones M, et al. Genomic alterations in uterine leiomyosarcomas: potential markers for clinical diagnosis and prognosis. *Genes Chromosomes Cancer.* 2001;31:117–124.
34. Levy B, Mukherjee T, Hirschhorn K. Molecular cytogenetic analysis of uterine leiomyoma and leiomyosarcoma by comparative genomic hybridization. *Cancer Genet Cytogenet.* 2000;121:1–8.
35. Packenham JP, du Manoir S, Schrock E, et al. Analysis of genetic alterations in uterine leiomyomas and leiomyosarcomas by comparative genomic hybridization. *Mol Carcinogen.* 1997;19:273–279.

36. Svarvar C, Larramendy ML, Blomqvist C, et al. Do DNA copy number changes differentiate uterine from non-uterine leiomyosarcomas and predict metastasis? *Mod Pathol.* 2006;19:1068–1082.
37. Cho YL, Bae S, Koo MS, et al. Array comparative genomic hybridization analysis of uterine leiomyosarcoma. *Gynecol Oncol.* 2005;99:545–551.
38. Matsumura N, Mandai M, Miyanishi M, et al. Oncogenic property of acrogranin in human uterine leiomyosarcoma: direct evidence of genetic contribution in in vivo tumorigenesis. *Clin Cancer Res.* 2006;12:1402–1411.
39. Quade BJ, Wang TY, Sornberger K, et al. Molecular pathogenesis of uterine smooth muscle tumors from transcriptional profiling. *Genes Chromosomes Cancer.* 2004;40:97–108.
40. Skubitz KM, Skubitz AP. Differential gene expression in leiomyosarcoma. *Cancer.* 2003;98:1029–1038.
41. de Vos S, Wilczynski SP, Fleischhacker M, et al. p53 alterations in uterine leiomyosarcomas versus leiomyomas. *Gynecol Oncol.* 1994;54:205–208.
42. Zhai YL, Nikaido T, Orii A, et al. Frequent occurrence of loss of heterozygosity among tumor suppressor genes in uterine leiomyosarcoma. *Gynecol Oncol.* 1999;75:453–459.
43. Atkins KA, Arronte N, Darus CJ, et al. The use of p16 in enhancing the histologic classification of uterine smooth muscle tumors. *Am J Surg Pathol.* 2008;32:98–102.
44. Chen L, Yang B. Immunohistochemical analysis of p16, p53, and Ki-67 expression in uterine smooth muscle tumors. *Int J Gynecol Pathol.* 2008;27:326–332.
45. O'Neill CJ, McBride HA, Connolly LE, et al. Uterine leiomyosarcomas are characterized by high p16, p53 and MIB1 expression in comparison with usual leiomyomas, leiomyoma variants and smooth muscle tumours of uncertain malignant potential. *Histopathology.* 2007;50:851–858.
46. Lee CH, Turbin DA, Sung YC, et al. A panel of antibodies to determine site of origin and malignancy in smooth muscle tumors. *Mod Pathol.* 2009;22:1519–1531.
47. Ip PP, Cheung AN, Clement PB. Uterine smooth muscle tumors of uncertain malignant potential (STUMP): a clinicopathologic analysis of 16 cases. *Am J Surg Pathol* 2009;33:992–1005.
48. Esposito NN, Hunt JL, Bakker A, et al. Analysis of allelic loss as an adjuvant tool in evaluation of malignancy in uterine smooth muscle tumors. *Am J Surg Pathol.* 2006;30:97–103.
49. Xing D, Scangas G, Nitta M, et al. A role for BRCA1 in uterine leiomyosarcoma. *Cancer Res.* 2009;69:8231–8235.
50. Moinfar F, Gogg-Kamerer M, Sommersacher A, et al. Endometrial stromal sarcomas frequently express epidermal growth factor receptor (EGFR, HER-1): potential basis for a new therapeutic approach. *Am J Surg Pathol.* 2005;29:485–489.
51. Mitsuhashi T, Nakayama M, Sakurai S, et al. KIT-negative undifferentiated endometrial sarcoma with the amplified epidermal growth factor receptor gene showing a temporary response to imatinib mesylate. *Ann Diagn Pathol.* 2007;11:49–54.
52. Moinfar F, Regitnig P, Tabrizi AD, et al. Expression of androgen receptors in benign and malignant endometrial stromal neoplasms. *Virchows Arch.* 2004;444:410–414.
53. Ferguson SE, Gerald W, Barakat RR, et al. Clinicopathologic features of rhabdomyosarcoma of gynecologic origin in adults. *Am J Surg Pathol.* 2007;31:382–389.
54. Rivasi F, Botticelli L, Bettelli SR, et al. Alveolar rhabdomyosarcoma of the uterine cervix. A case report confirmed by FKHR break-apart rearrangement using a fluorescence in situ hybridization probe on paraffin-embedded tissues. *Int J Gynecol Pathol.* 2008;27:442–446.
55. San Miguel-Fraile P, Carrillo-Gijon R, Rodriguez-Peralto JL, et al. DNA content and proliferative activity in pediatric genitourinary rhabdomyosarcoma. *Pediatr Pathol Mol Med.* 2003;22:143–152.
56. De Zen L, Sommaggio A, d'Amore ES, et al. Clinical relevance of DNA ploidy and proliferative activity in childhood rhabdomyosarcoma: a retrospective analysis of patients enrolled onto the Italian Cooperative Rhabdomyosarcoma Study RMS88. *J Clin Oncol.* 1997;15:1198–1205.
57. Rottenberg S, Jaspers JE, Kersbergen A, et al. High sensitivity of BRCA1-deficient mammary tumors to the PARP inhibitor AZD2281 alone and in combination with platinum drugs. *Proc Natl Acad Sci U S A.* 2008;105:17079–17084.

SECTION V

Staging

▶ **CHAPTER 10:** Staging and Issues Related to Staging of Endometrial Carcinoma

Staging and Issues Related to Staging of Endometrial Carcinoma

Anna Sienko, MD

The accurate evaluation of hysterectomy specimens resected for endometrial carcinoma is crucial for the accurate staging of the tumor. Tumor staging impacts patient care directly as the main basis for selection of treatment options and prognosis. The most important factors that have to be assessed by histologic examination, besides classification of tumor cell type and tumor nuclear grade, are the depth of tumor invasion of myometrium, involvement of the cervix, and lymphovascular space invasion.

In 2009, the staging system for endometrial carcinoma was revised on evidence-based data that showed that stage IA, grade 1 or 2, endometrial carcinoma and stage IB, grade 1 or 2, endometrial carcinoma had a similar 5-year survival rate. Based on these findings, the International Federation of Gynecology and Obstetrics (FIGO) committee recommended that these two stages be combined into the new stage IA, which now comprises only endometrial involvement by tumor and/or less than 50% of myometrial invasion, and stage IB, which has ≥50% of myometrial invasion (Table 10-1).[1,2] The new staging also merged stage IIA and stage IIB (tumor limited to glandular epithelium of endocervix with no evidence of stromal invasion and invasion of endocervical stroma, respectively) into stage II (invasion of endocervical stroma without extension beyond the uterus). Therefore, endocervical glandular involvement in the new staging does not upstage the tumor to stage II. An additional change in the new staging system is that positive cytology of ascites or peritoneal washings is not included in the staging and does not alter the stage; however, the findings should be included in the pathology report.[3] Issues concerning staging are discussed in this chapter.

HISTOLOGY

One of the issues that arises in pathologic staging of resected specimens is related to histopathologic assessment of tumor grade and tumor cell type, with several grading systems that have been proposed including use of special stains.[4] Generally, it has been accepted that in histologic grading of endometrial carcinomas, high nuclear grade that is inappropriate for the architectural grade raises the overall grade of a tumor to the next highest grade (e.g., architectural grade 2 with nuclear grade 3 results in an overall grade of 3). Serous carcinomas, clear cell carcinomas, and carcinosarcomas (Mixed Müllerian Tumor) are all considered high-risk tumors and considered to be grade 3. This topic is discussed in greater detail in Chapter 4.

Table 10-1 Comparison of "Old" and "New" Staging for Endometrial Carcinoma*

"Old" System

TNM	FIGO	Definition
TX		Primary tumor cannot be assessed
T0		No evidence of primary carcinoma
Tis	0	Carcinoma in situ
T1	I	Carcinoma confined to corpus uteri
T1a	*IA*	*Tumor limited to endometrium*
T1b	*IB*	*Tumor invades less than one-half of myometrium*
T1c	*IC*	*Tumor invades one-half or more of myometrium*
T2	II	Tumor invades cervix but does not extend beyond uterus
T2a	*IIA*	*Tumor limited to glandular epithelium of endocervix with no stromal invasion*
T2b	IIB	Tumor invades endocervical stroma
T3	III	Local and/or regional spread
T3a	IIIA	Tumor involves serosa and/or adnexa (direct extension or metastasis) and/or cancer cells in ascites or peritoneal washings
T3b	IIIB	Vaginal involvement (direct extension or metastasis) or parametrial involvement

"New" System

TNM	FIGO	Definition
TX		Primary tumor cannot be assessed
T0		No evidence of primary carcinoma
Tis	0	*Carcinoma in situ (no longer included)*
T1	I	Carcinoma confined to corpus uteri
T1a	*IA*	*Tumor limited to endometrium and/or invades less than one-half of myometrium*
T1b	*IB*	*Tumor invades more than one-half of myometrium*
T2	II	*Tumor invades stroma of endocervix but does not extend beyond uterus*
T3a	IIIA	Tumor involves serosa and/or adnexa (direct extension or metastasis)
T3b	IIIB	Vaginal involvement (direct extension or metastasis) or parametrial involvement
T4	IV	Tumor invades bladder mucosa and/or bowel mucosa

FIGO, International Federation of Gynecology and Obstetrics; TNM, tumor-node-metastasis.
*Changes in the "old" and "new" staging are set in italics.

DEPTH OF MYOMETRIAL INVASION AND ADENOMYOSIS

One of the most important histopathologic assessments of the surgical resected uterus is the depth of myometrial invasion by tumor. Depth of myometrial invasion correlates with choice of patient treatment, increased risk of lymph node metastasis, overall patient prognosis, and rate of recurrence.[5,6]

Usually the histologic assessment of depth of myometrial invasion does not cause problems and is not a complicated procedure, with the "conventional" method for assessing depth of invasion measuring from the endomyometrial interface or junction to the deepest point of tumor invasion in the myometrium. However, problems arise when the tumor has a predominate exophytic growth pattern or endophytic growth pattern with deep invagination into the underlying myometrium, which can result in under- or overestimation of the actual depth of invasion.[6,7] Additional problems that may arise are an obscured, irregular, or difficult to ascertain endomyometrial interface; different patterns of myometrial invasion; and involvement of foci of adenomyosis by tumor.[7–10] Most of these problems can be overcome by submitting additional tissue sections and by being aware of the different patterns of myometrial invasion.[7,8,11,12] Careful and extensive sampling of the myometrium may be needed to confirm "true" invasion versus foci of adenomyosis involved by tumor because adenomyosis has been found to occur in 10% to 70% of hysterectomy specimens.[7,13,14]

ENDOCERVICAL INVOLVEMENT

The new revised 2009 FIGO staging of endometrial carcinoma eliminated endocervical glandular involvement from the staging, and this finding no longer upstages the patient to stage II. The most important feature for stage II disease and the endocervix is tumor involvement of the connective tissue of the stroma. This usually does not cause problems in the histologic evaluation of surgically resected uteri with careful examination of the lower uterine and endocervical junction of the resected specimen and appropriate tissue section submission. Problems can arise when the tumor is located in the lower portion of the uterus or area of lower uterine segment, obscuring the landmarks of the junction. If the tumor is friable, added problems may arise from tumor "carryover" or "floaters," resulting in misinterpretation of "positive" involvement of the endocervix. Difficulties may also arise in interpretation of "bona fide" endocervical stromal involvement versus endocervical glandular involvement, which may be compounded by inflammation and metaplastic changes of the nonneoplastic cervix.[15] Some of these issues can once again be resolved by careful reexamination of the specimen and submission of additional tissue sections.

LYMPH NODE RESECTION

Usually, the primary treatment for FIGO stage I or II endometrial carcinoma is surgical resection, consisting most often of total abdominal hysterectomy with bilateral salpingo-oophorectomy. Extent of pelvic lymph node resection includes pelvic and para-aortic lymphadenectomy. Whether or not the lymph nodes are involved with tumor is the most important prognostic factor in carcinomas clinically confined to the uterine corpus. Currently, more advanced preoperative diagnostic imaging has raised the question of the need for invasive endometrial sampling procedures and extensive lymph node resection.[16-18] Controversy exists whether lymph node resection should include the para-aortic lymph nodes as well as the pelvic lymph nodes. Studies comparing patient outcome after only pelvic lymph node resection versus pelvic and para-aortic lymph node resection showed that patients with intermediate and high risk of tumor recurrence benefited from para-aortic lymph node resection, whereas no benefit was seen with para-aortic lymph node resection in patients with low risk of recurrence.[19,20] However, there appears to be no consensus because many gynecologic oncologists perform lymph node resection on all patients undergoing surgical resection for endometrial carcinoma.[21]

Lymph node staging was also revised in 2009, with the "new" staging separating pelvic from para-aortic lymph node metastatic disease, resulting in a higher grade if the para-aortic lymph nodes are involved (Table 10-2).[1,3]

Unfortunately, not all of the issues associated with staging that have been briefly discussed are resolved by reexamination of the resected specimen or by submission of additional tissue sections. Problems with staging arising from difficulties in histologic interpretation should be communicated to the clinicians/oncologists with details provided as to where or what the problem involves (e.g., depth of invasion in a tumor with an exophytic growth pattern). Because, as previously discussed, staging impacts on choice of treatment, prognosis, and rate of recurrence, recommendation is made to consult colleagues with more experience in gynecologic pathology or to consult specialist gynecology pathologists regarding difficult cases.

Table 10-2 Comparison of "Old" and "New" Staging for Regional Lymph Nodes*

TNM	FIGO	Definition
"Old" System		
NX		Regional lymph nodes cannot be assessed
N0		No regional lymph node metastatic disease
N1	IIIC	Regional lymph node metastatic disease present in pelvic and/or para-aortic lymph nodes
"New" System		
NX		Regional lymph nodes cannot be assessed
N0		No regional lymph node metastatic disease
N1	IIIC1	*Regional lymph node metastasis to pelvic lymph nodes*
N2	IIIC2	*Regional lymph node metastasis to para-aortic lymph nodes, with or without positive pelvic lymph nodes*

FIGO, International Federation of Gynecology and Obstetrics; TNM, tumor-node-metastasis.
*Changes in the "old" and "new" staging are set in italics.

References

1. Creasman W. Revised FIGO staging for carcinoma of the endometrium. *Int J Gynaecol Obstet.* 2009;105:109.
2. Petru E, Luck HJ, Stuart G, et al. Gynecologic Cancer Intergroup (GCIG) proposals for changes in the current FIGO staging system. *Eur J Obstet Gynaecol Reprod Biol.* 2009;143:69–74.
3. American Joint Committee on Cancer. *AJCC Cancer Staging Manual.* 7th ed. New York: Springer; 2010:403–418.
4. Clarke BA, Gilks BC. Endometrial carcinoma: controversies in histopathological assessment of grade and tumor cell type. *J Clin Pathol.* 2010;63:410–415.
5. Mountzios G, Pectasides D, Bournakis E, et al. Developments in the systemic treatment of endometrial cancer. *Crit Rev Oncol Hematol.* 2011;79:278–292.
6. Holland C. Unresolved issues in the management of endometrial cancer. *Expert Rev Anticancer Ther.* 2011;11:57–69.
7. Goff BA, Rice LW. Assessment of depth of myometrial invasion in endometrial adenocarcinoma. *Gynecol Oncol.* 1990;38:46–48.
8. Ali A, Black D, Soslow RA. Difficulties in assessing the depth of myometrial invasion in endometrial carcinoma. *Int J Gynecol Pathol.* 2007;26:115–123.
9. Hanley KZ, Dustin SM, Stoler MH, et al. The significance of tumor involved adenomyosis in otherwise low-stage endometrioid adenocarcinoma. *Int J Gynecol Pathol.* 2010;29:445–451.
10. Ismiil N, Rasty G, Ghorag Z, et al. Adenomyosis involved by endometrial adenocarcinoma is a significant risk factor for deep myometrial invasion. *Ann Diag Pathol.* 2007;11:252–257.
11. Longacre TA, Hendrickson MR. Diffusely infiltrative endometrial adenocarcinoma: an adenoma malignum pattern of myoinvasion. *Am J Surg Pathol.* 1999;23:69–78.
12. Marshall DS, Hummer A, Thaler H, et al. Myometrial invasion patterns are associated with lymphovascular invasion in endometrial adenocarcinomas of the endometrium [abstract 911]. *Mod Pathol.* 2003;16:200A.
13. Bergolt T, Eriksen L, Berendt N, et al. Prevalence and risk factors of adenomyosis at hysterectomy. *Hum Reprod.* 2001;16:2418–2421.
14. Ferenczy A. Pathophysiology of adenomyosis. *Hum Reprod Update.* 1998;4:312–322.
15. McCluggage WG, Hirschowitz L, Wilson GE, et al. Significant variation in the assessment of cervical involvement in endometrial carcinoma: an interobserver variation study. *Am J Surg Pathol.* 2011;35:289–294.
16. Dietl J. Is lymphadenectomy justified in endometrial cancer? *Int J Gynecol Cancer.* 2011;21:507–510.
17. Kaneda S, Fujii S, Fukunaga T, et al. Myometrial invasion by endometrial carcinoma: evaluation with 3.0T MR imaging. *Abdom Imaging.* 2011;36:612–618.
18. Ballester M, Koskas M, Coutant C, et al. Does the use of the 2009 FIGO classification of endometrial cancer impact on indications of the sentinel lymph node biopsy? *Cancer.* 2010;10:465
19. Chan JK, Cheung MK, Huh WK, et al. Therapeutic role of lymph node resection in endometrioid corpus cancer: a study of 12,333 patients. *Cancer.* 2006;107:1823–1830.
20. Todo Y, Kato H, Kaneuchi M, et al. Survival effect of para-aortic lymphadenopathy in endometrial cancer (SEPAL study): a retrospective cohort analysis. *Lancet.* 2010;375:1165–1172.
21. Soliman PT, Frumovitz M, Spannuth W, et al. Lymphadenectomy during endometrial cancer staging: practice patterns among gynaecological oncologists. *Gynecol Oncol.* 2010;119:291–294.

SECTION VI

Role of Cytology

- **CHAPTER 11:** Glandular Cell Abnormalities in Pap Tests
- **CHAPTER 12:** Peritoneal Washings
- **CHAPTER 13:** Endometrial Biopsy versus Curettings versus Cytology

Glandular Cell Abnormalities in Pap Tests

11

▶ Ognjen Kosarac, MD, and
Dina Mody, MD

The Papanicolaou (Pap) smear/test is a screening test for cervical squamous cell carcinoma and its precursors. It is not and was never meant to be a screening test for endometrial cancer or its precursors. Based on published data, only about half of Pap smears/tests prior to the histologic diagnosis of endometrial cancers show any significant abnormal findings. However, endometrial carcinomas and hyperplasias may shed cells or bleed, and this may be picked up on a Pap test. Hence, every attempt should be made to identify these on Pap tests and report them using consistent terminology. The 2001 Bethesda System does just that, and the details follow below.

ENDOMETRIAL CELLS IN PAP TESTS

Benign-appearing endometrial glandular cells are seen in exfoliative gynecologic preparations obtained from premenopausal women during the first half of the menstrual cycle (cutoff day 10 to 14).[1,2] A small association of benign endometrial cells with endometrial neoplasia has been found, according to some authors in the range of 1% to 11%.[3-6] Because the endometrial carcinomas mostly occur in postmenopausal women, the presence of benign endometrial cells in Pap tests in those women warrants further follow up. It is also known that the sensitivity of the Pap test for endometrial carcinoma is low.[7] The most current reporting system, the 2001 Bethesda System, recommends reporting benign/normal endometrial cells in women aged 40 years or older.

Exfoliated endometrial cells occur in ball-like clusters and rarely as single cells. Abraded endometrial cells and fragments from the lower uterine segment and stromal and histiocytic cells should not be reported because they are not associated with endometrial pathology. In the first half of the menstrual cycle, endometrial cells often have a double contour, with glandular cells surrounding a core of stromal cells ("exodus" pattern; Fig. 11-1). Endometrial cell nuclei are about the size of an intermediate cell nucleus and are either round or bean-shaped. The chromatin pattern may be difficult to discern in the cell groups, but nucleoli are usually inconspicuous, and nuclei may be degenerated. Cytoplasm is scant, basophilic, and occasionally vacuolated. Cell borders are ill defined, and the cells frequently appear to be packed together. The background is often bloody and may contain histiocytes and endometrial stromal cells. In liquid-based preparations, three-dimensional cell clusters are common, with the plane of focus often above the plane of the normal squamous cells (Fig. 11-2). Single cells may be more commonly seen, and the background is usually cleaner with less blood. Nuclear chromatin detail may be more easily discerned, and single-cell necrosis (apoptosis) is common within exfoliated cell groups.[8]

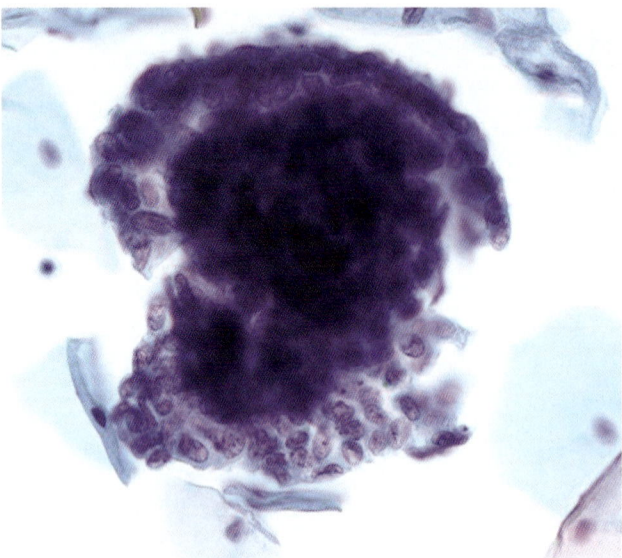

FIGURE 11-1: Exodus pattern. Three-dimensional group with central, dark endometrial cells surrounded by paler glandular cells.

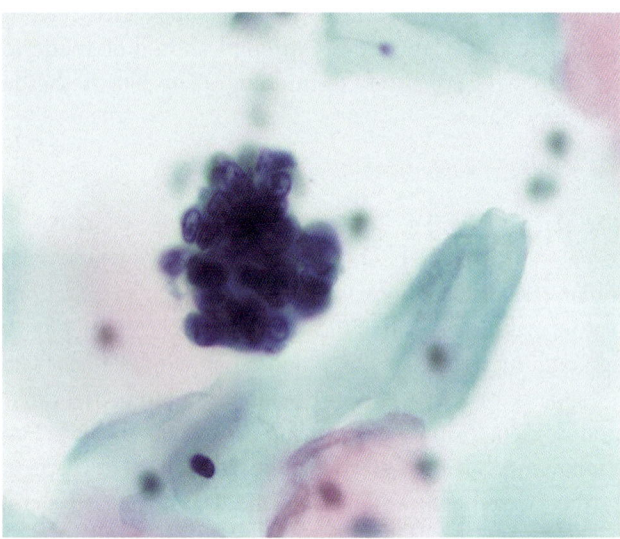

FIGURE 11-2: Endometrial cells. Exfoliated three-dimensional cluster of endometrial cells with small, round nuclei; inconspicuous nucleoli; and scant cytoplasm.

EPITHELIAL CELL ABNORMALITIES IN PAP TESTS—GLANDULAR CELL TYPE

The glandular cell abnormalities on Pap tests are divided into endocervical, endometrial, or generic glandular cells if one cannot tell with certainty if the cells are endocervical or endometrial in origin. For the purposes of this chapter, only endometrial cell abnormalities will be discussed.

Atypical Endometrial Cells

Atypical endometrial cells generally occur in small groups, with 5 to 10 cells in each group (Fig. 11-3). In contrast to normal endometrial cells, nuclei are slightly enlarged with mild hyperchromasia and more prominent nucleoli. Cell borders are usually ill defined,

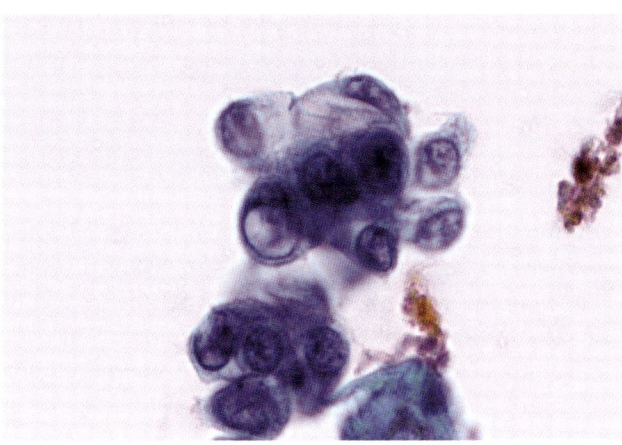

FIGURE 11-3: Atypical endometrial cells. Small clusters of cells with slightly enlarged nuclei, more prominent nucleoli, and occasionally vacuolated cytoplasm.

and cytoplasm may be vacuolated.[8] Atypical cells may be associated with dysfunctional uterine bleeding, use of an intrauterine device, endometrial polyps, endometrial hyperplasia, or endometrial adenocarcinoma.[9] Several studies addressed the incidence of atypical endometrial cells in cervicovaginal smears (Table 11-1).[4,10–18] Cherkis et al.[4] showed a prevalence rate of atypical endometrial cells of 1 in 1,700 from a screening pool of 300,000 smears, resulting in a frequency of 0.06%. Another study found atypical endometrial cells in 5 (6.2%) of 81 cervicovaginal smears with a diagnosis of atypical glandular cells of undetermined significance (AGUS), and 40% (2 of 5 cases) had a significant uterine lesion on follow-up.[10] More recently, Chhieng et al.[17] reported atypical endometrial cells in 5.25% of smears with a diagnosis of AGUS or in 0.03% of all smears. In their study, 31% of patients with histologic follow-up had a significant uterine lesion.

Table 11-1 AGUS Reporting Rates and Follow-up with a Significant Uterine Lesion (%)

First Author, Year of Publication	Number of Pap Smears	AGUS Rate (%)	EMH (%)	ECA (%)
Cherkis, 1987[4]	300,000	0.06*	11.0	20.0
Goff, 1992[10]	21,930	0.46	3.2	3.2
Nasu, 1993[11]	34,384	1.80	NA	4.0
Zweizig, 1997[12]	46,804	0.27	11.8	9.4
Eddy, 1997[13]	177,715	0.63	1.1	6.0
Duska, 1998[14]	120,338	0.17	NA	8.2
Veljovich, 1998[15]	84,442	0.53	2.5	4.0
Soofer, 2000[16]	87,632	0.11	18.0	12.0
Chhieng, 2001[17]	211,220	0.56	11.0	12.0
Saad, 2006[18]	25,777	0.34	15.0	18.0

AGUS, atypical glandular cells of undetermined significance; ECA, endometrial adenocarcinoma; EMH, endometrial hyperplasia; NA, not available.
*Rate of atypical endometrial cells.

Saad et al.,[18] in their study, demonstrated an AGUS rate of 0.34%, and 40% of patients with atypical glandular cells, favoring endometrial origin, had significant uterine lesions on histologic follow-up.

Endometrial Adenocarcinoma

Endometrial carcinoma is the most common cancer of the female genital tract in the United States, with an estimated 42,160 new cases and 7,780 estimated deaths in 2009.[19] It occurs predominantly in postmenopausal women in the late fifth and early sixth decades of life. In 1983, the hypothesis of two distinctly different forms of endometrial carcinoma and their associated differences in risk factors and prognosis was proposed.[20] Type 1, or endometrioid carcinoma, represents an estrogen-stimulated progression, often arising in the setting of endometrial hyperplasia. Endometrioid carcinomas are associated with increased exposure to estrogen (nulliparity, early menarche, chronic anovulation, and unopposed exogenous estrogen) and obesity, and they are responsive to progesterone therapy. Patients more often are white, are younger in age, and have a better prognosis than their type 2 counterparts. On the other hand, type 2, or nonendometrioid, carcinoma often arises in those who are black, multiparous, and not obese. These tumors do not respond as well to progesterone therapy, and their prognosis is worse.

Approximately 90% of women present with postmenopausal bleeding. At the present time, there is no cost-effective screening tool for this tumor.[21] Koss et al.,[22] in their cohort study on endometrial screening in asymptomatic women, found an incidence rate of endometrial cancer of 6.96 per 1,000. In another study, Hayashi et al.[23] reported only one patient with endometrial carcinoma of 1,283 asymptomatic women. In recent study, Jobo et al.[24] found a 4.7% incidence rate of asymptomatic endometrial carcinoma, and they concluded that detection in asymptomatic women was not related to a reduced mortality rate and, therefore, screening was not recommended. The diagnostic rate of endometrial cancer by Pap smear is extremely low.[25] Endometrial cells are not exfoliated at an early stage from the endometrium as they are from the cervix, and this is the main reason for the low detection rate. It is generally accepted that direct endometrial sampling is the best diagnostic approach.

Endometrioid carcinoma is the most common form (90%) of endometrial carcinoma. The cells exfoliate singly or in small, three-dimensional clusters. In well-differentiated carcinoma, nuclei are slightly enlarged with mild anisonucleosis, loss of polarity, and mild hyperchromasia. Nucleoli are small to medium in size; cytoplasm is typically scant, cyanophilic, and vacuolated; and intracytoplasmic neutrophils are often present (Fig. 11-4). In higher grade carcinoma, there is an increase in nuclear size with nuclear irregularity, irregular chromatin distribution, parachromatin clearing, and prominent nucleoli. A finely granular or watery tumor diathesis is sometimes present as a diagnostic clue (Table 11-2).

Nonendometrioid Carcinomas

The most common forms of nonendometrioid carcinomas are papillary serous carcinoma (10%), clear cell carcinoma (2% to 4%), mucinous carcinoma (0.6% to 5%), and squamous cell carcinoma (0.1% to 0.5%).[26] Other rare types include villoglandular, secretory, ciliated, and adenosquamous carcinoma.

Papillary serous carcinoma is associated with aggressive behavior and pure prognosis. It has a propensity for vascular or lymphatic invasion, extensive myometrial invasion, and early peritoneal dissemination.[27,28] In contrast to endometrioid carcinoma, abnormal cervical

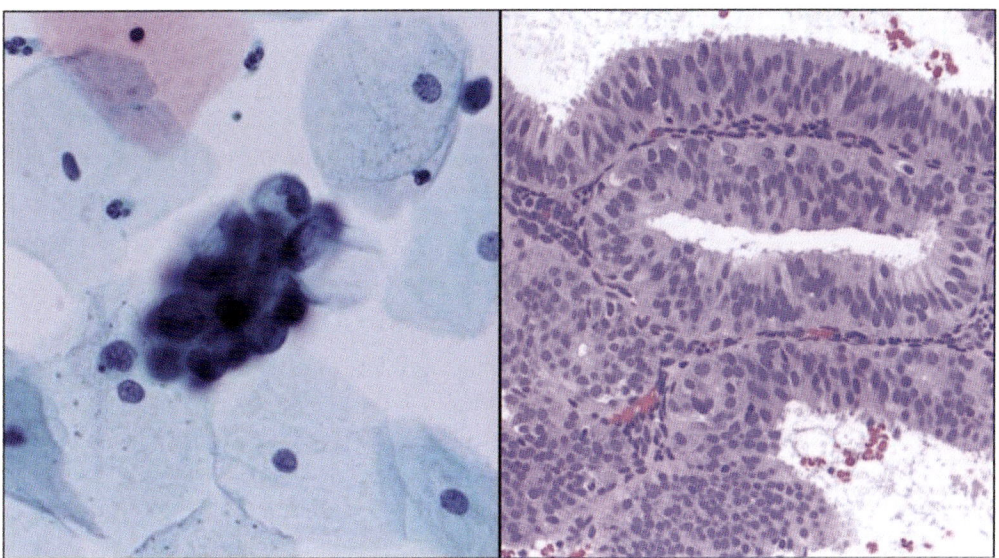

FIGURE 11-4: Endometrial endometrioid adenocarcinoma. **A:** Small, three-dimensional group of cells with enlarged hyperchromatic nuclei, small nucleoli, and scant vacuolated cytoplasm (ThinPrep Papanicolaou test). **B:** Follow-up histology was endometrioid adenocarcinoma International Federation of Gynecology and Obstetrics (FIGO) grade 1.

cytologic findings are more likely to be identified in papillary serous carcinoma, perhaps due to the papillary nature of the lesion and the frequent exfoliation of tumor cells.[29] The smears are typically hypercellular, with frequent papillae, single tumor cells with large pleomorphic nuclei and prominent nucleoli, and bulky dense cytoplasm.[30–32] The presence of numerous bare nuclei in a background tumor diathesis is a distinctive diagnostic feature.[33]

Clear cell carcinoma occurs in older women, is predominantly associated with atrophic endometrium, has not been found to be associated with hormone replacement therapy, and

Table 11-2 Cytomorphology of Endometrioid Adenocarcinoma	
Well-Differentiated Adenocarcinoma	**High-Grade Adenocarcinoma**
Low cellularity	Usually more cellular, especially in endocervical involvement
Single-rounded cells or three-dimensional clusters	Single-rounded cells or three-dimensional clusters
Nuclei slightly enlarged	Nuclei markedly enlarged and irregular
Mild hyperchromasia	Marked hyperchromasia, irregular chromatin
Nucleoli small to medium	Nucleoli prominent
Cytoplasm scant, cyanophilic, vacuolated	Cytoplasm scant, cyanophilic, vacuolated
Intracytoplasmic neutrophils	Intracytoplasmic neutrophils
Finely granular or watery diathesis*	Finely granular or watery diathesis*

*Best appreciated on conventional smears.

most often presents at high stage.[34] Prominent exfoliation is not present, and tumor cells usually have relatively uniform nuclei, prominent nucleoli, and clear cytoplasm.

Papillary endometrioid or villoglandular adenocarcinoma is a relatively common type of endometrial adenocarcinoma.[35] Several studies reported similar prognosis to that of typical endometrioid carcinoma.[35-37] The cervical smear demonstrates papillae and tumor cells with lower nuclear grade compared with those from serous carcinoma.

Malignant Mixed Müllerian Tumor

Malignant mixed müllerian tumor (MMMT) is a rare and highly aggressive neoplasm that represents less than 5% of malignant neoplasms of the uterine corpus.[37] It occurs most frequently in postmenopausal women and is characterized histologically by a mixture of malignant epithelial and sarcomatous components.[38,39] A recent study showed that the majority of patients with MMMT do not present with abnormal Pap smears. The presence of malignant cells in the Pap smear is related to advanced-stage disease involving the lower uterine segment or the cervix.[40] The presence of both malignant epithelial and sarcomatous components suggests MMMT diagnosis. However, several studies demonstrated an absence of mesenchymal cells in smears and confirm that the sarcomatous component of this neoplasm rarely sheds cells.[41-44] The most consistent features on smears are high-grade epithelial malignant cells in a necrotic background.[40]

In summary, the presentation of endometrial cancers on Pap smears/tests will depend on the type, grade, and stage of the tumor. The higher the grade and stage of the tumor, the more likely it is to exfoliate or involve the lower uterine segment or endocervical canal and hence be picked up on Pap testing. The type of cells on cytology can vary from atypical endometrial cells, which fall short of a diagnosis of cancer in the low-grade endometrioid carcinomas, to cells that are easily recognized as malignant in cases of high-grade serous papillary or clear cell types.

MIMICS OF ENDOMETRIAL CANCERS ON PAP TESTS

A variety of conditions can mimic endometrial cancers on Pap tests. These are listed in Table 11-3. The history helps differentiate some of the conditions, whereas the morphology is helpful in others. However, endometrial polyps frequently present as atypical endometrial cells and, depending on the degree of atypia, may be misinterpreted as malignant.

Table 11-3 Mimics of Endometrial Adenocarcinoma

Hyperplasia
Arias-Stella reaction and pregnancy
Endometrial and endocervical polyps
Cervical small-cell carcinoma
Intrauterine device changes
Fixation and staining artifacts
Radiation changes
Postmenopausal atrophy and bare nuclei

HUMAN PAPILLOMAVIRUS TESTING IN ENDOMETRIAL CANCERS

There is no association between human papillomavirus (HPV) infection and endometrial cancers; hence, HPV testing has no role in the diagnosis of endometrial cancers other than to exclude endocervical primary because most endocervical adenocarcinomas are high-risk HPV positive.

References

1. Brogi E, Tambouret R, Bell DA. Classification of benign endometrial glandular cells in cervical smears from postmenopausal women. *Cancer Cytopathol*. 2002;96:60–66.
2. Karim BO, Burroughs FH, Rosenthal DL, et al. Endometrial-type cells in cervico-vaginal smears: Clinical significance and cytopathologic correlates. *Diagn Cytopathol*. 2002;26:123–127.
3. Ashfaq R, Sharma S, Dulley T, et al. Clinical relevance of benign endometrial cells in postmenopausal women. *Diagn Cytopathol*. 2001;25:235–238.
4. Cherkis RC, Patten SF, Dickinson JC, et al. Significance of atypical endometrial cells detected by cervical cytology. *Obstet Gynecol*. 1987;69:786–789.
5. Cherkis RC, Patten SF, Andrews TJ, et al. Significance of normal endometrial cells detected by cervical cytology. *Obstet Gynecol*. 1988;71:242–244.
6. Gondos B, King EB. Significance of endometrial cells in cervicovaginal smears. *Ann Clin Lab Sci*. 1977;7:486–490.
7. Raab SS. Can glandular lesions be diagnosed in Pap smear cytology? *Diagn Cytopathol*. 2000;23:127–133.
8. Moriarty AT, Cibas ES. Endometrial cells: the how and when of reporting. In: Solomon D, Nayar R, eds. *The Bethesda System for Reporting Cervical Cytology*. 2nd ed. New York: Springer-Verlag; 2004:57–65.
9. Wilbur DC, Henry MR. Atypical glandular cells: endometrial. In: *College of American Pathologists Practical Guide to Gynecologic Cytopathology: Morphology, Management, and Molecular Methods*. Washington, DC: College of American Pathologists; 2008;99–100.
10. Goff BA, Atanasoff P, Brown E, et al. Endocervical glandular atypia in Papanicolaou smears. *Obstet Gynecol*. 1992;79:101–104.
11. Nasu I, Meurer W, Fu YS. Endocervical glandular atypia and adenocarcinoma: a correlation of cytology and histology. *Int J Gynecol Pathol*. 1993;12:208–218.
12. Zweizig S, Noller K, Reale F, et al. Neoplasia associated with atypical glandular cells of undetermined significance on cervical cytology. *Gynecol Oncol*. 1997;65:314–318.
13. Eddy GL, Strumpf KB, Wojtowycz MA, et al. Biopsy findings in 531 patients with atypical glandular cells of uncertain significance as defined by the Bethesda System. *Am J Obstet Gynecol*. 1997;177:1188–1195.
14. Duska LR, Flynn CF, Chen A, et al. Clinical evaluation of atypical glandular cells of undetermined significance on cervical cytology. *Obstet Gynecol*. 1998;91:278–282.
15. Veljovich DS, Stoler MH, Anderson WA, et al. Atypical glandular cells of undetermined significance: a five year retrospective histopathologic study. *Am J Obstet Gynecol*. 1998;179:382–390.
16. Soofer SB, Sidawy MK. Atypical glandular cells of undetermined significance: clinically significant lesions and means of patient follow-up. *Cancer Cytopathol*. 2000;90:207–214.
17. Chhieng DC, Elgert P, Cohen JM, et al. Clinical implications of atypical glandular cells of undetermined significance, favor endometrial origin. *Cancer Cytopathol*. 2001;93:351–356.

18. Saad RS, Takei H, Liu YL, et al. Clinical significance of a cytologic diagnosis of atypical glandular cells, favor endometrial origin, in Pap smears. *Acta Cytol.* 2006;50:48–54.
19. Jemal A, Siegel R, Ward E, et al. Cancer statistics, 2009. *CA Cancer J Clin.* 2009;59:225–249.
20. Bokhman JV. Two pathogenetic types of endometrial carcinoma. *Gynecol Oncol.* 1983;15:10–17.
21. Zhou J, Tomashefski J, Khiyami A. Diagnostic value of the thin-layer liquid-based Pap test in endometrial carcinoma: a retrospective study with emphasis on cytomorphologic features. *Acta Cytol.* 2007;51:735–741.
22. Koss LG, Schreiber K, Oberlander SG, et al. Detection of endometrial carcinoma and hyperplasia in asymptomatic women. *Obstet Gynecol.* 1984;64:1–11.
23. Hayashi R, Jobo T, Kuramato H. Screening of asymptomatic women for endometrial carcinoma. *J Jpn Soc Clin Cytol.* 1987;26:1–6.
24. Jobo T, Arai T, Sato R, et al. Clinicopathologic relevance of asymptomatic endometrial carcinoma. *Acta Cytol.* 2003;47:611–615.
25. Gray J, Nguyen G. Cytologic detection of endometrial pathology by Pap smears. *Diagn Cytopathol.* 1999;20:181–182.
26. Mendevil A, Schuler KM, Gehrig PA. Non-endometrioid adenocarcinoma of the uterine corpus: a review of selected histological subtypes. *Cancer Control.* 2009;16:46–52.
27. Hendrickson M, Ross J, Eifel P, et al. Uterine papillary serous carcinoma: a highly malignant form of endometrial adenocarcinoma. *Am J Surg Pathol.* 1982;6:93–108.
28. Walker AN, Mills SE. Serous papillary carcinoma of the endometrium. A clinicopathologic study of 11 cases. *Diagn Gynecol Obstet.* 1982;4:261–267.
29. Kuebler DL, Nikrui N, Bell DA. Cytologic features of endometrial papillary serous carcinoma. *Acta Cytol.* 1989;33:120–126.
30. Wright CA, Leiman G, Burgess SM. The cytomorphology of papillary serous carcinoma of the endometrium in cervical smears. *Cancer Cytopathol.* 1999;87:12–18.
31. Hagiwara T, Kaku T, Kobayashi H, et al. Clinico-cytological study of uterine papillary serous carcinoma. *Cytopathology.* 2005;16:125–131.
32. Park JY, Kim HS, Hong SR, et al. Cytologic findings of cervicovaginal smears in women with uterine papillary serous carcinoma. *J Korean Med Sci.* 2005;20:93–97.
33. Lax SF, Pizer ES, Ronnett BM, et al. Clear cell carcinoma of the endometrium is characterized by a distinctive profile of p53, Ki-67, estrogen, and progesterone receptor expression. *Human Pathol.* 1998;29:551–558.
34. Zaino RJ, Kurman RJ, Brunneto VL, et al. Villoglandular adenocarcinoma of the endometrium: a clinicopathologic study of 61 cases: a Gynecologic Oncology Group study. *Am J Surg Pathol.* 1998;22:1379–1385.
35. Chen J, Trost D, Wilkinson E. Endometrial papillary adenocarcinoma: two clinicopathological types. *Int J Gynecol Pathol.* 1985;4:279–288.
36. Ward BG, Wright RG, Free K. Papillary carcinoma of the endometrium. *Gynecol Oncol.* 1990;39:347–351.
37. Silverberg SG, Major FJ, Blessing JA, et al. Carcinosarcoma (malignant mixed mesodermal tumor) of the uterus: a Gynecologic Oncology Group pathologic study of 203 cases. *Int J Gynecol Pathol.* 1990;9:1–19.
38. Norris HJ, Roth E, Taylor HB. Mesenchymal tumors of the uterus: II. A clinical and pathologic study of 31 mixed mesodermal tumors. *Obstet Gynecol.* 1966;28:57–63.
39. Salazar OM, Bonfiglio TA, Patten SF, et al. Uterine sarcomas: natural history, treatment, and prognosis. *Cancer.* 1978;42:1152–1160.
40. Casey MB, Caudill JL, Salomão DR. Cervicovaginal (Papanicolaou) smear findings in patients with malignant mixed müllerian tumors. *Diagn Cytopathol.* 2003;28:245–248.
41. Costa MJ, Tidd C, Willis D. Cervicovaginal cytology in carcinosarcoma [malignant mixed mullerian (mesodermal) tumor] of the uterus. *Diagn Cytopathol.* 1992;8:33–40.

42. An-Foraker SH, Kawada CY. Cytodiagnosis of endometrial malignant mixed mesodermal tumor. *Acta Cytol.* 1985;29:137–141.
43. Massoni EA, Hajdu SI. Cytology of primary and metastatic uterine sarcomas. *Acta Cytol.* 1984;28:93–100.
44. Parker JE. Cytologic findings associated with primary uterine malignancies of mixed cell types (malignant mixed Müllerian tumor). *Acta Cytol.* 1964;57:316–320.

Peritoneal Washings

▸ Ognjen Kosarac, MD, and
Dina Mody, MD

ENDOMETRIAL ADENOCARCINOMA FIGO TUMOR STAGE

Peritoneal washings, when collected, continue to be considered in the prognosis of endometrial carcinoma. However, controversy exists as to the connection between positive peritoneal washings and adverse impact on prognosis, with further study and follow-up needed. The 2008 International Federation of Gynecology and Obstetrics (FIGO) staging system recommends that positive peritoneal washings should be reported. However, a "positive washing" in the new 2008 FIGO staging system is no longer used to "upstage" the patient.

ENDOMETRIAL ADENOCARCINOMA IN PERITONEAL WASHING CYTOLOGY

Peritoneal washings are collected in saline at the time of surgery. Hence, they need to be quickly delivered to the cytology laboratory for processing before serious artifacts and degeneration of the cells set in. Artifacts and degeneration can make interpretation of an already difficult specimen nearly impossible. A negative peritoneal washing consists of a few mesothelial cells, usually in flat sheets, admixed with some blood and blood elements, which can be easily lysed prior to preparation. Peritoneal washings for the most common endometrioid type of endometrial carcinoma show single tumor cells and three-dimensional clusters. Nuclei are enlarged with course chromatin and prominent nucleoli. Cytoplasm is usually scant to moderate. Nuclear pleomorphism is marked in high-grade tumors. Yanoh et al.[1] found in their study that patients with endometrial adenocarcinoma and positive peritoneal cytology were exhibiting microscopic features such as high cellularity, scalloped edges of cell clusters, and isolated cells in peritoneal fluids; thus, these microscopic features were associated with the presence of intra-abdominal macroscopic metastatic lesions. Papillary serous (Fig. 12-1) and clear cell types of endometrial adenocarcinoma are more aggressive and spread to the peritoneum more often than endometrioid type. Cytomorphologic features of these tumors are marked nuclear pleomorphism, prominent nucleoli, and abnormal mitoses. Malignant mixed müllerian tumors usually show an adenocarcinoma component only (Fig. 12-2) and rarely a sarcomatous component or a combination of both.[2] The differential diagnosis of various subtypes of endometrial adenocarcinoma in peritoneal fluids includes ovarian and primary peritoneal carcinomas, but there are no reliable cytomorphologic features to distinguish among them.

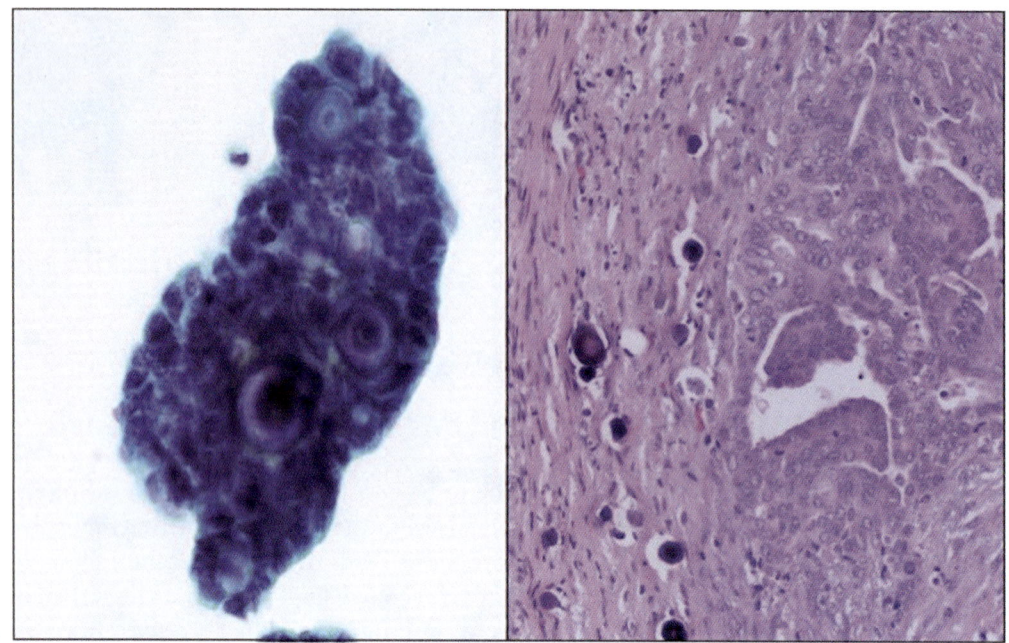

FIGURE 12-1: Papillary serous carcinoma in peritoneal washing. **A:** A cluster of cells with marked nuclear pleomorphism, prominent nucleoli, and psammoma bodies. **B:** Follow-up histology with numerous psammoma bodies and papillary structures with markedly atypical cells.

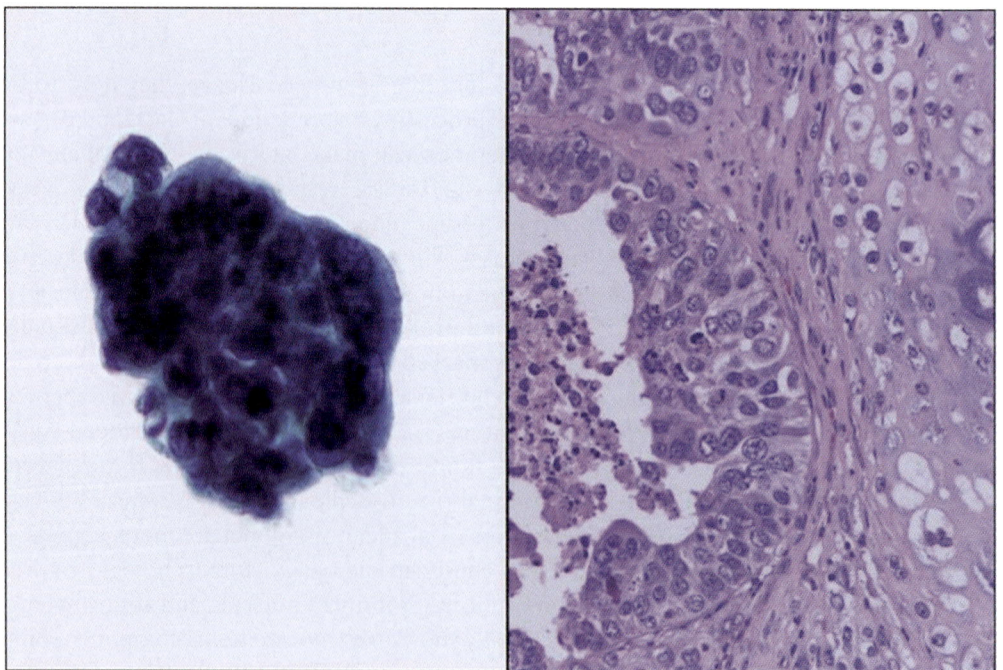

FIGURE 12-2: Malignant mixed müllerian tumor in peritoneal washing. **A:** High-grade adenocarcinoma component with marked pleomorphism, course chromatin, and scant cytoplasm. **B:** Follow-up histology with adenocarcinoma and chondrosarcoma components.

SIGNIFICANCE OF POSITIVE PERITONEAL CYTOLOGY

Endometrial carcinoma malignant cells may appear in the peritoneal cavity by direct extension through the myometrium and serosa, lymphatic and vascular invasion, migration through fallopian tubes, or reflection of multifocal peritoneal occult spread.[3,4] The transtubal transport seems to have the greatest attention. In several earlier studies, the presence of tumor cells within the fallopian tubes of patients with endometrial carcinoma was found.[5,6] Another more recent study demonstrated that 41% of women with endometrial cancer had malignant cells in the lumen of the fallopian tubes.[5]

The clinical significance and management of a woman with endometrial carcinoma and positive peritoneal cytology are still controversial. Since 1981, many studies have found that positive cytology is an independent adverse prognostic factor, whereas other studies have not confirmed this finding; thus, postoperative adjuvant chemotherapy was or was not recommended, respectively (Table 12-1).[7–34] This difference may be due to the following: (1) the number of cases was small, and the reported incidence was about 10%; (2) it was not always clear whether surgical or clinical stage was used; (3) various pre- and/or postoperative therapies were performed; (4) multivariate analysis was not always applied; (5) objectivity of peritoneal cytology was not warranted; and (6) prospective studies were not performed. (31) McLellan et al.[3] reported that positive peritoneal cytology was associated with other prognostic factors such as the depth of myometrial invasion, tumor grade, and lymph node metastasis. Other studies found that positive peritoneal cytology has an adverse effect only if endometrial cancer has spread to adnexae, peritoneum, or lymph nodes, but not if cancer is confined to the uterus.[22,23] The majority of patients with endometrial carcinoma have good prognosis, especially with early-stage cancer, and a 5-year survival rate of 80% to 90% can be expected.[34]

IMMUNOHISTOCHEMISTRY OF ENDOMETRIAL ADENOCARCINOMA IN PELVIC/PERITONEAL WASHINGS

Immunohistochemical stains are potentially useful as a cytologic adjunct to distinguish endometrial adenocarcinoma in pelvic/peritoneal washings from other metastatic adenocarcinomas or reactive mesothelial cells and malignant mesothelioma. Endometrial adenocarcinoma, particularly endometrioid type, typically express estrogen receptor (ER), progesterone receptor (PR), and vimentin.[35–37] Strong p53 immunoreactivity and p16 expression are seen in more than 80%[38,39] and in 90%[35] of papillary serous carcinomas, respectively, whereas these carcinomas lack expression of ER and PR (Table 12-2). Another subtype of endometrial adenocarcinoma, clear cell carcinoma, overexpresses p53 and p16 in approximately 25%[40] and 45%[36] of cases, respectively; has a high Ki-67 proliferation index; and lacks expression of ER and PR. Deavers[41] recently found 16% immunoreactivity of thyroid transcription factor-1 in endometrioid adenocarcinomas, and one must be cautious regarding potential misdiagnosis of metastatic lung adenocarcinoma.

In summary, peritoneal fluid cytology is an important part of endometrial and adnexal carcinoma staging with prognostic and therapeutic implications.

Table 12-1. Significance of Positive Peritoneal Cytology as Independent Prognostic Factor in Women with Endometrial Carcinoma

First Author	Year of Publication	No. of Patients	FIGO Stage	Positive Cytology (%)	Prognostic Significance
Creasman[7]	1981	167	Clinical I	16.0	Yes
Szpak[8]	1981	54	Surgical I	22.0	Yes
Yazigi[9]	1983	93	Clinical I	11.0	No
Ide[10]	1984	94	Clinical I	30.0	Yes
Konski[11]	1988	134	Clinical I	14.0	No
Heath[12]	1988	190	Clinical I	13.0	Yes
Imachi[13]	1988	35	Clinical I	14.0	No
Hirai[14]	1989	173	Clinical I	15.0	No
Turner[15]	1989	567	Surgical I	5.0	Yes
Brewington[16]	1989	335	Clinical I	6.0	Yes
Grimshaw[17]	1990	305	Surgical I	2.0	No
Sutton[18]	1990	276	Clinical I	17.0	Yes
Lurain[19]	1991	230	Clinical I	17.0	No
Gal[20]	1991	93	Clinical I	19.0	Yes
Morrow[21]	1991	895	Clinical I, II	11.0	Yes
Kadar[22]	1992	269	Clinical I, II	13.0	No
Ebina[23]	1997	114	Surgical I, II, III, IV	35.0	No
Kashimura[24]	1997	199	Clinical I, II, III, IV	15.0	Yes
Descamps[25]	1997	144	Clinical I, II	9.7	Yes
Takeshima[26]	2001	534	Non-FIGO groups	22.0	No
Obermair[27]	2001	369	Clinical I	3.5	Yes
Ming-Liang[28]	2001	115	Surgical I, II, III, IV	15.7	Yes
Hirai[29]	2001	50	Clinical I, II	10.0	Yes
Mariani[30]	2002	51	Surgical IIIA	82.0	No
Kasamatsu[31]	2003	280	Surgical I, II, IIIA	17.0	No
Santala[32]	2003	43	Surgical II, III, IV	35.0	Yes
Fadare[33]	2005	220	Surgical I, II	8.6	No
Saga[34]	2006	307	Surgical I, II, IIIA	10.4	Yes

Table 12-2. Immunohistochemistry of Endometrial Adenocarcinoma

	ER	PR	Vimentin	p53	p16	Ki-67
Endometrioid carcinoma	(+)	(+)	(+)	(−)	(−)*	Low
Papillary serous carcinoma	(−)	(−)	(+)	(+)	(+)	High
Clear cell carcinoma	(−)	(−)	(+)	(+/−)	(+/−)	High

*FIGO grade 3 endometrioid adenocarcinomas positive up to 25%.[36]

References

1. Yanoh K, Takeshima N, Hirai Y, et al. Morphologic analysis of positive peritoneal cytology in endometrial carcinoma. *Acta Cytol*. 1999;43:814–819.
2. Kanbour AI, Buchsbaum HJ, Hall A, et al. Peritoneal cytology in malignant mixed Müllerian tumors of the uterus. *Gynecol Oncol*. 1989;33:91–95.
3. McLellan R, Dillon MB, Currie JL. Peritoneal cytology in endometrial cancer: a review. *Obstet Gynecol Surv*. 1989;44:711–719.
4. Creasman WT, Lukeman J. Role of the fallopian tube in dissemination of malignant cells in corpus cancer. *Cancer*. 1972;29:456–457.
5. Menczer J, Modan M, Goor E. The significance of positive tubal cytology in patients with endometrial carcinoma. *Gynecol Oncol*. 1980;10:249–252.
6. Mulvany NJ, Arnstein M, Ostor AG. Fallopian tube cytology: a histocorrelative study of 150 washings. *Diagn Cytopathol*. 1997;16:483–488.
7. Creasman WT, Disaia PJ, Blessing J, et al. Prognostic significance of peritoneal cytology in patients with endometrial cancer and preliminary data concerning therapy with intraperitoneal radiopharmaceuticals. *Am J Obstet Gynecol*. 1981;141:921–929.
8. Szpak CA, Creasman WT, Vollmer RT, et al. Prognostic value of cytologic examination of peritoneal washings in patients with endometrial carcinoma. *Acta Cytol*. 1981;25:640–646.
9. Yazigi R, Piver MS, Blumenson L. Malignant peritoneal cytology as prognostic indicator in stage I endometrial cancer. *Obstet Gynecol*. 1983;62:359–362.
10. Ide P. Prognostic value of peritoneal fluid cytology in patients with endometrial cancer stage I. *Eur J Obstet Gynecol Reprod Biol*. 1984;18:343–349.
11. Konski A, Poulter C, Keys H, et al. Absence of prognostic significance, peritoneal dissemination and treatment advantage in endometrial cancer patients with positive peritoneal cytology. *Int J Radiat Oncol Biol Phys*. 1988;14:49–55.
12. Heath R, Rosenman J, Varia M, et al. Peritoneal fluid cytology in endometrial cancer: its significance and the role of chromic phosphate (32P) therapy. *Int J Radiat Oncol Biol Phys*. 1988;15:815–822.
13. Imachi M, Tsukamoto N, Matsuyama, et al. Peritoneal cytology in patients with endometrial carcinoma. *Gynecol Oncol*. 1988;30:76–86.
14. Hirai Y, Fujimoto I, Yamauchi K, et al. Peritoneal fluid cytology and prognosis in patients with endometrial carcinoma. *Obstet Gynecol*. 1989;73:335–338.
15. Turner DA, Gershenson DM, Atkinson N, et al. The prognostic significance of peritoneal cytology for stage I endometrial cancer. *Obstet Gynecol*. 1989;74:775–780.
16. Brewington KC, Hughes RR, Coleman S. Peritoneal cytology as a prognostic indicator in endometrial carcinoma. *J Reprod Med*. 1989;34:824–826.
17. Grimshaw RN, Tupper WC, Fraser RC, et al. Prognostic value of peritoneal cytology in endometrial carcinoma. *Gynecol Oncol*. 1990;36:97–100.

18. Sutton GP. The significance of positive peritoneal cytology in endometrial cancer. *Oncology.* 1990;4:21–26.
19. Lurain JR, Rice BL, Rademaker AW, et al. Prognostic factors associated with recurrence in clinical stage I adenocarcinoma of the endometrium. *Obstet Gynecol.* 1991;78:63–69.
20. Gal D, Recio FO, Zamurovic D, et al. Lymphovascular space involvement: a prognostic indicator in endometrial carcinoma. *Gynecol Oncol.* 1991;42:142–145.
21. Morrow C, Bundy BB, Kurman RJ, et al. Relationship between surgical-pathological risk factors and outcome in clinical stage I and II carcinoma of the endometrium: a Gynecologic Oncology Group study. *Gynecol Oncol.* 1991;40:55–65.
22. Kadar N, Homesley HD, Malfetano JH. Positive peritoneal cytology is an adverse factor in endometrial carcinoma only if there is other evidence of extrauterine disease. *Gynecol Oncol.* 1992;46:145–149.
23. Ebina Y, Hareyama H, Sakuragh N, et al. Peritoneal cytology and its prognostic value in endometrial carcinoma. *Int Surg.* 1997;82:244–248.
24. Kashimura M, Sugihara K, Toki N, et al. The significance of peritoneal cytology in uterine cervix and endometrial cancer. *Gynecol Oncol.* 1997;67:285–290.
25. Descamps P, Calais G, Moire C, et al. Predictors of distant recurrence in clinical stage I or II endometrial carcinoma treated by combination surgical and radiation therapy. *Gynecol Oncol.* 1997;64:54–48.
26. Takeshima N, Nishida H, Tabata T, et al. Positive peritoneal cytology in endometrial cancer: enhancement of other prognostic indicators. *Gynecol Oncol.* 2001;82:470–473.
27. Obermair A, Geramou M, Tripcony L, et al. Peritoneal cytology: impact on disease-free survival in clinical stage I endometrioid adenocarcinoma of the uterus. *Cancer Lett.* 2001;164:105–110.
28. Ming-Liang L, Sakuragi N, Shimizu M, et al. Prognostic significance of combined conventional and immunocytochemical cytology for peritoneal washings in endometrial carcinoma. *Cancer Cytopathol.* 2001;93:115–123.
29. Hirai Y, Takeshima N, Kato T, et al. Malignant potential of positive peritoneal cytology in endometrial cancer. *Obstet Gynecol.* 2001;97:725–728.
30. Mariani A, Weeb MJ, Keeney GL, et al. Assessment of prognostic factors in stage IIIA endometrial cancer. *Gynecol Oncol.* 2002;86:38–44.
31. Kasamatsu T, Onda T, Katsumata N, et al. Prognostic significance of positive peritoneal cytology in endometrial carcinoma confined to the uterus. *Br J Cancer.* 2003;88:245–250.
32. Santala M, Talvensaari-Mattila A, Kaupilla A. Peritoneal cytology and preoperative serum CA 125 level are important prognostic indicators of overall survival in advanced endometrial cancer. *Anticancer Res.* 2003;23:3097–3103.
33. Fadare O, Mariappan MR, Hileeto D, et al. Upstaging based solely on positive peritoneal washing does not affect outcome in endometrial cancer. *Mod Pathol.* 2005;18:673–680.
34. Saga Y, Imai M, Jobo T, et al. Is peritoneal cytology a prognostic factor of endometrial cancer confined to the uterus? *Gynecol Oncol.* 2006;103:277–280.
35. Mittal K, Soslow R, McCluggage WG. Application of immunohistochemistry to gynecologic pathology. *Arch Pathol Lab Med.* 2008;132:402–423.
36. Reid-Nicholson M, Iyenger P, Hummer AJ, et al. Immunophenotypic diversity of endometrial adenocarcinomas: implications for differential diagnosis. *Mod Pathol.* 2006;19:1091–1100.
37. Kuonelis S, Kapranos N, Kouri E, et al. Immunohistochemical profile of endometrial adenocarcinoma: a study of 61 cases and review of the literature. *Mod Pathol.* 2000;13:379–388.
38. Lax SF, Kendell B, Tashiro H, et al. The frequency of p53, K-ras mutations, and microsatellite instability differs in uterine endometrioid and serous carcinoma: evidence of distinct molecular genetic pathway. *Cancer.* 2000;88:814–824.
39. Sherman ME, Bur ME, Kurman RJ. p53 gene mutation in endometrial cancer and its putative precursors: evidence for diverse pathways of tumorigenesis. *Hum Pathol.* 1995;26:1268–1274.
40. Lax SF, Pizer ES, Ronnett BM, et al. Clear cell carcinoma of the endometrium is characterized by a distinctive profile of p53, Ki-67, estrogen, and progesterone receptor expression. *Hum Pathol.* 1998;29:551–558.
41. Deavers MT. Immunohistochemistry in gynecologic pathology. *Arch Pathol Lab Med.* 2008;132:175–180.

Endometrial Biopsy versus Curettings versus Cytology

13

▶ Anna Sienko, MD

Greater than 90% of patients with endometrial lesions, either nonneoplastic or neoplastic, present clinically with abnormal uterine bleeding and postmenopausal bleeding. Assessing the cause for the abnormal uterine bleeding or postmenopausal bleeding necessitates endometrial tissue sampling for histopathologic evaluation and appropriate treatment planning. In patients with postmenopausal bleeding, approximately 10% will be diagnosed with endometrial carcinoma upon further investigation.[1] Tissue sampling of the endometrium includes invasive and noninvasive methods. Invasive procedures include endometrial curetting (dilatation and curettage [D&C]), endometrial biopsy or hysteroscopy, and directed biopsy.[2] Evaluation of the endometrium by noninvasive methods includes procedures performed by transvaginal ultrasound and endometrial cytology (direct sampling). In 5% of asymptomatic women, endometrial cells will be found in Papanicolaou (Pap) tests in routine cervical screening as an incidental finding. Follow-up and additional investigations are recommended in patients with "abnormal endometrial cells" in a Pap test and in all patients 40 years of age and older (see Chapter 11).[3,4]

DILATATION AND CURETTAGE

In the past, endometrial tissue sampling was most often performed as a D&C procedure, and D&C is still considered the "gold standard" for investigation of abnormal uterine bleeding, especially in postmenopausal patients and patients with endometrium thickness of 5 mm or more by transvaginal ultrasonography.[5,6] D&C is an invasive procedure that requires operating room time with general anesthesia. Although many different types of sampling devices are available, the procedure is similar and entails insertion of a curette into the endometrial cavity through a vaginal speculum and gradual dilatation of the cervix. The curette has a hollow head, which is often "spoon shaped." Some curetting devices may also have a longitudinal slot through which the endometrial sample is suctioned into the curetting head. The sample is obtained by rotating the curette and scraping the top layer of endometrium (Figs. 13-1 and 13-2).

Sampling Issues with Dilatation and Curettage

D&C sampling is performed "blind," without direct visualization of the uterine cavity, and is limited, with only 30% to 60% of the endometrial cavity sampled.[5] Comparison studies of endometrial tissue sampling obtained by D&C and hysterectomy specimen showed that

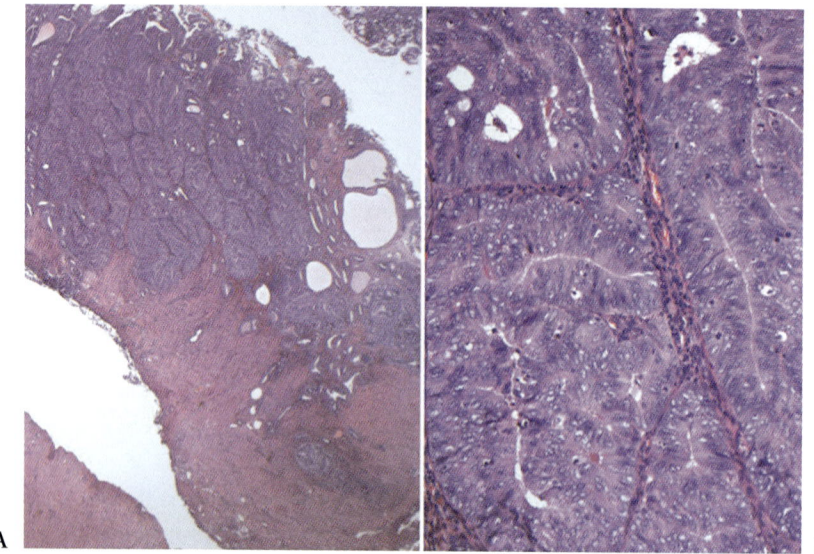

FIGURE 13-1: Curettings from a 63-year-old female with postmenopausal abnormal uterine bleeding (AUB). **A:** Endometrial curettings showing endometrioid, well-differentiated adenocarcinoma classified as International Federation of Gynecology and Obstetrics (FIGO) stage I (magnification, ×2). Tumor invades underlying portions of myometrium. **B:** Higher power view demonstrating endometrioid adenocarcinoma classified as FIGO stage I (magnification, ×20).

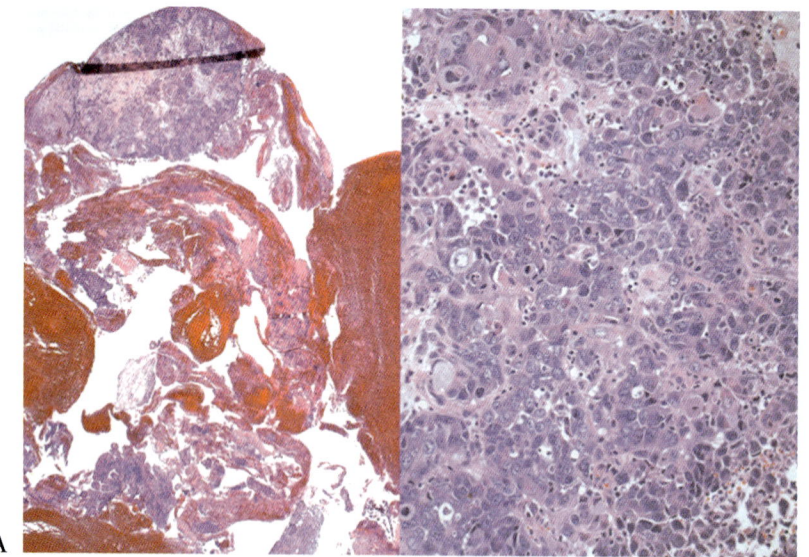

FIGURE 13-2: Curettings from a 64-year-old female with postmenopausal abnormal uterine bleeding (AUB). **A:** Endometrial curettings showing very bloody background with pieces of tumor (magnification, ×2). **B:** Higher power view showing high-grade pleomorphic carcinoma with mesenchymal malignant component (carcinosarcoma) (magnification, ×20).

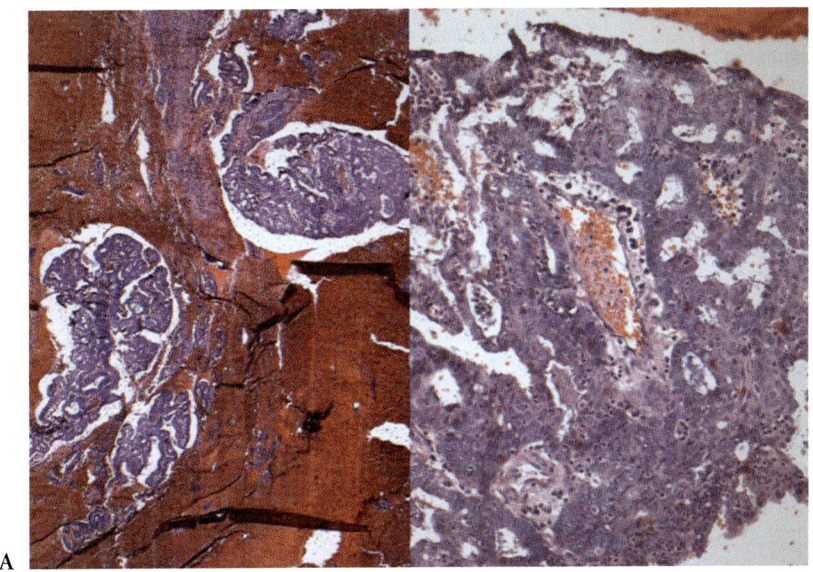

FIGURE 13-3: Curettings from a 61-year-old female with postmenopausal abnormal uterine bleeding (AUB). **A:** Endometrial curettings showing bloody background with pieces of tumor (magnification, ×2). **B:** Higher power view showing one piece of endometrioid well-differentiated adenocarcinoma classified as International Federation of Gynecology and Obstetrics (FIGO) stage I (magnification, ×20).

D&C undersampling can occur with lesions that are focal, exophytic, or endophytic.[7,8] In endometrial lesions that were diffuse, D&C had a high yield, with a greater than 92% to 94% detection rate of hyperplasia and carcinoma (Fig. 13-3).[5] D&C tissue sampling was also found to be limited in patients with endometrial thickness of ≤4 mm by transvaginal ultrasonography (Fig. 13-4).[6] Because D&C only "scrapes" the top layer of endometrium for sampling, depth of tumor invasion cannot be ascertained, and accurate staging cannot be performed by this method. Thus, the tissue sample obtained by D&C sampling and the tumor grading of that sample would be the most measurable and heavily used parameter for preoperative

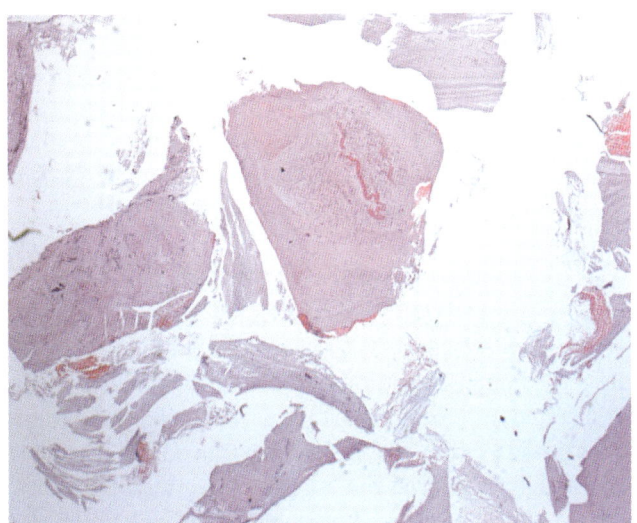

FIGURE 13-4: Curettings from a 51-year-old female with abnormal uterine bleeding (AUB). Unsatisfactory specimen showing mostly mucous and scattered inflammatory cells (magnification, ×2).

evaluation in surgical planning and staging. However, the tumor grade has been found to be underestimated in tissue sampling by D&C in more than 25% of patients, with a higher grade found on hysterectomy specimen in more than 10% of patients.[5,9,10]

ENDOMETRIAL BIOPSY (PIPELLE)

Many different types of instruments for endometrial sampling have been developed as an alternative to inpatient procedures for evaluation of abnormal uterine bleeding. These office outpatient procedures do not require operating room time or general anesthesia and are more cost effective than a D&C procedure. All are based on aspiration sampling of the endometrium. The sample is obtained by introducing into the uterine cavity, through a vaginal speculum, a flexible or rigid hollow sheath (Pipelle; Unimar, Wilton, CT) inserted up to the fundus; suction is generated (via internal piston, vacuum syringe, or vacuum pump), and the sheath is rotated and moved back and forth as it is withdrawn. Tissue is "sucked" into openings at the "head tip" of the sheath and into lumen of the sheath.[11,12]

Issues with Endometrial Biopsy

The Pipelle is currently the most commonly used and most studied device for office outpatient endometrial sampling.[1] The problems and issues with the Pipelle and similar devices are predominately based on sample tissue size. Adequate samples consisting of one or more pieces large enough and intact enough for histopathologic interpretation were obtained in 87% to 99% of patients according to several studies.[5,13,14] A diagnosis of endometrial adenocarcinoma was made in 67% to 98% of samples.[1,13,14] Inadequate specimens with scant tissue for evaluation were obtained from 12% to 22% of patients who were menopausal or had cervical stenosis, with an overall false-negative rate of up to 15%.[1,13,15] The same disadvantages as with D&C sampling were also found with the Pipelle and similar sampling devices in that focal lesions of the endometrium, exophytic lesions, and endophytic lesions were either not sampled or undersampled.[15,16] The Pipelle and similar devices were found to provide a better tissue sample than D&C when sampling endometrial tissue with thicknesses of less than 7 mm and between 4 and 6 mm, but with increasing endometrial thickness of ≥7 mm, these sampling devices were found to be less reliable and less suitable than samples obtained by D&C.[15]

A depth of tumor invasion also cannot be determined or predicted based on these sampling methods. As with D&C, the accuracy of tumor grading based on sampled tissue was found to correlate in only 85% of cases to the final tumor grading based on corresponding hysterectomy specimens, with almost 9% of cases showing higher tumor grade.[16] An inadequate office-based endometrial sampling procedure requires additional follow-up with tissue studies. Suggested recommended follow-up is illustrated in Figure 13-5.

HYSTEROSCOPY AND DIRECTED BIOPSY/CURETTAGE

Hysteroscopy is an invasive procedure based on visualization of the whole uterine cavity by a flexible "telescope-like" instrument inserted into the uterine cavity. For the procedure, the uterine cavity is usually infused with a liquid (saline, sorbitol, or dextran solution) or gas (carbon dioxide). The hysteroscope has a light source at the "tip," and macroscopic evaluation of the uterine cavity is made. Any visually detected abnormalities can be sampled or

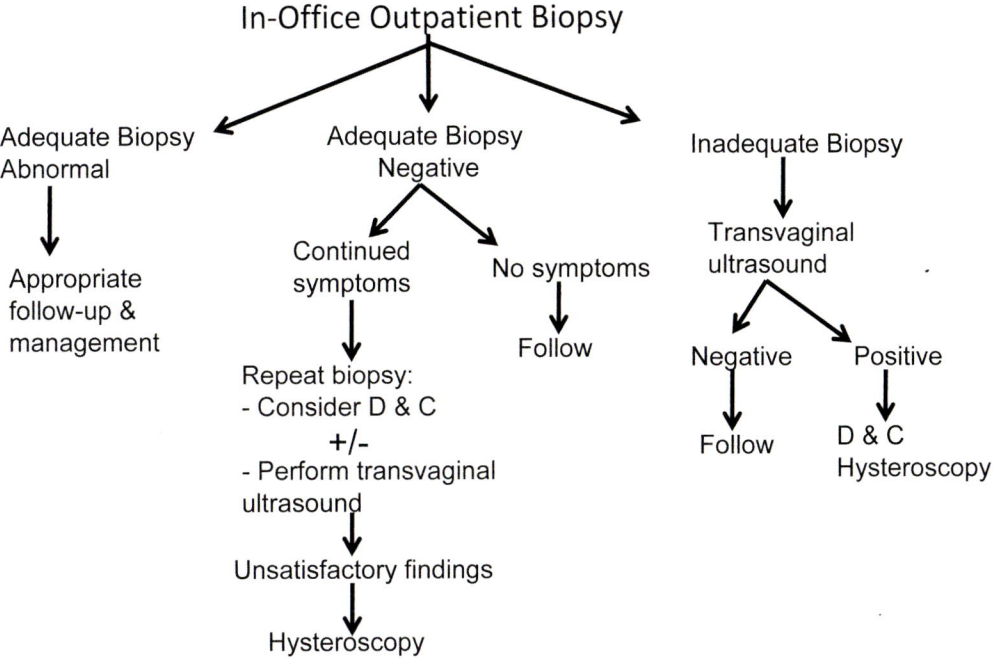

FIGURE 13-5: Abnormal uterine bleeding. Algorithm showing necessary diagnostic procedures. (Modified from van Doom HC, Opmeer BC, Burger CW, et al. Inadequate office endometrial biopsy sample requires further evaluation in women with postmenopausal bleeding and abnormal ultrasound results. *Int J Gynaecol Obstet*. 2007;99:100–104; and Brand A. Diagnosis of endometrial cancer in women with abnormal vaginal bleeding. *SOGC Clin Pract Guide*. 2000;86:1–3, with permission.)

surgically removed by allowing additional instruments to be inserted into a special channel in the instrument. Currently, newer more flexible hysteroscopy devices of variable diameters allow for in-office procedures.

Sampling Issues with Hysteroscopy

Although hysteroscopy does allow visualization of the uterine cavity, sampling of the lesion and obtaining adequate tissue for evaluation are the main shortcomings. Focal lesions may not be sampled, and in one study, the sensitivity of this procedure was comparable with that of D&C.[17] In another study, the failure rate of adequate hysteroscopy was found to be 3.4%, with an overall specificity of 96% for hysteroscopic diagnosis of uterine abnormalities (86% in premenopausal women and 99% in postmenopausal women).[18,19]

TRANSVAGINAL ULTRASOUND

Transvaginal ultrasound (TVU) is a noninvasive procedure that has been advocated as the initial investigative procedure in abnormal uterine bleeding, avoiding the need for tissue sampling in up to 40% of patients.[6,15] The procedure is used to indirectly visualize the thickness of the endometrium by measuring the maximum thickness by echocardiography of the long-axis transvaginal view in the anterior-posterior aspect of the uterus.[6] Although there is no firm agreement and controversy exists as to the "cutoff" for a "positive" finding, most studies recommend an endometrial thickness of greater than 4 mm as a positive finding; however, this is not indicative of any specific pathology.[6,20,21] When TVU was paired with either an office-based outpatient endometrial sampling or a D&C procedure, a sensitivity of 96% to 98% and a specificity of 36% to 68% were found for evaluation and diagnosis of an endometrial abnormality.[1] An endometrial thickness of 5 to 7 mm in postmenopausal patients presenting with abnormal bleeding correlated with a specificity of 64% and a sensitivity of 100% for significant pathology on biopsy.[20,22] The problem among different studies evaluating TVU is the variable endometrial thickness that is used as the "baseline" for normal endometrial thickness. The cutoff used in most studies for postmenopausal women is 4 to 5 mm, and no abnormality, including exclusion of endometrial carcinoma, was found in postmenopausal patients with an endometrial thickness of less than 4 mm.[14,22] However, no guideline or consensus as to "normal" thickness in premenopausal women has been established, with studies using a thickness cutoff ranging from 5 to 22 mm and with endometrial thickness being greater in symptomatic patients.[20,22] In one study, four of five premenopausal women with an endometrial thickness of ≥22 mm on follow-up tissue sampling showed endometrial adenocarcinoma.[22]

Issues with Transvaginal Ultrasound

Case reports exist of postmenopausal patients presenting with no symptoms and an endometrial thickness of 18 mm and of symptomatic patients with an endometrial thickness of ≤4 mm who have demonstrated adenocarcinomas with additional investigation and sampling.[22,23] The false-negative rate for TVU has been reported to range from 44% to 56%, with inadequate or limited measurements due to patient obesity, leiomyomas, or previous uterine surgery.[1,6] In high-risk patients (e.g., patients on tamoxifen or hormone replacement, or nulliparous, diabetic, or obese patients), a "negative" TVU should triage these patients for additional investigation and endometrial biopsy.[1,21] A scant insufficient biopsy or an unsatisfactory biopsy procedure in a symptomatic patient should be investigated further, with TVU advocated to triage between the low-risk and high-risk patient (see Fig. 13-1).[20,24]

ENDOMETRIAL CYTOLOGY (DIRECT SAMPLING)

Conventional Pap tests, including liquid-based Pap tests, are well established as procedures for cervical screening but are not used as screening or evaluation procedures for abnormal uterine bleeding and have minimal impact on detection of endometrial carcinomas. The finding of endometrial cells in a Pap test with a diagnosis of "abnormal endometrial glandular cells" is an incidental finding with a pick-up rate of 0.1%[25] and requires further follow-up (see Chapter 11).[3,4]

However, follow-up and additional investigation for "normal" endometrial cells found on Pap tests of asymptomatic premenopausal women were not found to be cost effective.[26] The direct cytologic sampling of the endometrium is a new and evolving technique. The noninvasive procedure is similar to cervical cytologic sampling. A flexible plastic tube or guide is inserted into the endometrial cavity through the cervical os. Various cytologic endometrial sampling devices are then introduced ("unsheathed") through the plastic tube or guide, such as a stiff wire brush (Endo brush, Tao Brush), dart-like sampler (Endopap), or spatula-like sampler (Mi-Mark).[27] The brush or sampler "brushes" the endometrium, with the sample processed similar to a conventional Pap smear or a liquid-based Pap test.[27,28]

Issues with (Direct) Endometrial Cytology

Studies comparing other sampling techniques to direct endometrial cytology found that endometrial cytology provided comparable diagnostic results[28–32] and, in postmenopausal patients with atrophy, better results with higher sensitivity and specificity.[32,33] When paired with a TVU cutoff of ≥4 mm for endometrial thickness, endometrial direct cytology sampling was shown to have a sensitivity of 95% and specificity of 98%.[34] Direct endometrial cytology shares common problems with the other sampling techniques discussed in this chapter. The procedure is performed "blind," similar to endometrial biopsy and endometrial curetting. Criteria for interpretation of endometrial cytology are different than those for cervical cytology, and it is advocated that interpretation be performed by experienced pathologists.[27,28] Undersampling can occur with focal endometrial lesions, endophytic lesions, and exophytic lesions, where "brushing" may not represent the lesional tissue.[28] Interpretation problems can arise when the sampling devices that have a sheath must be resheathed to prevent contamination of the sample by endocervical cells as the sampling device is removed from the uterine cavity, creating problems in differentiating endocervical cells from endometrial cells.[29] Blood and excess cell overlapping is an additional factor contributing to difficulty in interpretation; however, according to several studies, this difficulty was much improved when the "brush sample" was processed as a liquid-based gynecologic cytology specimen.[28,30] However, neither direct endometrial cytology technique nor screening for endometrial carcinoma is widely accepted,[26,32] and neither is currently routinely performed and frequently used for endometrial evaluation of abnormal uterine bleeding.

References

1. Brand A. Diagnosis of endometrial cancer in women with abnormal vaginal bleeding. *SOGC Clin Pract Guide*. 2000;86:1–3.
2. Seamark CJ. Endometrial sampling in general practice. *Br J Gen Pract*. 1998;48:1597–1598.
3. Jones E, Frain BM, Crabtree W. Clinical significance of reporting benign-appearing endometrial cells in Pap tests in women aged 40 years and over. *Acta Cytol*. 2009;53:18–23.
4. Greenspan DL, Cardillo M, Davey DD, et al. Endometrial cells in cervical cytology: review of cytological features and clinical assessment. *J Low Genit Tract Dis*. 2006;10:111–122.
5. Yarandi F, Izad-Mood N, Eftekhar Z, et al. Diagnostic accuracy of dilatation and curettage for abnormal uterine bleeding. *J Obstet Gynaecol Res*. 2010;36:1049–1052.
6. ACOG Committee on Gynecologic Practice. ACOG Committee Opinion No. 426: the role of transvaginal ultrasonography in the evaluation of postmenopausal bleeding. *Obstet Gynecol*. 2009;113:462–464.
7. Valle RF. Hysteroscopic evaluation of patients with abnormal uterine bleeding. *Surg Gynecol Obstet*. 1981;153:521–526.
8. Epstein E, Ramirez A, Skoog L, et al. Dilatation and curettage fails to detect most focal lesions in the uterine cavity in women with postmenopausal bleeding. *Acta Obstet Gynecol Scand*. 2001;80:1131–1136.

9. Obeidat B, Mohtaseb A, Matalka I. The diagnosis of endometrial hyperplasia on curettage: how reliable is it? *Arch Gynecol Obstet*. 2009;279:489–492.
10. Larson DM, Johnson KK, Broste SK, et al. Comparison of D & C and office endometrial biopsy in predicting final histopathological grade in endometrial cancer. *Obstet Gynecol*. 1995;86:38–42.
11. Cornier E. The Pipelle: a disposable device for endometrial biopsy. *Am J Obstet Gynecol*. 1984;148:109–110.
12. Jiménez-Ayala M, Jiménez-Ayala Portillo B. Techniques of endometrial histopathology. In: Orell SR, ed. *Monographs in Clinical Cytology*. Vol. 17. New York: Karger; 2008.
13. Youssif SNM, McMillan DL. Outpatient endometrial biopsy: the pipelle. *Br J Hosp Med*. 1995;54:198–201.
14. Fakhar S, Saeed G, Khan AK, et al. Validity of pipelle endometrial sampling in patients with abnormal uterine bleeding. *Ann Saudi Med*. 2008;28:188–191.
15. Epstein E, Skoog L, Valentin L. Comparison of Endorette and dilatation and curettage for sampling the endometrium in women with postmenopausal bleeding. *Acta Obstet Gynecol Scand*. 2001;80:959–964.
16. Leitao MM Jr, Kehoe S, Barakat RR, et al. Comparison of D&C and office endometrial biopsy accuracy in patients with FIGO grade 1 endometrial adenocarcinoma. *Gynecol Oncol*. 2009;113:105–108.
17. Ben-Yehuda OM, Kim YB, Leuchter RS. Does hysteroscopy improve the sensitivity of dilatation and curettage in the diagnosis of endometrial hyperplasia or carcinoma? *Gynecol Oncol*. 1998;68:4–7.
18. Clark TJ, Voit D, Gupta JK, et al. Accuracy of hysteroscopy in the diagnosis of endometrial cancer and hyperplasia: a systematic quantitative review. *JAMA*. 2002;288:1610–1621.
19. Van Hanegem N, Breijer MC, Khan KS, et al. Diagnostic evaluation of the endometrium in postmenopausal bleeding: an evidence-based approach. *Maturitas*. 2011;68:155–164.
20. Williams SC, Lopez C, Yoong A, et al. Developing a robust and efficient pathway for the referral an investigation of women with post-menopausal bleeding using a cut-off of ≤ 4mm for normal thickness. *Br J Radiol*. 2007;80:719–723.
21. Van den Bosch T, Van Schoubroeck D, Domali E, et al. A thin and regular endometrium on ultrasound is very unlikely in patients with endometrial malignancy. *Ultrasound Obstet Gynecol*. 2007;29:674–679.
22. Minagawa Y, Sato S, Ito M, et al. Transvaginal ultrasonography and endometrial cytology as a diagnostic schema for endometrial cancer. *Gynecol Obstet Invest*. 2005;59:149–154.
23. Ferrazzi E, Torri V, Trio D, et al. Sonographic endometrial thickness: a useful test to predict atrophy in patients with postmenopausal bleeding. *Ultrasound Obstet Gyecol*. 1996;7:315–321.
24. van Doom HC, Opmeer BC, Burger CW, et al. Inadequate office endometrial biopsy sample requires further evaluation in women with postmenopausal bleeding and abnormal ultrasound results. *Int J Gynaecol Obstet*. 2007;99:100–104.
25. Mathers ME, Johnson SJ, Wadehra V. How predictive is a cervical smear suggesting glandular neoplasia? *Cytopathology*. 2002;13:83–91.
26. Kapali M, Agaram NP, Dabbs D, et al. Routine endometrial sampling of asymptomatic premenopausal women shedding endometrial cells in Papanicolaou tests is not cost effective. *Cancer Cytopathol*. 2007;111:26–33.
27. Jiménez-Ayala M, Jiménez-Ayala Portillo B. Techniques of endometrial cytopathology. In: Orell SR, ed. *Monographs in Clinical Cytology*. Vol. 17. New York: Karger; 2008.
28. Buccoliero AM, Castiglione F, Gheri CF, et al. Liquid-based endometrial cytology: its possible value in postmenopausal asymptomatic women. *Int J Gynecol Cancer*. 2007;17:182–187.
29. Buccoliero AM, Resta L, Napoli A, et al. Liquid-based endometrial cytology: the Florence and Bari experience. *Pathologica*. 2009;101:80–84.
30. Mossa B, Ebano V, Marziani R. Reliability of outpatient endometrial brush cytology vs biopsy in postmenopausal symptomatic women. *Eur J Gynaecol Oncol*. 2010;31:621–626.
31. Buccoliero AM, Gheri CF, Castiglione F, et al. Liquid-based endometrial cytology: cyto-histological correlation in a population of 917 women. *Cytopathology*. 2007;18:241–249.

32. Papaefthimiou M, Symiakaki H, Mentzelopoulou P, et al. The role of liquid-based cytology associated with curettage in the investigation of endometrial lesions from postmenopausal women. *Cytopathology*. 2005;16:32–39.
33. Williams ARW, Brechin S, Porter AJL, et al. Factors affecting adequacy of Pipelle and Tao Brush endometrial sampling. *BJOG*. 2008;115:1028–1036.
34. Buccoliero AM, Gheri CF, Castiglione F, et al. Liquid-based endometrial cytology in the management of sonographically thickened endometrium. *Diagn Cytopathol*. 2007;35:398–402.

Index

Page numbers followed by *f* and *t* indicate figures and tables, respectively.

A

α-fetoprotein (AFP) level, in hepatoid carcinoma, 81
ACTH. *See* adrenocorticotropic hormone
activin A, inhibin α loss and, 113
adenomyosis
 carcinomas arising in, 94
 myometrial invasion, assessment of, and, 90, 195
adjuvant therapy for endometrial cancer
 advanced-stage disease, 139
 anthracyclines for, 9
 carcinosarcoma, 139–140
 chemotherapy in, 138–140
 debulking surgery in, 136
 hormones in, 9–10
 issues in, 9–10
 radiation in, 8, 137–140
adrenocorticotropic hormone (ACTH), pretreatment serum marker evaluation, 112–113
age, endometrial carcinoma incidence and, 3, 5, 93
American Brachytherapy Society, 136
American Society for Colposcopy and Cervical Pathology, 107
androstenedione, elevated, risk factor and, 7
anthracyclines, in adjuvant chemotherapy, 9
APA. *See* atypical polypoid adenomyomas
APA of low malignant potential (APA-LMP), 94
Apo-megestrol. *See* megestrol
Arias-Stella reaction, clear cell carcinoma *vs.*, 70
ASTEC trial, 135
atypia
 artifactual changes in, 21–22*f*, 23*f*
 in endometrial hyperplasia, 20, 24
 in endometrial polyps, 206
 PAP smear result, 107, 202–204, 203*t*
atypical polypoid adenomyoma (APA), 58, 94

B

biomarkers, of endometrial cancer, 112–113, 185
biopsy
 endometrial, issues with, 220, 221*f*
 pathologist's responsibility and, 11
bleeding
 in papillary syncytia metaplasia, 34
 postmenopausal, as presenting symptom
  of endometrial carcinoma, 6
  endometrial tissue sampling, 217
  of endometrioid adenocarcinoma, 10
  in small-cell carcinoma, 75
  in transitional cell carcinoma, 73
 uterine, abnormal, 10
  diagnostic procedures for, 221*f*
  endometrial tissue sampling, 217
brachytherapy, 136, 138–140
Brenner tumors, 73

C

cancer antigen 125 (CA-125), 112
carboplatin, in chemotherapy, 9, 139, 140
carcinoembryonic antigen (CEA)
 immunohistochemical demonstration of, 49
 levels of in postoperative evaluation, 111–112
carcinoma with trophoblastic differentiation, 82–83, 82*f*, 87
carcinosarcoma
 adjuvant therapy of, 139–140
 histology and clinical correlation, 132
 molecular pathology, 175–176
CDKN2A. *See* cyclin-dependent kinase inhibitor 2A
CEA. *See* carcinoembryonic antigen
cervical involvement, assessment of, 92–93, 92*f*
CGH. *See* comparative genomic hybridization
chemotherapy
 adjuvant, 138–140
 anthracyclines in, 9
 carboplatin in, 9, 139, 140
 cisplatin in, 9, 139, 140, 174
 doxorubicin in, 9, 138, 139, 140
 in endometrial carcinoma, positive cytology and, 213
 etoposide in, 174
 ifosfamide in, 139
 issues in, 9–10
 mesna in, 139
 in neuroendocrine carcinomas, 174
 ongoing trials, 140
 paclitaxel in, 9, 139, 140, 174
 platinum-based agents in, 9, 138–139
 response, subpopulations of cancer cells and, 177
ciliated (tubal) metaplasia, 34, 35*f*
cisplatin, in chemotherapy, 9, 139, 140, 174
clear cell carcinoma
 differential diagnosis, 70
 molecular pathology, 167–168, 168*f*
 overview, 68–69*f*, 68–70
 prognostic factors and behavior of, 86
clear cell metaplasia, 36
comparative genomic hybridization (CGH), 184
complex hyperplastic papillary proliferation, 27
computed tomography (CT), 118, 119*f*, 120*f*, 121*f*, 122*f*
Cowden syndrome, 149
CT. *See* computed tomography
CTNNB1 gene, mutation in endometrioid carcinomas, 145, 146*t*, 147*f*, 149–151, 150*f*, 164*t*, 169, 170*f*, 171*t*
cyclin-dependent kinase inhibitor 2A (CDKN2A), in endometrial serous carcinomas, 167
cytology, role of
 glandular cell abnormalities in Pap tests, 201
  endometrial cells, 201–202, 202*f*
  epithelial cell abnormalities, 202–206, 203*f*, 203*t*, 205*f*, 205*t*
  HPV, 207
  mimics of endometrial cancers, 206, 206*t*
 peritoneal washings
  endometrial adenocarcinoma FIGO tumor stage, 211
  endometrial adenocarcinoma in, 211, 212*f*
  immunohistochemistry of endometrial adenocarcinoma in, 213, 215*t*
  significance of, 213, 214*t*

D

D&C. *See* dilation and curettage
"debulking" surgery, advanced-stage disease, 136
dedifferentiated carcinoma, 174–175
diabetes
  importance of, in preoperative evaluation, 106
  PET imaging for endometrial carcinoma and, 125
  risk of endometrial cancer and, 7, 108
diagnostic modalities for endometrial carcinoma
  general medical evaluation, 105, 106f
  pretreatment evaluation and diagnosis, 105–106
    dilation and curettage, 109–111
    endocervical curettage, 107–108
    endometrial sampling, 108–109
    PAP smear, 106–107
  pretreatment imaging modalities, 114, 115f
    CT scan, 118, 119f, 120f, 121f, 122f
    MRI, 122–124, 123f
    PET scan, 124–126, 125f, 126f
    ultrasound, 114–117, 115f
  pretreatment serum marker evaluation, 111–113
Dickkopf-1 (DKK-1), overexpression in endometrioid carcinomas, 151
diet, fat-rich, risk factors for endometrial carcinoma and, 7
dilation and curettage (D&C)
  diagnosis of endometrial cancer, 109–111, 217
  sampling issues with, 217–220, 219f
disordered proliferative endometrium, 25, 26f
DKK-1. *See* Dickkopf-1
Doppler ultrasonography, 116–117
doxorubicin
  in adjuvant chemotherapy, 9, 138, 139
  in ongoing trials for endometrial cancer, 140

E

early menarche, risk factors for endometrial carcinoma, 7
ECC. *See* endocervical curettage
EGFR. *See* epidermal growth factor receptor
EIC. *See* endometrial intraepithelial carcinoma
18-fluoro-2-deoxy-D-glucose (FDG), 124–126, 125f, 126f
EIN. *See* endometrial intraepithelial neoplasia
EmGD. *See* endometrial glandular dysplasia
endocervical curettage (ECC), 107–108
endocervical involvement, staging and, 195
endometrial adenocarcinoma
  FIGO tumor stage, 211
  immunohistochemistry of, in pelvic/peritoneal washings, 213, 214t, 215t
  PAP smear/test, 204, 205f, 205t
  in peritoneal washing cytology, 211, 212f
endometrial atrophy with cystic change, 24, 24f
endometrial biopsy (Pipelle), 11, 220, 221f
endometrial carcinoma
  adenocarcinoma (*See* endometrial adenocarcinoma)
  epidemiology of, 5, 6t
  etiology of, 5–7, 6t
  high-risk, 163
    carcinosarcomas, 175–176
    clear cell carcinomas, 167–168, 168f
    diagnostic markers, 168–173, 170f, 171f, 171t, 172f
    grade 3 endometrioid carcinomas, 163–164, 164t
    malignant mixed müllerian tumors, 175–176
    mixed endometrial carcinomas, 173, 174f
    outlook, 176–177
    rare tumor types, 174–175
    serous carcinoma, 164–167, 166f
  histologic classification of, 42t
  carcinoma with trophoblastic differentiation, 82–83, 82f
  clear cell carcinoma, 68–69f, 68–70
  endometrioid adenocarcinoma (*See* endometrioid adenocarcinoma)
  giant-cell carcinoma, 80–81, 80f
  hepatoid carcinoma, 81, 81f
  large-cell neuroendocrine carcinoma, 77–78, 78f
  lymphoepithelioma-like carcinoma, 78–80, 79f
  metastatic carcinoma, 83–84
  mucinous adenocarcinoma, 71–72, 71f
  small-cell carcinoma, 74–76, 75f
  squamous carcinoma, 72–73, 73f
  transitional cell carcinoma, 73–74, 74f
  undifferentiated carcinoma, 76–77, 77f
  management (*See* management, issues in)
  pathogenetic classification of, 41, 42t
  pathologist's responsibility, 11
  pregnancy and, 93
  prognostic factors and behavior of
    histotypes, 84f, 84–87, 85f
    staging, 87–93, 87t, 88–92f
  risk factors for, 5–7
  staging of (*See* staging, of endometrial carcinoma)
  surgery for (*See* surgery for endometrial carcinoma)
  survival rates, tumor stage distribution and, 10
  treatment (*See* treatment, of endometrial carcinoma)
  WHO classification of, 42t
endometrial cells
  atypical, in endometrial polyps, 206
  in PAP tests, 201
    atypical, 107, 202–204, 203f, 203t
endometrial cytology (direct sampling), 222–223
endometrial glandular dysplasia (EmGD), 165
endometrial hyperplasia, 6, 17, 18t
  atypical, 20–24, 20f, 21–22f, 23f
  clinical implications, 29–31
  complex, 20, 21f
  differential diagnosis
    artifacts and contaminants, 29
    disordered proliferative endometrium, 25, 26f
    endometrial atrophy with cystic change, 24, 24f
    endometrial polyp, 25
    endometrioid adenocarcinoma, FIGO grade 1, 26
    endometritis, 25, 25f
    hyperplastic papillary proliferation of endometrium, 27, 28f
    secretory endometrium, 26
    serous carcinoma, 26–27, 27f
  gland-to-stroma ratio, shift of, 18, 18f, 19f
  histology and clinical correlation, 130
  misdiagnosis of, artifacts and contaminants and, 29, 29f, 30f
  simple, 20, 20f
  WHO classification, 17, 18t, 31, 32t
endometrial intraepithelial carcinoma (EIC), 165
endometrial intraepithelial neoplasia (EIN), 31–33, 32t
endometrial metaplasias
  ciliated (tubal) metaplasia, 34, 35f
  clear cell metaplasia, 36
  eosinophilic metaplasia, 34, 35f
  hobnail metaplasia, 36, 37f
  mucinous metaplasia, 36, 37f
  papillary syncytial metaplasia, 34–36, 36f
  squamous metaplasia, 33, 34f
endometrial polyps
  atypia, 206
  carcinoma in, 93–95
  endometrial hyperplasia, differential diagnosis, 25
endometrial sampling, 108–109

Index

endometrial sarcomas, 181, 182t
  endometrial stromal sarcoma, 181–184, 183f
  rhabdomyosarcoma, 186
  undifferentiated endometrial/uterine sarcoma, 186
  uterine leiomyosarcoma, 185
endometrial stromal sarcoma (ESS), 181
  molecular genetics and biology, 181–184, 182t, 183f
  potential biologically oriented therapies, 184
endometrioid adenocarcinoma, 41, 43f, 44f, 45f
  differential diagnosis
    complex endometrial hyperplasia vs., 52, 53f, 54f
    in endometrium vs. in uterine cervix, 58, 61, 62–63f
    FIGO grade 1, with myometrial invasion vs. atypical polypoid adenomyoma, 58, 61f
    glandular variant of serous carcinoma vs., 52, 57f
    glycogenated squamous differentiation vs. clear cell carcinoma, 52, 57f
    International FIGO grade 1, 26
    primitive neuroectodermal tumor vs. malignant mixed müllerian tumor, 58, 59–60f
    prognostic factors and behavior of, 84–86, 84f, 85f
    sarcomatoid (spindle cell) features vs. malignant mixed müllerian tumor, 52, 58
    sex cord-like pattern/hyalinization vs. malignant mixed müllerian tumor, 52
    squamous differentiation vs. clear cell carcinoma, 52, 57f
    villoglandular pattern vs. papillary endometrial adenocarcinoma of intermediate grade vs. serous carcinoma, 52, 55f, 56f
  variants of
    ciliated variant, 45, 47f
    clear cell changes, 49
    microglandular hyperplasia-like pattern, 49, 49f
    oxyphilic (oncocytic) changes, 51, 51f
    sarcomatoid (spindle cell) features, 48–49, 48f
    secretory variant, 45, 47f
    sertoliform pattern, 50
    sex cord-like pattern and hyalinization, 50, 51f
    small nonvillous papillae, 50, 50f
    variant with squamous differentiation, 45, 46f
    villoglandular variant, 45, 46f
endometrioid carcinogenesis, model of, 155–156, 155f
endometrioid carcinoma
  histology and clinical correlation, 130–132, 131t
  prognostic factors and behavior, 83–86, 84f, 85f
endometritis, 25, 25f
endometrium
  appearance on ultrasound, 114–116
  normal thickness values, 222
  tissue sampling techniques, 217
endometrium, preneoplastic conditions of
  differential diagnosis, 24–29, 24f, 25f, 26f, 27f, 28f
  endometrial hyperplasia, 17, 18t
    atypia, 20–24, 21–22f, 23f
    clinical implications, 29–31, 30f
    gland-to-stroma ratio, shift of, 18, 18f, 19f
    simple vs. complex, 20, 20f, 21f
    WHO classification of, 31
  endometrial intraepithelial neoplasia, 32t, 33f
  endometrial metaplasias, 33–36, 34f, 35f, 36f, 37f
EORTC. See European Organisation for Research and Treatment of Cancer
eosinophilic metaplasia, 34, 35f
epidermal growth factor receptor (EGFR), 186
ESS. See endometrial stromal sarcoma
estrogen, risk of endometrial adenocarcinoma and
  excess, 6–7
  unopposed, 6–7
etoposide, in chemotherapy for neuroendocrine carcinomas, 174
European Organisation for Research and Treatment of Cancer (EORTC), 140
external-beam radiation therapy, for endometrial cancer, 136

F

FDG. See 18-fluoro-2-deoxy-D-glucose
FIGO. See International Federation of Gynecology and Obstetrics

G

GCDFP-15. See gross cystic disease fluid protein
general medical evaluation for endometrial carcinoma, 105, 106f
giant-cell carcinoma
  differential diagnosis, 80–81
  overview, 80, 80f
  prognostic factors and behavior of, 87
gland-to-stroma ratio, shift in, endometrial hyperplasia, 18, 18f, 19f
glycogen synthase kinase 3 (GSK3), 149–151, 150f
GOG. See Gynecologic Oncology Group
grade 3 endometrioid carcinomas, molecular pathology, 163–164, 164t
gross cystic disease fluid protein (GCDFP-15), 83
GSK3. See glycogen synthase kinase 3
Gynecologic Oncology Group (GOG), 130

H

hepatoid carcinoma, 81, 81f, 87
hereditary nonpolyposis colorectal cancer (HNPCC), 5, 95
  mismatch repair deficiency and, 151–154, 154f
  pretreatment evaluation and diagnosis, 105–106, 109
high intermediate risk endometrioid histology, adjuvant therapy, 137–138
histology, clinical correlation of endometrial carcinoma
  carcinosarcoma, 132
  endometrial hyperplasia, 130
  endometrioid carcinoma, 130–132, 131t
  high-risk histologies, 132
HK. See human kallikrein
HNPCC. See hereditary nonpolyposis colorectal cancer
hobnail metaplasia, 36, 37f
hormonal therapy for endometrial carcinoma
  adjuvant, 9–10
  initial, 136–137
hormone replacement therapy (HRT), 7
  PET scanning and, 126
  ultrasound accuracy and, 116
HPV. See human papillomavirus
human kallikrein (HK), 113
human papillomavirus (HPV)
  PAP smear/test, 207
  in situ hybridization, 61, 93
  squamous carcinoma and, 72
  transitional cell carcinoma and, 73
hyperplastic papillary proliferation of endometrium, 27, 28f
hysterectomy
  for atypical endometrial hyperplasia, endometrial cancer and, 130
  with bilateral salpingo-oophorectomy for endometrial carcinoma, 195–196
  laparoscopic, 133–134
  pelvic lymphadenectomy vs. nodal sampling, 135

hysteroscopy
  D&C and, 110–111
  directed biopsy/curettage and, 220–221
  sampling issues with, 221

I

ifosfamide, in adjuvant chemotherapy for carcinosarcoma, 139
IGF2BP3 gene, reexpression in endometrial serous carcinomas, 169
IL-6. *See* interleukin-6
imaging modalities, pretreatment, for endometrial carcinoma, 114, 115*f*
  CT scan, 118, 119*f*, 120*f*, 121*f*, 122*f*
  MRI, 122–124, 123*f*
  PET scan, 124–126, 125*f*, 126*f*
  ultrasound, 114–117, 115*f*
immunohistochemistry, in diagnoses of endometrial carcinoma, 176
immunoperoxidase studies, metastatic carcinoma, 83
inhibins, prognostic factor in endometrial cancer, 113
interleukin-6 (IL-6), biomarkers of endometrial cancer, 112
International Federation of Gynecology and Obstetrics (FIGO)
  revised staging, endometrial carcinoma, 2009, 132, 133*t*, 193
  surgical staging, endometrioid carcinoma, 130
  updated staging, endometrial carcinoma, 87*t*

J

JAZF1 gene, in endometrial stromal sarcoma, 183–184, 183*f*

K

KRAS-BRAF-MAPK pathway, alteration in endometrioid carcinomas, 154–155
KRAS proto-oncogene, in type I endometrial carcinoma, 6

L

laparoscopy, 133–134
laparotomy, 133–134
large-cell neuroendocrine
  differential diagnosis, 78*f*
  overview, 77–78, 78*f*, 79*f*
Linmegestrol. *See* megestrol
lower uterine segment (uterine isthmus), 94
lymph node resection, 8–9, 195–196, 196*t*
lymph nodes
  metastasis, finding of, imaging modalities, 124
  metastatic spread of endometrial carcinoma to, 130, 131*t*
  staging, 196, 196*t*
lymphadenectomy, 130, 132, 134–135
lymphadenopathy, surgical staging and, 130
lymphoepithelioma-like carcinoma, 78–80
Lynch syndrome, 5, 95
  mismatch repair deficiency and, 151–154, 154*f*
  pretreatment evaluation and diagnosis, 105–106, 109
Lynch II syndrome, 5

M

magnetic resonance imaging (MRI), 9, 118, 122–124, 123*f*, 136
malignant mixed müllerian tumor (MMMT)
  molecular pathology, 175–176
  PAP smear/test, 206
mammalian target of rapamycin (mTOR), 146–147
management strategies, 129
  adjuvant therapy
    carcinosarcoma, 139–140
    chemotherapy in, 138–140
    hormones in, 9–10
    radiation in, 137–140
  FIGO staging, endometrial cancer, 132, 133*t*
  histology and clinical correlation
    carcinosarcoma, 132
    endometrial hyperplasia, 130
    endometrioid carcinoma, 130–132, 131*t*
    high-risk histologies, 132
  initial treatment
    hormonal therapy, 136–137
    radiation therapy, 136
    surgery, 133–136
  issues in, 8–10, 10*t*
  ongoing trials, 140
massively parallel DNA sequencing, 176–177
matrix metalloproteinase (MMP), elevation in endometrial cancer, 112–113
medroxyprogesterone (Provera), in adjuvant hormonal therapy, 9
Megace. *See* megestrol
megestrol (Megace, Apo-megestrol, Nu-megestrol, Linmegestrol), in adjuvant hormonal therapy, 9
MELF pattern. *See* microcystic, elongated, and fragmented pattern
menopause, late, risk factor for endometrial carcinoma, 7
menstrual cycle
  appearance of endometrial cells in first half, 201, 202*f*
  appearance of endometrium throughout, 114
  FDG uptake, PET scanning and, 125–126
  prolactin production during secretory phase, 112
mesna, in chemotherapy for carcinosarcoma, 139
metastatic carcinoma, 83–84, 83*f*
microcystic, elongated, and fragmented (MELF) pattern
  serous carcinoma, differential diagnosis, 66
  staging for endometrial carcinoma, 88
mimics of endometrial cancers, PAP smear/test, 206, 206*t*
mismatch repair deficiency (MMR), 151–152
  Lynch syndrome, 153–154, 154*f*
  oncogenic consequences, 152–153
mixed endometrial carcinomas, molecular pathology, 173, 174*f*
MMMT. *See* malignant mixed müllerian tumor
MMP. *See* matrix metalloproteinase
MMR. *See* mismatch repair deficiency
molecular pathogenesis of endometrial carcinoma, 145–146, 146*t*
  low-grade endometrial carcinoma
    model of endometrioid carcinogenesis, 155–156, 156*f*
    molecular pathways, 146–155, 147*f*, 148*f*, 150*f*, 154*f*
  molecular prognostic markers, 157–158
  targeted therapy, 158–159
MRI. *See* magnetic resonance imaging
mTOR. *See* mammalian target of rapamycin
mucinous adenocarcinoma
  differential diagnosis, 71–72
  overview, 71, 71*f*
  prognostic factors and behavior, 86
mucinous metaplasia, 36, 37*f*
myometrial invasion, in staging of endometrial carcinoma
  assessment of, 87–90, 88*f*, 89*f*, 90*f*
  depth of, adenomyosis and, 195

N

neuroendocrine carcinomas, 174–175
nonendometrioid carcinomas, PAP smear/test and, 204–206

Index

Nu-megestrol. See megestrol
nulliparity, risk factors for endometrial carcinoma, 7

O

obesity
    CT scanning and, 118
    risk factor for endometrial carcinoma, 7, 129
ongoing trials, for endometrial cancer, 140
oral contraceptives, unopposed estrogen and, 7

P

p53 protein
    endometrioid adenocarcinoma differential diagnosis, 52
    in type II endometrial carcinomas, 6, 6t
paclitaxel, in chemotherapy, 9, 139, 140
Papanicolaou (PAP) smear/test, 106–107
    endometrial cells in, 201, 202f
    epithelial cell abnormalities in
        atypical endometrial cells, 202–204, 203t
        endometrial adenocarcinoma, 204, 205f, 205t
        malignant mixed müllerian tumor, 206
        nonendometrioid carcinomas, 204–206
    HPV testing, 207
    mimics of endometrial cancers on, 206, 206t
papillae, small nonvillous pattern, 50, 50f
papillary proliferation, 27
papillary syncytial metaplasia, 34–36, 36f
pathologist, responsibility of, 11
peritoneal cytology, 93, 213, 214t
peritoneal washings
    endometrial adenocarcinoma FIGO tumor stage, 211
    endometrial adenocarcinoma in, 211, 212f
    immunohistochemistry of endometrial adenocarcinoma in, 213, 214t, 215t
    positive peritoneal cytology, significance of, 213, 214t
PET. See positron emission tomography
phosphatase and tensin homolog (PTEN)
    in endometrial intraepithelial neoplasia, 32–33, 33f
    endometrioid adenocarcinoma differential diagnosis, 52
    loss of, in endometrioid carcinogenesis, model of, 155
    mutations in, endometrioid carcinomas, 146–149, 147f, 148f
    in type I endometrial carcinomas, 6, 6t
phosphatidylinositol 3-kinase (PI3K), 146–149, 147f
phosphatidylinositol-3,4,5-triphosphate (PIP3), 146
Pipelle device, 108–109, 220
placental site trophoblastic tumor (PSTT), 80–81
platinum-based agents, in chemotherapy, 9
PNET. See primitive neuroectodermal tumor
polycystic ovary syndrome, 7
PORTEC-1 trial, 138
PORTEC-2 trial, 138
positive peritoneal cytology, 93, 213, 214t
positron emission tomography (PET), 118, 124–126, 125f, 126f
pregnancy, endometrial carcinoma and, 93
pretreatment evaluation and diagnosis, of endometrial carcinoma, 105–106
    dilation and curettage, 109–111
    endocervical curettage, 107–108
    endometrial sampling, 108–109
    Papanicolaou smear, 106–107
pretreatment imaging modalities, for endometrial carcinoma, 114, 115f
    CT scan, 118, 119f, 120f, 121f, 122f
    MRI, 122–124, 123f
    PET scan, 124–126, 125f, 126f
    ultrasound, 114–117, 115f
pretreatment serum marker evaluation, 111–113

primitive neuroectodermal tumor (PNET), 58, 59–60f, 76
progestin
    in hormonal therapy, 137
    in hormone replacement therapy, 70
    targeted therapy and, 158
prolactin, as biomarker for endometrial cancer, 112–113
Protocol 150, 139
Provera. See medroxyprogesterone
PSTT. See placental site trophoblastic tumor
PTEN. See phosphatase and tensin homolog
PTEN/PI3K pathway, 146–149, 148f

R

radiation therapy, 8, 137–140
ras pathway, alteration, in endometrioid carcinomas, 154–155
resistance index (RI), 116–117
rhabdomyosarcoma (RMS), 186
RI. See resistance index
risk factors, for endometrial carcinoma, 5–7
RMS. See rhabdomyosarcoma

S

saline infusion sonography (SIS), 114–116
SCGB2A gene, endometrioid cell lineage marker, 169
secretory endometrium, 26
serous carcinoma
    differential diagnosis
        clear cell carcinoma vs., 66
        endometrial adenocarcinoma, FIGO grade 1, and complex endometrial hyperplasia vs., 66
        endometrial hyperplasia vs., 26–27, 27f
        endometrioid adenocarcinoma, villoglandular variant vs., 64
        papillary endometrial adenocarcinoma of intermediate grade vs., 64, 66, 66f, 67f
        papillary syncytial metaplasia vs., 66
    molecular pathology, characteristics, 164–167, 166f
    molecular prognostic markers, 167
    overview, 61, 64, 64–65f
    prognostic factors and behavior of, 86
SIS. See saline infusion sonography
small-cell carcinoma
    differential diagnosis, 76
    overview, 74–75, 75f
sonohysterosalpingogram, 116
squamous carcinoma
    differential diagnosis, 72–73
    molecular pathology, 174–175
    overview, 72, 73f
    prognostic factors and behavior of, 86
squamous metaplasia, 33, 34f
staging, of endometrial carcinoma, 193
    cervical involvement, assessment of, 92–93, 92f
    endocervical involvement, 195
    FIGO, 87t, 132, 133t, 193
    histology, 193
    lymph node resection, 195–196, 196t
    myometrial invasion, assessment of, 87–90, 88f, 89f, 90f
    myometrial invasion and adenomyosis, depth of, 195
    old vs. new, 194t
    peritoneal cytology, 93
    vascular/lymphatic invasion, assessment of, 90–92, 91f
surgery for endometrial carcinoma, 7–8, 133
    "debulking," advanced-stage disease, 136
    lymphadenectomy, 134–135
    minimally invasive, 133–134

survival rates, tumor stage distribution and, 10, 10*t*
SUZ12 gene, in endometrial stromal sarcoma, 183–184
synchronous ovarian, endometrial primaries and, 94, 95*t*

T

TAH-BSO. *See* total abdominal hysterectomy and bilateral salpingo-oophorectomy
tamoxifen
   cancer pretreatment evaluation and diagnosis and, 109
   endometrial thickness measurement and, 117
   PET scanning and, 126
   risk of endometrial carcinomas and, 7, 158
   serous carcinoma and, 64
   transvaginal ultrasound, issues with, 222
TAP regimen, 139
targeted therapy, 158–159
telescoping, in endometrium, 29, 30*f*
three-dimensional (3D) ultrasonography, 117
thrombomodulin, in transitional cell carcinoma, 73
thyroid-stimulating hormone (TSH), alteration in endometrial cancer, 112–113
Toronto Sunnybrook Regional Cancer Center (TSRCC), 134
total abdominal hysterectomy and bilateral salpingo-oophorectomy (TAH-BSO), 8
TP53 mutation, 145, 146*t*, 157
   in carcinosarcomas/malignant mixed müllerian tumors, 175
   in clear cell carcinomas, 167
   diagnostic markers, 169, 171*t*
   in grade 3 endometrioid carcinomas, 163–164, 164*t*
   in serous carcinoma, 164–165, 166*f*, 167
transabdominal ultrasound, 114
transitional cell carcinoma
   differential diagnosis, 74
   overview, 73, 74*f*
   prognostic factors and behavior of, 86
transvaginal ultrasound (TVU), 114, 115*f*, 117, 221–222
treatment, of endometrial carcinoma, 7–8, 129
   adjuvant therapy
      advanced-stage disease, 139
      carcinosarcoma, 139–140
      chemotherapy in, 138–140
      early-stage, high-risk histology, 138–139
      high intermediate risk endometrioid histology, 137–138
      hormones in, 9–10
      issues in, 9–10
      radiation in, 137–140
   FIGO staging for, 132, 133*t*
   histology and clinical correlation
      carcinosarcoma, 132
      endometrial hyperplasia, 130, 131*t*
      endometrioid carcinoma, 131*t*
      high-risk histologies, 132
   initial treatment
      hormonal therapy, 136–137
      radiation therapy, 136
      surgery, 133–136
   issues in, 8–10, 10*t*
   ongoing trials, 140
trials
   ASTEC trial, 135
   ongoing, 140
   PORTEC-1 trial, 138
   PORTEC-2 trial, 138
TSH. *See* thyroid-stimulating hormone
TSRCC. *See* Toronto Sunnybrook Regional Cancer Center
TVU. *See* transvaginal ultrasound
type I endometrial carcinomas, 5–6, 6*t*, 41, 42*t*, 129, 145
type II endometrial carcinomas, 5–6, 6*t*, 41, 42*t*, 129, 145

U

UES. *See* undifferentiated endometrial/uterine sarcoma
ULMS. *See* uterine leiomyosarcoma
ultrasound, 114–117, 115*f*
undifferentiated carcinoma
   differential diagnosis, 76–77
   molecular pathology, 174–175
   overview, 76, 77*f*
   prognostic factors and behavior of, 86
undifferentiated endometrial/uterine sarcoma (UES), 185
   biomarker expression, 186
   molecular genetics and biology, 186
unopposed estrogen, 6–7
unopposed exogenous hormones, 7
uterine leiomyosarcoma (ULMS), 184
   diagnostic markers, 185
   molecular genetics and biology, 185
   potential biologically oriented therapies, 185

V

Vabra Aspirator, 108
vaginal brachytherapy, 138–140
vascular/lymphatic invasion, prognostic factor in endometrial carcinoma, 90–92, 91*f*
verrucous carcinoma, 72, 86

W

WAR. *See* whole abdominal radiation
well-differentiated endometrioid adenocarcinoma, 26
WHO. *See* World Health Organization
whole abdominal radiation (WAR), 139
Wnt/CTNNB1 pathway, in endometrioid carcinomas, 149–151, 150*f*
World Health Organization (WHO)
   endometrial carcinoma, classification of, 42*t*
   endometrial hyperplasia, classification of, 17, 18*t*, 31, 32*t*